Thieme

Techniques and Key Points for Endoscopic Cranial Base Reconstruction

Carlos D. Pinheiro-Neto, MD, PhD
Associate Professor
Department of Otorhinolaryngology/Head and Neck Surgery
Mayo Clinic
Rochester, Minnesota, USA

Maria Peris-Celda, MD, PhD
Associate Professor
Department of Neurosurgery
Mayo Clinic
Rochester, Minnesota, USA

250 illustrations

Thieme
New York • Stuttgart • Delhi • Rio de Janeiro

Library of Congress Cataloging-in-Publication Data is available from the publisher.

Thieme Medical Publishers, Inc.
333 Seventh Avenue, 18th Floor,
New York, NY 10001, USA
www.thieme.com
+1 800 782 3488, customerservice@thieme.com

Illustrations: Jennifer Pryll
Cover design: © Thieme
Cover images source: © Carlos D. Pinheiro-Neto and
Maria Peris-Celda
(© to all artwork in the book remains with the authors. All reproductions of the artwork will need to have permission from the authors to publish or use it in any form.)
Typesetting by DiTech Process Solutions, India

Printed in USA by King Printing Company, Inc. 5 4 3 2 1

ISBN: 978-1-68420-232-4

Also available as an e-book:
eISBN: 978-1-68420-233-1

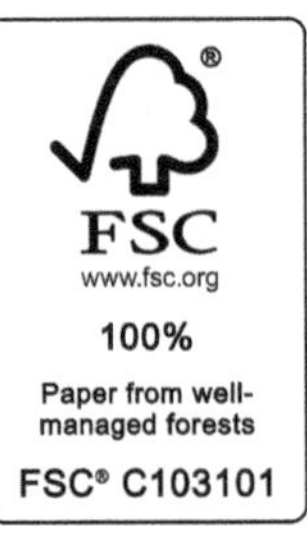

To my father, Dr. Sebastião Diógenes Pinheiro, for being an example of father, friend, physician, and professor. Thank you for showing me the fascinating world of the otorhinolaryngology and being the ultimate model of dedication to the patients.

To my mother, Erineide, for the love, constant presence, and major efforts in my early education.

To my family for the unconditional love and support.

Carlos D. Pinheiro-Neto, MD, PhD

To my past, present, and future patients for the immense privilege to be involved in their care.

To those who donate their bodies for the study of anatomy and their families for their generosity that allows us to train, develop, and perfect new and safer surgical techniques.

To the memory of Professor A.L. Rhoton and his legacy to strive for more accurate, gentle, and safe surgeries.

To my beloved family, especially my parents Antonio and Maria, whose generosity and support are beyond comprehension.

Maria Peris-Celda, MD, PhD

Contents

Videos

Video 3.1: Nasoseptal flap harvest and inset for reconstruction after anterior cranial base resection.

Video 3.2: Reconstruction of suprasellar defect after resection of craniopharyngioma using inlay–onlay fascia lata button graft and onlay nasoseptal flap.

Video 3.3: Nasoseptal flap incision along the nasal dorsum mucosa using endoscopic microscissors.

Video 4.1: Rescue flap incision during a transsphenoidal approach.

Video 5.1: Extended nasoseptal flap.

Video 6.1: Nasoseptal flap pedicle release into the pterygopalatine fossa and dissection of the maxillary artery.

Video 6.2: Nasoseptal flap pedicle release for reconstruction after partial rhinectomy.

Video 7.1: Composite cartilagomucosal nasoseptal flap for reconstruction of suprasellar defect.

Video 8.1: Inferior meatal flap to resurface the septum donor site after harvest of nasoseptal flap.

Video 10.1: Posterior-based lateral nasal wall flap.

Video 10.2: Inferior turbinate/lateral nasal wall flap for reconstruction of clival osteoradionecrosis with exposed carotid stent and coil.

Video 11.1: Anterior-based lateral nasal wall flap.

Video 15.1: Anatomical dissection of temporalis muscle flap.

Video 17.1: Nasal floor free mucosal graft for reconstruction of sellar defect after pituitary tumor resection.

Video 17.2: Nasal floor free mucosal graft for repair of chronic post-traumatic CSF leak.

Video 18.1: Preparation of the fascia lata button graft on the surgical back table and inset of the graft for reconstruction of suprasellar defect.

Video 19.1: Vastus lateralis free tissue transfer for endoscopic reconstruction of anterior cranial base defect.

Video 20.1: Endoscopic anterior cranial base reconstruction with vastus lateralis muscle free flap. Inset through a maxillotomy approach.

Video 26.1: Endoscopic cranial base reconstruction with vastus lateralis muscle free flap. Inset through a retropharyngeal corridor.

Foreword

Endoscopic endonasal surgery has become the new paradigm for the management of a variety of neoplastic and non-neoplastic conditions of the cranial base. The techniques have been widely adopted by skull base surgeons across surgical disciplines. As skull base teams gain experience and ascend the learning curve, they are more able to address large and complex pathologies that need more robust reconstruction of dural defects.

The early years of endoscopic endonasal surgery were plagued by a high postoperative cerebrospinal fluid leak rate. The advent of the vascularized nasoseptal flap for reconstruction was a major advance, with a dramatic and sudden decrease in postoperative cerebrospinal fluid leak rates. The initial publication describing the Hadad-Bassagasteguy flap in 2006 continues to be one of the most highly cited papers in skull base surgery. Subsequent literature reviews have confirmed the benefit of vascularized reconstruction of skull base defects. Multiple variations and refinements of the nasoseptal flap have been introduced subsequently along with a greater appreciation for other vascularized flaps, both local and regional. The lateral nasal wall flap (inferior turbinate flap) and extracranial pericranial flap are examples of local and regional flaps that were developed to provide a reconstructive alternative when a nasoseptal flap is not available while minimizing morbidity.

Carlos D. Pinheiro-Neto and Maria Peris-Celda have succeeded in bringing together all the reconstructive techniques that are needed by the modern skull base surgeon, whether they are doing an open or endoscopic or combined approach. The chapters are organized in a succinct bulleted format that highlights essential information efficiently but still captures nuanced description of surgical technique. This format is optimal for quick reference and most conducive to learning. The chapters are lavishly illustrated with superb anatomical dissections using fully injected specimens from the laboratory of Pinheiro-Neto and Celda. The drawings are beautifully rendered and provide clear illustrations of reconstructive concepts. An added feature of this book is inclusion of *challenging cases* that anticipate the complications and reconstructive dilemmas born out of experience. This textbook is an essential addition to the bookshelf of every skull base surgeon.

Carl Snyderman, MD, MBA

Preface

In the past two decades, endoscopic endonasal cranial base surgery has become part of the surgical armamentarium to successfully treat a variety of cranial base pathologies. Currently, it is considered the gold standard surgical technique for many types of tumors. The evolution of a completely new surgical approach was only possible because of the close collaboration between otorhinolarygologists and neurosurgeons. A key limiting factor encountered early during this process was the high rates of postoperative cerebrospinal fluid (CSF) leak. In 2006, Gustavo Hadad and Luis Bassagasteguy from Argentina in association with Ricardo Carrau, Amin Kassam, and Carl Snyderman from the University of Pittsburgh published the first vascularized flap for endoscopic cranial base reconstruction. The nasoseptal flap revolutionized the field and allowed further advance in endoscopic skull base surgery, decreasing dramatically the postoperative CSF leak rates. Since then, numerous other flaps and modifications of techniques in endoscopic cranial base reconstruction have been published in the literature.

This project aims to compile in a unique book the most important endoscopic reconstructive surgical techniques published in the past two decades. This book is composed of 26 chapters divided into 7 sections. Section I provides an overview of general principles to be followed in endoscopic cranial base reconstruction and resources to help decide the best technique for each type of skull base defect. Sections II to VI provide descriptions of each surgical technique, step-by-step, in a bullet format to make the reading more productive and to the point. Each chapter starts with a brief review of the important anatomical concepts for the surgical technique. Every nuance of each surgical step is described in detail and alternatives are provided. The surgical description is enriched with high-quality pictures and drawings illustrating the steps of the operation. Narrated videos are provided to demonstrate the technique and consolidate the learning. After reviewing the most important surgical techniques currently available for cranial base reconstruction, the reader will be able to acquire some practical clinical experience from difficult clinical examples in Section VII. This final section provides description of seven challenging cases managed by different and experienced skull base teams.

We hope this work serves as a practical reconstructive resource to the endoscopic skull base surgeon.

Carlos D. Pinheiro-Neto, MD, PhD
Maria Peris-Celda, MD, PhD

Acknowledgments

We are indebted to Jennifer Pryll for her effort and dedication to perform illustrations that make complex techniques easier to understand.

We would like to thank Shipra Sehgal and the rest of the Thieme team for their dedication and commitment to the publication of this book.

Carlos D. Pinheiro-Neto, MD, PhD
Maria Peris-Celda, MD, PhD

Contributors

Adedamola Adepoju, MD
Neurosurgeon
Department of Neurosurgery
CHI St. Vincent Arkansa Neuroscience Institute
Sherwood, Arkansas, USA

Amit Agrawal, MD
Associate Professor
Department of Otolaryngology – Head and Neck Surgery
The James Cancer Hospital and Solove Research Institute
The Ohio State University Wexner Medical Center
Columbus, Ohio, USA

Abdulaziz Alrasheed, MD
Clinical Fellow
Department of Otolaryngology – Head and Neck Surgery
The James Cancer Hospital and Solove Research Institute
The Ohio State University Wexner Medical Center
Columbus, Ohio, USA

Serdar Aydin, MD
Research Fellow
Department of Neurosurgery, Albany Medical Center
Albany, New York, USA

Courtney Carpenter, MD
Assistant Professor of Plastic Surgery
Albany Medical Center
Albany, New York, USA

Ricardo L. Carrau, MD, MBA
Professor
Department of Otolaryngology – Head and Neck Surgery;
Lynne Shepard Jones Chair in Head and Neck Oncology;
Director of the Comprehensive Skull Base Surgery Program
The Ohio State University Medical Center;
Co-Director
Anatomy Laboratory Toward Visuospatial Surgical Innovations in Otolaryngology and Neurosurgery (*ALT-VISION*)
The Ohio State University Wexner Medical Center
Columbus, Ohio, USA

Garret W. Choby, MD
Associate Professor
Rhinology and Skull Base Surgery;
Chair of Quality
Department of Otolaryngology – Head and Neck Surgery, Joint Appointment
Department of Neurologic Surgery
Mayo Clinic
Rochester, Minnesota, USA

Salomon Cohen Cohen, MD
Resident
Department of Neurosurgery
Mayo Clinic
Rochester, Minnesota, USA

Felipe S. G. Fortes, MD, PhD
Otolaryngologist and Facial Plastic Surgeon, Clinica Fortes
São Paulo, Brazil

Paul A. Gardner, MD
Professor and Peter J. Janetta Endowed Chair
Department of Neurological Surgery
University of Pittsburgh School of Medicine;
Co-Director
Center for Cranial Base Surgery
University of Pittsburgh Medical Center
Pittsburgh, Pennsylvania, USA

Stephen Y. Kang, MD
Head and Neck Surgeon
Department of Otolaryngology – Head and Neck Surgery
The James Cancer Hospital and Solove Research Institute
The Ohio State University Wexner Medical Center
Columbus, Ohio, USA

Tyler Kenning, MD
Neurosurgeon
Piedmont Heathcare
Atlanta, Georgia, USA

Luciano C. P. C. Leonel, PhD
Research Fellow
Department of Neurosurgery
Mayo Clinic
Rochester, Minnesota, USA

Michael J. Link, MD
Professor
Departments of Neurologic Surgery and Otorhinolaryngology
Mayo Clinic
Rochester, Minnesota, USA

Ramon Moreno-Luna, MD, PhD
Otolaryngologist
Rhinology and Skull Base Unit
University Hospital Virgen de la Macarena
Seville, Spain

Mathew Old, MD
Associate Professor
Department of Otolaryngology – Head and Neck Surgery
The James Cancer Hospital and Solove Research Institute
The Ohio State University Wexner Medical Center
Columbus, Ohio, USA

Enver Ozer, MD
Professor
Department of Otolaryngology – Head and Neck Surgery
Wexner Medical Center
The James Cancer Hospital and Solove Research Institute, The Ohio State University
Columbus, Ohio, USA

Maria Peris-Celda, MD, PhD
Associate Professor
Department of Neurosurgery
Mayo Clinic
Rochester, Minnesota, USA

Carlos D. Pinheiro-Neto, MD, PhD
Associate Professor
Department of Otorhinolaryngology/Head and Neck Surgery
Mayo Clinic
Rochester, Minnesota, USA

Daniel Prevedello, MD
Professor
Department of Neurological Surgery
The James Cancer Hospital and Solove Research Institute
The Ohio State University Wexner Medical Center
Columbus, Ohio, USA

Natalia C. Rezende, MD
Research Fellow
Department of Neurosurgery
Mayo Clinic
Rochester, Minnesota, USA

Laura Salgado-Lopez, MD
Research Fellow
Department of Neurosurgery
Mount Sinai Hospital
New York, New York, USA

Nolan Seim, MD
Assistant Professor
Department of Otolaryngology – Head and Neck Surgery
The James Cancer Hospital and Solove Research Institute
The Ohio State University Wexner Medical Center
Columbus, Ohio, USA

Carl H. Snyderman, MD, MBA
Professor
Department of Otolaryngology
University of Pittsburgh School of Medicine;
Co-Director
Center for Cranial Base Surgery
University of Pittsburgh Medical Center
Pittsburgh, Pennsylvania, USA

C. Arturo Solares, MD, FACS, MD, FACS
Professor of Otolaryngology and Neurosurgery;
Director, Skull Base Surgery
Emory University
Atlanta, Georgia, USA

Roberto M. Soriano, MD
Research Fellow
Department of Otolaryngology – Head and Neck Surgery
Emory University
Atlanta, Georgia, USA

Janalee Stokken, MD
Associate Professor
Department of Otolaryngology – Head and Neck Surgery
Mayo Clinic
Rochester, Minnesota, USA

Akina Tamaki, MD
Assistant Professor
Department of Otolaryngology
Case Western Reserve University
University Hospitals Cleveland Medical Center
Cleveland, Ohio, USA

Jamie J. Van Gompel, MD, FAANS
Professor in Neurosurgery and Otorhinolaryngology;
Program Director
International Neurosurgery Fellowship;
Associate Program Director
Neurosurgical Skull Base Oncology Fellowship
Mayo Clinic
Rochester, Minnesota, USA

Section I

Introduction

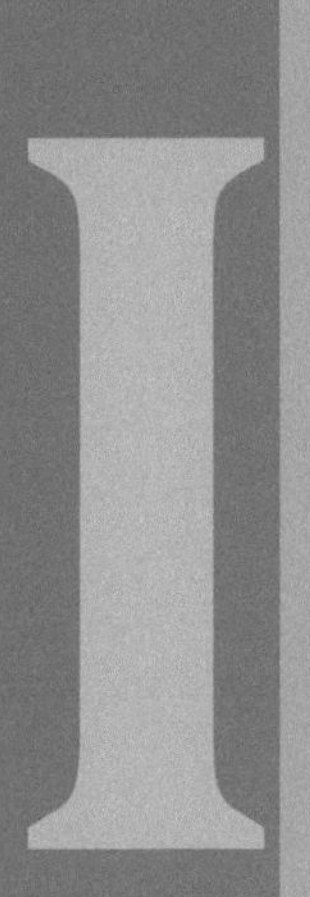

1 Principles of Endoscopic Cranial Base Reconstruction

Tyler Kenning, Laura Salgado-Lopez, Maria Peris-Celda, and Carlos D. Pinheiro-Neto

1.1 Introduction

- Endonasal approaches to the cranial base have not only permitted access to an increasingly vast range of pathology but have also brought new surgical challenges.
- Reconstruction after cranial base surgery separates the sinonasal and intracranial compartments, preventing postoperative cerebrospinal fluid (CSF) fistulas, and limiting the morbidity and mortality.
- The goals for repair of the cranial base include the elimination of dead space, providing structural support, contour and function of the cranial base, and protection and preservation of intracranial and orbital contents.
- Beyond the need for reoperation and further repair, reconstruction failures have the potential for significant morbidity: meningitis, subdural hemorrhage, intracranial abscess, hydrocephalus, pneumocephalus, and even death.[1] Delayed complications include epistaxis, chronic rhinosinusitis, and sinonasal mucocele formation.[2]
- Advances in cranial base repair may be the most critical factor allowing for the increasing use of endoscopic endonasal surgery of the cranial base.

1.2 Fundamentals of Endonasal Reconstruction

- The principles of endonasal cranial base reconstruction remain similar to transcranial approaches.
- Challenges for endonasal reconstruction include the lack of supporting structures and the effects of gravity.
- Reconstruction in purely transsellar surgery can be accomplished with greater than 99% success rate with nonvascularized mucosal grafts alone.[3]
- Initially, dural and osseous defects were largely repaired with nonvascular tissue grafts in expanded endonasal approaches. Postoperative CSF leaks occurred in up to 15% of the cases.[4,5]
- The utility of vascularized tissue for cranial base coverage becomes evident when extending beyond the sella (success rates over 95% in the anterior cranial base vs. 67–93% with nonvascularized grafts).[6]
- Resection of tumors with large mass effect in the frontal lobes creates a large surgical cavity intracranially which makes the endonasal reconstruction of the anterior cranial base more challenging. The absence of adequate support of the frontal lobes for the reconstruction and the column of CSF that forms between the brain and the reconstruction increases the risk of failure. Partial filling of the intracranial surgical cavity with absorbable sponges and/or fat graft, particularly along the anterior edge of the defect, may prevent intracranial displacement of the flap and CSF leak.
- Defects in the posterior fossa with transclival approaches are the most problematic to repair. Nonvascularized tissues have proven ineffective with postoperative CSF leaks occurring in nearly 40% of the cases. Conversely, with flap repair and use of postoperative lumbar drain, the rates of CSF fistulas in these cases can be reduced to less than 5%.[5,6,7]
- Certain pathologies and comorbidities are associated with increased risk for postoperative CSF leaks, and more robust reconstructions should be considered for these patients.[8,9,10]
  - Meningiomas—treatment involves osseous and dural resection, as well as disruption of the arachnoid.
  - Craniopharyngiomas—with potential extension through the basilar cisterns and into the ventricular system.
  - Cushing's disease—compromised healing due to endocrinopathy, likely obesity with associated intracranial hypertension, possible obstructive sleep apnea requiring continuous positive airway pressure (CPAP).
  - Morbid obesity—associated with intracranial hypertension.
  - Obstructive sleep apnea—requirement of CPAP postoperatively.
  - Idiopathic CSF leaks/encephaloceles/meningoencephaloceles—associated with obesity and increased intracranial pressure.
  - History of or need for radiotherapy—vascularized flaps are more likely to withstand long-term effects of radiotherapy.
  - Immunosuppression/steroid use/diabetes—compromised healing.

1.3 Repair Options

- There is a wide variety of options available for endoscopic cranial base reconstruction, including free mucosal grafts, autologous fat, muscle, and fascia lata, allograft dural substitutes, and vascularized flaps.
- Synthetic rigid materials (titanium meshes, porous polyethylene implants, etc.) should be avoided due to the higher risk of infections and/or extrusions. If a more rigid reconstruction is desired, vascularized composite flaps are recommended.
- The selection of the repair option is based on the anatomic location and extent of the defect, the degree and type of intraoperative CSF leak, the underlying pathology, and patient comorbidities.
- Any dural defect is usually repaired with an intradural graft, especially if there is an accompanying arachnoid opening. In cases where the arachnoid is exposed and contains the CSF flow, an onlay mucosal reconstruction may be enough to repair the defect.
- Autologous vascularized flaps have the greatest success rates in preventing postoperative CSF leaks. However, their use is commonly accompanied by additional morbidity. When effective alternatives are available, "non-flap" repairs may be considered.[6]
- Absorbable sealants and glues are useful for holding multilayered repairs in position. These should be applied over top of the repair and then supported by nasal packing. If sealants/glues are placed between layers of the repair, a gap will develop with their absorption, preventing appropriate healing of the repair.
- Dissolvable packs are preferred to limit patient discomfort with removal. When greater pressure is needed to the cranial base repair, nonabsorbable packing should be considered.[9]

- Improvements in reconstruction materials and techniques have allowed moving away from lumbar CSF drains in the majority of the cases.
- An exception may be in posterior cranial fossa surgery/large transclival approaches where the postoperative use of lumbar drains has been shown to be a more effective adjunct to the direct repair.[11]
- Early surgical reexploration and repair revision is advocated instead of only lumbar drainage for treatment of postoperative CSF leaks.
- If a postoperative CSF fistula is suspected, direct bedside nasal endoscopy is performed, and if a defect is evident or still unclear, proceed to evaluation in the operating room.[12] With attempts at lumbar drainage alone in this setting, the failure rate and associated morbidity (infection, overdrainage, subdural hematomas, tension pneumocephalus, etc.) are high.

1.4 Vascularized Reconstruction

- The use of vascularized flaps revolutionized the field of endoscopic endonasal surgery and broadly widened its applicability.
- The most commonly used flaps are summarized in ▶ Table 1.1 and ▶ Table 1.2. Each of the different options will be detailed in latter chapters.
- The perichondrial or periosteal surface of intranasal flaps must contact bone along its entire length. This contact is essential circumferentially not only around the cranial base defect but also along the proximal portion of the flap.
- If the proximal portion of the flap does not contact bone or other nonmucosal surface, the contraction during the healing process intensifies, pulling the flap away from the defect and increasing the risk of CSF leak.
- In order to maximize the length of the flap, all bone ridges and septations within the sinuses should be removed to optimize the bone contact of the flap. If excess bone is left, the folds of the flap along the septations will shorten its "usable" area and increase the risk of dead space underneath the flap.[13]
- When possible, intranasal flaps should have their donor site covered with a second vascularized flap or mucosal graft to optimize healing and minimize donor site morbidity, including crusting and repeated postoperative debridements. Covering the nasal septum donor site will also help in limiting septal perforations and collapse of the dorsum.
- A previously used pedicled flap can be carefully dissected respecting the vascular pedicle and reused for reoperations, avoiding harvest of additional flaps.
- During the harvesting of the healed flap to the skull base, attention should be given to the neurovascular structures possibly previously exposed and not covered by bone (such as internal carotid arteries and optic nerves).
- The healed flap will often maintain the shape acquired during the healing process along the cranial base. This "memory" of the flap may lead to some difficulties during the new inset, particularly if a larger approach was required and the previous flap turned to be short for the new defect.

1.5 Reconstruction Decalogue

1. Perform a preoperative nasal endoscopy to evaluate the quality of the sinonasal mucosa, concurrent inflammatory disease, and options available for reconstruction.
2. Review imaging examinations to estimate the size of the defect and the size and availability of the flap/graft.
3. Always try to preserve both middle turbinates and pedicles for the nasoseptal flap during the approach (including anterior cranial base resection).
4. Try to preserve the roof and posterior wall of the nasopharynx if possible in transclival approaches.
5. Remove all bony septations in order to leave the surface flushed to receive the flap/graft.
6. Remove all mucosa around the defect and along the course of the flap toward the defect. Lay the flap always in contact with a surface in order to minimize flap contraction.
7. Use multilayer reconstruction with an inlay dural substitute and onlay flap/graft. Avoid synthetic rigid implants.
8. Do not interpose dural sealant, oxidized cellulose, gelatin foam, or any other synthetic material between the flap and the bone or dural substitute.
9. Support the reconstruction with absorbable packing when possible. The preservation of sinonasal structures during the approach improves the support to the packing and minimizes the need for nonabsorbable nasal packing.
10. Take into account risk factors and preoperative morbidity, and modify reconstruction options accordingly.

Table 1.1 Intranasal flaps[9,13]

Nasoseptal flap	• *Pedicle*: Posterior septal artery—branch of the sphenopalatine artery—branch of the maxillary artery • *Uses*: All ventral cranial base defects • *Advantages*: It has a long pedicle with robust mucosa, has great arch of rotation, and is customizable/adaptable • *Limitations*: For extreme anterior defects/frontal sinus and lower clivus/craniovertebral junction, it may need to be modified (augmented and/or elongated)
Middle turbinate flap	• *Pedicle*: Middle turbinate branch of the posterior lateral nasal artery—branch of the sphenopalatine artery • *Uses*: Limited defects of cribriform plate, fovea ethmoidalis, planum, and sella • *Advantages*: Proximity to the ethmoid roof and cribriform plate • *Limitations*: Large defects
Lateral wall flap—posteriorly based	• *Pedicle*: Inferior turbinate artery—branch of posterior lateral nasal artery—branch of sphenopalatine artery • *Uses*: Clival defects. Back-up intranasal flap when the nasoseptal flap is not available • *Advantages*: Robust flap, well-vascularized flap • *Limitations*: Nasolacrimal duct; disruption of the lateral wall with risk of atrophic rhinitis
Lateral wall flap—anteriorly based	• *Pedicle*: Anterior lateral nasal artery—branch of facial artery and lateral branch of the anterior ethmoidal artery • *Uses*: Anterior cranial base defects, especially when cranialization of the frontal sinus is needed • *Advantages*: Robust and well-vascularized flap • *Limitations*: nasolacrimal duct; broad pedicle and less favorable arch of rotation; disruption of the lateral wall with risk of atrophic rhinitis

Table 1.2 Extranasal flaps and free flaps[9,13]

Extranasal flaps	Large, robust, can reach most of the cranial base but require extra time to harvest using external incisions
Pericranial flap	• *Pedicle*: Supraorbital artery and supratrochlear artery • *Uses*: Large anterior cranial base defects • *Advantages*: Large and well-vascularized flap • *Limitations*: Bicoronal incision and need for intranasal transposition through a nasionectomy
Temporoparietal fascia flap	• *Pedicle*: Superficial temporal artery • *Uses*: Clival defects, craniovertebral junction, infratemporal fossa • *Advantages*: Large vascularized flap, usually out of the radiation field in patients with prior radiation • *Limitations*: Hemicoronal incision, time-consuming separation of the flap from the subcutaneous tissue of the scalp, risk of alopecia, transposition through the infratemporal fossa
Osteotemporoparietal fascia and osteopericranial flaps	• *Pedicle*: Superficial temporal artery (osteotemporoparietal). Supraorbital artery and supratrochlear artery (osteopericranial) • *Uses*: Reconstruction of zygomatic prominence, orbit, anterior cranial base • *Advantages*: Rigid reconstruction • *Limitations*: Time-consuming harvesting, risk of trauma to the inner cortical of the diploe, possible CSF leak, brain or vascular injury
Temporalis muscle flap	• *Pedicle*: Deep temporal arteries (anterior and posterior)—branches of the maxillary artery and middle temporal artery—branch of the superficial temporal artery • *Uses*: Orbital reconstruction and clival defects • *Advantages*: Large vascularized bulky flap • *Limitations*: Temporal howling, transposition through the infratemporal fossa or through a lateral orbitotomy

Other extranasal flaps (buccinator, palatal)	• *Pedicle*:
	  ○ Buccinator: Branches of the facial artery
	  ○ Palatal: Descending palatine artery
	• *Uses*:
	  ○ Buccinator: Orbital and anterior cranial base defects
	  ○ Palatal: Experimental
	• *Advantages*: Vascularized flaps and likely out of the radiation field in patients with prior radiation
	• *Limitations*:
	  ○ Buccinator: Risk of injury of the parotid duct or facial nerve terminal branches, requires transmaxillary approach for the flap transposition to the nasal cavity
	  ○ Palatal: High-risk of oronasal/oroantral fistula from transposition of the palatal flap, high donor site morbidity, risk of dentoalveolar injury or soft palate injury with possible velopharyngeal insufficiency

Free flaps	• *Flaps*: ALT flap or RFF. Microanastomosis performed through an open incision in the neck. Pedicle anastomosis to the facial artery and vein. Transposition into the nasal cavity through a transmaxillary approach. It requires fine manipulation endoscopically for the flap inset • *Uses*: All cranial base defects when intranasal and extranasal flap options are exhausted for endoscopic endonasal reconstruction • *Advantages*: Robust reconstruction with tissue not affected by radiation in patients with previous radiation treatment • *Limitations*: Requires a team with experience in microvascular reconstruction

Abbreviations: ALT, anterolateral thigh; RFF, radial forearm flap.

References

[1] Sokoya M, Mourad M, Ducic Y. Complications of skull base surgery. Semin Plast Surg. 2017; 31(4):227–230

[2] Naunheim MR, Sedaghat AR, Lin DT, et al. Immediate and delayed complications following endoscopic skull base surgery. J Neurol Surg B Skull Base. 2015; 76(5):390–396

[3] Scagnelli RJ, Patel V, Peris-Celda M, Kenning TJ, Pinheiro-Neto CD. Implementation of free mucosal graft technique for sellar reconstruction after pituitary surgery: outcomes of 158 consecutive patients. World Neurosurg. 2019; 122: e506–e511

[4] Harvey RJ, Parmar P, Sacks R, Zanation AM. Endoscopic skull base reconstruction of large dural defects: a systematic review of published evidence. Laryngoscope. 2012; 122(2):452–459

[5] Hegazy HM, Carrau RL, Snyderman CH, Kassam A, Zweig J. Transnasal endoscopic repair of cerebrospinal fluid rhinorrhea: a meta-analysis. Laryngoscope. 2000; 110(7):1166–1172

[6] Soudry E, Turner JH, Nayak JV, Hwang PH. Endoscopic reconstruction of surgically created skull base defects: a systematic review. Otolaryngol Head Neck Surg. 2014; 150(5):730–738

[7] Thorp BD, Sreenath SB, Ebert CS, Zanation AM. Endoscopic skull base reconstruction: a review and clinical case series of 152 vascularized flaps used for surgical skull base defects in the setting of intraoperative cerebrospinal fluid leak. Neurosurg Focus. 2014; 37(4):E4

[8] Clavenna MJ, Turner JH, Chandra RK. Pedicled flaps in endoscopic skull base reconstruction: review of current techniques. Curr Opin Otolaryngol Head Neck Surg. 2015; 23(1):71–77

[9] Sigler AC, D'Anza B, Lobo BC, Woodard TD, Recinos PF, Sindwani R. Endoscopic skull base reconstruction: an evolution of materials and methods. Otolaryngol Clin North Am. 2017; 50(3):643–653

[10] Zanation AM, Thorp BD, Parmar P, Harvey RJ. Reconstructive options for endoscopic skull base surgery. Otolaryngol Clin North Am. 2011; 44 (5):1201–1222

[11] Zwagerman NT, Wang EW, Shin SS, et al. Does lumbar drainage reduce postoperative cerebrospinal fluid leak after endoscopic endonasal skull base surgery? A prospective, randomized controlled trial. J Neurosurg. 2018; 1–7

[12] Conger A, Zhao F, Wang X, et al. Evolution of the graded repair of CSF leaks and skull base defects in endonasal endoscopic tumor surgery: trends in repair failure and meningitis rates in 509 patients. J Neurosurg. 2018; 130 (3):861–875

[13] Chakravarthi S, Gonen L, Monroy-Sosa A, Khalili S, Kassam A. Endoscopic endonasal reconstructive methods to the anterior skull base. Semin Plast Surg. 2017; 31(4):203–213

2 Operative Planning and Treatment Algorithm

Serdar Aydin, Carlos D. Pinheiro-Neto, and Maria Peris-Celda

2.1 Introduction

- The ultimate goal is to choose the optimal reconstruction for each case in order to reestablish a barrier between the sinonasal cavity and the central nervous system and avoid unnecessary nasal morbidity.[1]
- The most important complications that an effective reconstruction avoids include cerebrospinal fluid (CSF) leak, pneumocephalus, and infection.[2]
- Meticulous preoperative planning is important to anticipate the need of any additional sinonasal procedure during the surgery (septoplasty, turbinoplasty) and to detect sinus conditions that could potentially postpone the intradural work (bacterial sinusitis, fungus ball).
- Immediate postoperative care and compliance with postoperative restrictions are essential for a good outcome.[3]

2.2 Preoperative Planning

- It is essential to plan the reconstruction options before the surgery and be ready for an alternative plan in case of failure or unexpected findings.
- If the availability of the nasoseptal flap is uncertain due to possibility of tumor involvement, it is imperative to plan the possibility of harvesting an alternative flap for reconstruction.
- In cases where complex reconstruction is anticipated, it is recommended to prep multiple sites for flap/graft harvest, for example, bicoronal or hemicoronal incision for pericranial or temporoparietal fascia flap, the abdomen for fat/muscle grafts, and the thigh for fat/fascia lata/muscle grafts. It is important to have the site prepared and ready if needed during the surgery.
- Detailed clinical history, past surgical history, nasal endoscopy, and radiological examinations are essential for a successful reconstructive plan and outcomes.
- Computed tomography (CT) scan measurements of the flap are useful to predict its potential reach.[4,5]
- 3D reconstruction images from CT scans help to simulate the skull base defect configuration and dimensions. It can also be used to estimate the dimensions of the flap and simulate the arch of rotation.
- 3D printing models may also be useful for preoperative planning of the reconstruction.
- Preoperative angiography may be useful to demonstrate the vascularization status of the nasal cavity and extranasal flaps in selected cases.
- A comprehensive preoperative planning helps not only to establish a good strategy for the surgical procedure but also in preoperative counseling of the patients.

2.3 Perioperative and Intraoperative Considerations

- Antibiotic prophylaxis is usually second-generation cephalosporin or second-generation cephalosporin + vancomycin in case of expanded approaches starting within 1 hour prior to the operation and for 24 hours postoperatively.
- Total intravenous anesthesia (TIVA) is preferred to minimize vasodilatation of the nasal mucosa and decrease intraoperative bleeding.
- Neuromonitoring (somatosensory-evoked potential [SSEP], motor-evoked potential [MEP], electroencephalography [EEG], and cranial nerves depending on the location of the lesion).
- Perioperative corticosteroids (dexamethasone) in case of brain edema, compression of the optic nerves, or chiasm. Perioperative mineralocorticoids (hydrocortisone) stress dose in case of preoperative steroid treatment or hypocortisolism.

2.4 Treatment Algorithm

- A general algorithm for repair of skull base defects is presented based on low- or high-flow intraoperative CSF leak and size of the defect. It can be modified according to the pathology, patient conditions, and preoperative comorbidities (▸ Fig. 2.1).
- High-flow CSF leak is observed in cases with communication with intracranial cisterns/ventricles.
- ▸ Table 2.1 provides a simplified scheme of the recommended first-line reconstruction and alternatives according to the site of the defect.

2.5 Postoperative Considerations

2.5.1 Inpatient Care

- If lumbar drain is required for posterior fossa defects, 10 to 15 mL/h drainage for 3 days is usually appropriate.
- Keep normotension, with an upper limit of 140 mm Hg for at least 24 hours after the procedure.
- Remove arterial line 12 to 24 hours after the procedure.
- Keep head of the bed elevated at 30 to 60 degrees at all times for 3 days. The patient can ambulate as soon as tolerated.
- "No nasal intrusions" sign should be visible and highlighted at the bed of the patient. If nasogastric tube is required, it should be passed under endoscopic visualization.
- No bending over and nose blowing. Recommend sneezing with the mouth open.
- Avoid and treat constipation.
- Lifting restrictions: avoid lifting greater than 5 lbs for 4 to 6 weeks.
- Saline nasal sprays are not recommended during the first 48 hours after surgery to avoid misdiagnosis with early postoperative CSF leak.
- After 48 hours of the surgery, saline nasal sprays are initiated and maintained until the first postoperative visit.

2.5.2 Outpatient Care

- If nasal packing and/or nasal splints are used, antibiotic prophylaxis with a second-generation cephalosporin is maintained during the first week postoperative.

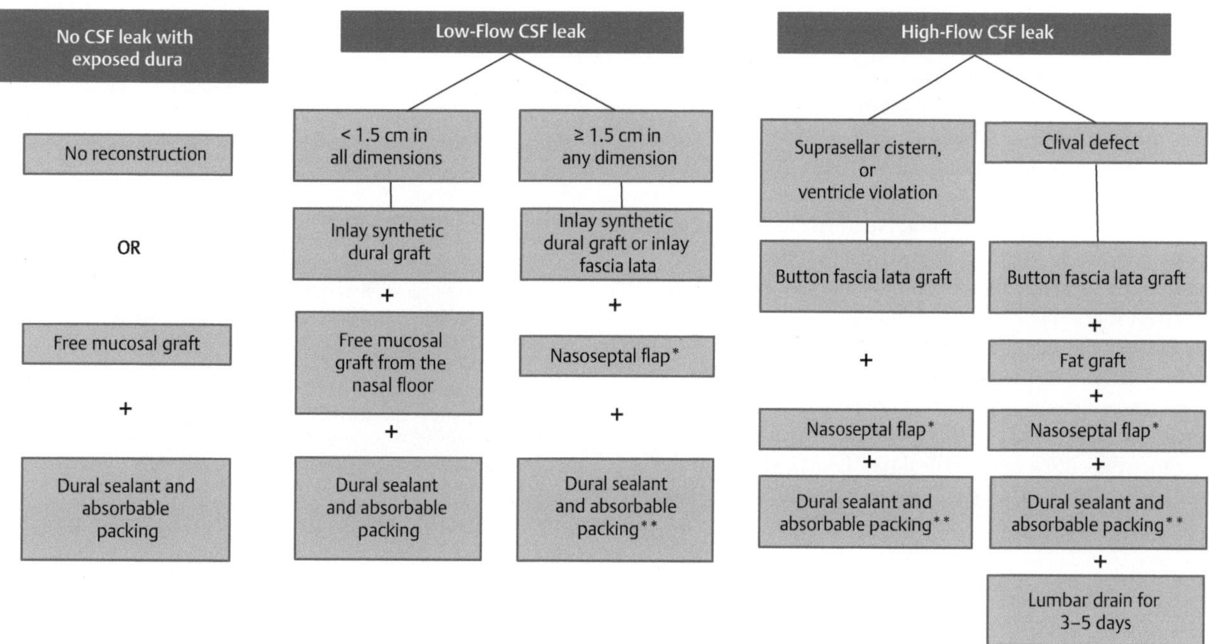

Fig. 2.1 Skull base defect reconstruction.
* If the nasoseptal flap is not available other flaps are indicated.
** Add nonabsorbable packing after placing the absorbable packing to improve support, particularly for large anterior cranial base or clival defects.

Table 2.1 Skull base reconstruction according to the site of the defect

Skull base defect	First option	Alternatives
Sella	Nasal floor FMG	Middle turbinate FMG Nasoseptal flap
Suprasellar space	Nasoseptal flap	Middle turbinate flap Pericranial flap
Lateral recess of the sphenoid	Nasal floor FMG	Nasoseptal flap
Anterior cranial base (< 1.5 cm)	Nasal floor FMG	Nasoseptal flap
Anterior cranial base (≥ 1.5 cm)	Nasoseptal flap	Pericranial flap
Posterior table frontal sinus (< 1.5 cm)	Nasal floor FMG[a]	Nasoseptal flap with pedicle release[a] Pericranial flap[b]
Posterior table frontal sinus (≥ 1.5 cm)	Nasoseptal flap with pedicle release[a]	Pericranial flap[b]
Clivus	Extended nasoseptal flap	Posterior-based lateral nasal wall flap Nasoseptal flap with pedicle release Temporoparietal fascia flap
Orbit	Temporalis muscle flap or free flap	

Abbreviation: FMG, free mucosal graft.
[a]With preservation of the frontal sinus outflow. [b]With obliteration or cranialization of the frontal sinus.

- One week after the surgery: First postoperative visit. Nasal splints are removed, and limited debridement is performed, focusing on removal of loose crusts to improve the nasal breathing. The sinus cavities are left alone and the reconstructed area is usually not visualized during the first debridement.
- After the first postoperative visit, large-volume saline rinses are indicated daily for 1 month to help the removal of absorbable packing and dural sealant.
- One month after surgery: Second nasal debridement. Deep cleaning of the sinuses is performed, with removal of the remnant packing and dural sealant. Great visualization of the flap/graft is obtained.
- Keep large-volume nasal saline rinses as needed.
- For very large anterior cranial base defects, large-volume saline rinses may be postponed to the second or third week postoperative.
- Four months after surgery: Third nasal debridement in the outpatient setting. After that, follow up for nasal debridement as needed and keep routine follow-up for the baseline pathology.

References

[1] Tien DA, Stokken JK, Recinos PF, Woodard TD, Sindwani R. Comprehensive postoperative management after endoscopic skull base surgery. Otolaryngol Clin North Am. 2016; 49(1):253–263

[2] Reuter G, Bouchain O, Demanez L, Scholtes F, Martin D. Skull base reconstruction with pedicled nasoseptal flap: technique, indications, and limitations. J Craniomaxillofac Surg. 2019; 47(1):29–32

[3] Tabaee A, Anand VK, Brown SM, Lin JW, Schwartz TH. Algorithm for reconstruction after endoscopic pituitary and skull base surgery. Laryngoscope. 2007; 117(7):1133–1137

[4] Pinheiro-Neto CD, Prevedello DM, Carrau RL, et al. Improving the design of the pedicled nasoseptal flap for skull base reconstruction: a radioanatomic study. Laryngoscope. 2007; 117(9):1560–1569

[5] Pinheiro-Neto CD, Ramos HF, Peris-Celda M, et al. Study of the nasoseptal flap for endoscopic anterior cranial base reconstruction. Laryngoscope. 2011; 121 (12):2514–2520

Section II

Nasoseptal Flap and Variations

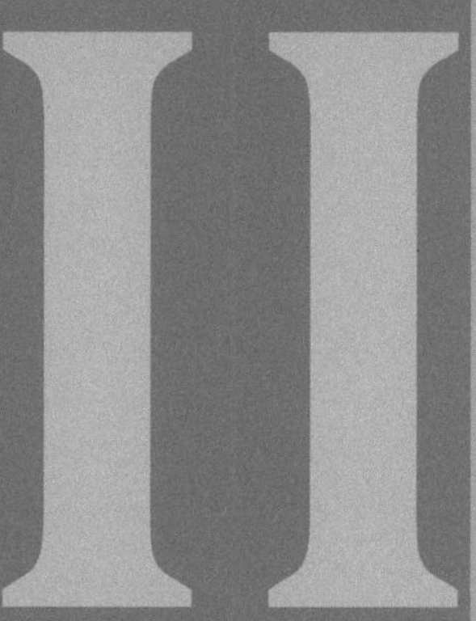

3 Standard Nasoseptal Flap

Carlos D. Pinheiro-Neto, Luciano C. P. C. Leonel, Natalia C. Rezende, and Maria Peris-Celda

3.1 Anatomy

- The nasal septum is formed by the septal cartilage (also known as quadrangular cartilage), perpendicular plate of the ethmoid, vomer, and maxillary crest.
- The septal cartilage anteriorly and the vomer posteriorly articulate with the maxillary crest, which is formed by the maxillary bone anteriorly and the palatine bone posteriorly (▶ Fig. 3.1).
- The septal cartilage is covered by mucoperichondrium. The perpendicular plate of the ethmoid, vomer, and maxillary crest are covered by mucoperiosteum. The mucoperichondrium is thicker than the mucoperiosteum.
- The septal mucosa is supplied by branches of the sphenopalatine artery (SPA), anterior and posterior ethmoidal arteries, and facial artery.
- The nasoseptal flap (NSF) is pedicled upon the posterior septal artery, which is a terminal branch of the SPA.[1]
- The posterior septal artery ascends from the SPA foramen and crosses the anterior wall of the sphenoid sinus between the sphenoid ostium and the arch of the choana to reach the nasal septum.[2]
- This artery has three branches that contribute to the septal circulation.[2]
- The superior branch supplies the anterior-superior area of the septum. In this region, the superior branch anastomoses with a branch from the facial artery and with collaterals of the anterior ethmoidal artery.[2]
- The two inferior branches of the septal artery supply the inferior septum.[2]
- The lowest branch enters the incisive canal to reach the hard palate. It anastomoses with branches of the greater palatine artery.[2]
- The posterior and superior area of the septum are supplied by the posterior ethmoidal artery and its branches.[2]
- In 40% of the cases, there are two branches of the posterior septal artery at the level of the SPA foramen, and in 70% of the cases, there are two branches crossing the anterior wall of the sphenoid sinus inferior to the sphenoid ostium.[3]
- The mean distance between the sphenoid ostium and the first branch crossing below the ostium is 9.3 mm (5–15 mm).[3] This and the presence of two branches crossing below the sphenoid ostium explain the potential availability of the septal flap pedicle in cases of prior sphenoidotomy.[4]

3.2 Fundamentals

- The NSF is the workhorse flap and the first option for vascularized endoscopic cranial base reconstruction.
- It provides transfer of sinonasal mucosa (ciliated pseudostratified columnar epithelium) to cover the nasal surface of the defect.
- The subperichondrial/subperiosteal surface of the flap is oriented toward the defect.
- The main axis of the flap is an imaginary line from the pedicle to the anterior border of the flap and parallel to the nasal floor. This concept is important to help understand the rotation and orientation of the flap during the inset.
- The NSF can be divided into three different regions according to their anatomofunctional characteristics: mucoperichondrium, mucoperiosteum, and vascular pedicle.
  - The mucoperichondrium that covers the septal cartilage is the thicker part and the most reliable for reconstruction (reconstructive area of the flap) (▶ Fig. 3.2a).
  - The mucoperiosteum that covers the vomer and part of the perpendicular plate of the ethmoid is usually used as a "bridge" connecting the pedicle to the reconstructive area (bridging area of the flap).
  - The vascular pedicle is a short area of the flap in close relation to the SPA foramen and the main pivot area for the rotation of the flap.
- These anatomofunctional divisions of the flap are valid for the majority of reconstruction cases and should be considered during the flap inset. It is recommended to always attempt to place the anterior part of the flap covering the defect. However, there are situations (large skull base defects) where the mucoperiosteum can be successfully used to cover the defect and serve as reconstructive area. In such cases, extended dissection of the pedicle area toward the pterygopalatine fossa can improve the reach of the flap and allow the bridging area to be effectively used as reconstructive area (Chapter 6).
- The flap can be harvested from either side of the nasal septum.
- Several factors should be considered before the decision of the harvesting side:
  - Presence of septal deviation: A spur increases the risk of a laceration in the septal mucosa during the harvest and consequently the risk of postoperative cerebrospinal fluid (CSF) leak through the laceration.
  - Preference to the side where less instrumentation is anticipated; particularly, the side where the high-speed drill will be used less.
  - Harvesting the flap on the contralateral side of the tumor or defect is desirable. For example, in cases of meningocele involving the right inferolateral recess of the sphenoid sinus, the left-sided NSF is preferred. This allows a more natural rotation of the flap positioning the thicker reconstructive area of the septal mucosa toward the right inferolateral recess.
  - More spacious side facilitates the harvest. If the harvest is still indicated in the narrow side, consider inferior turbinoplasty and outfracture of the inferior turbinate, resection of the middle turbinate and/or anterior-posterior ethmoidectomy to create more space for the harvest.
- A large sphenoidotomy can preclude the use of the NSF if the septal artery branches are injured during the procedure.[4]
- The availability of the vascular pedicle can be assessed intraoperatively with Doppler sonography in patients with prior sinus or septal surgery.[4]
- The use of intravenous indocyanine green (ICG) can also assess the vascular integrity of the flap intraoperatively.[5]

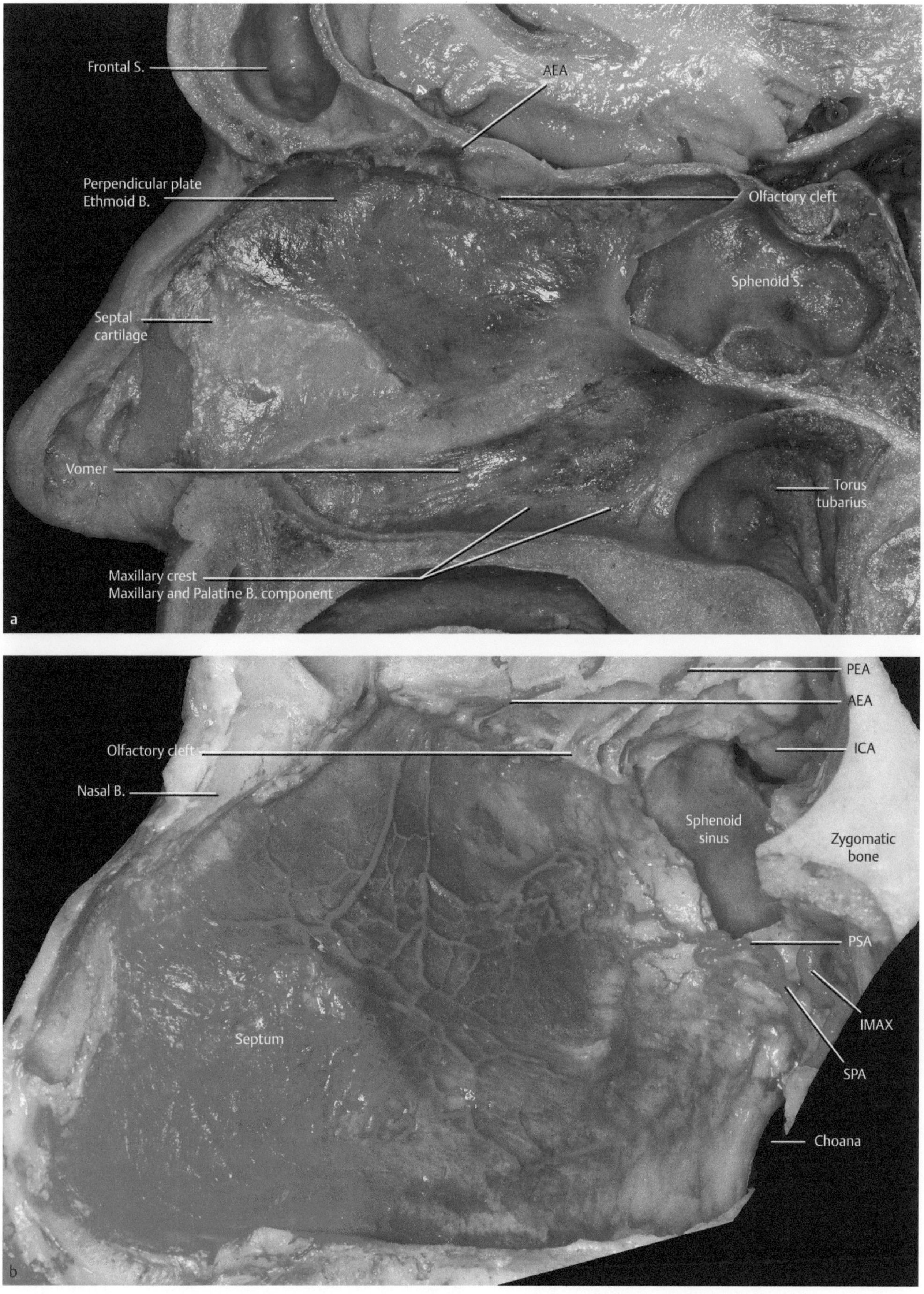

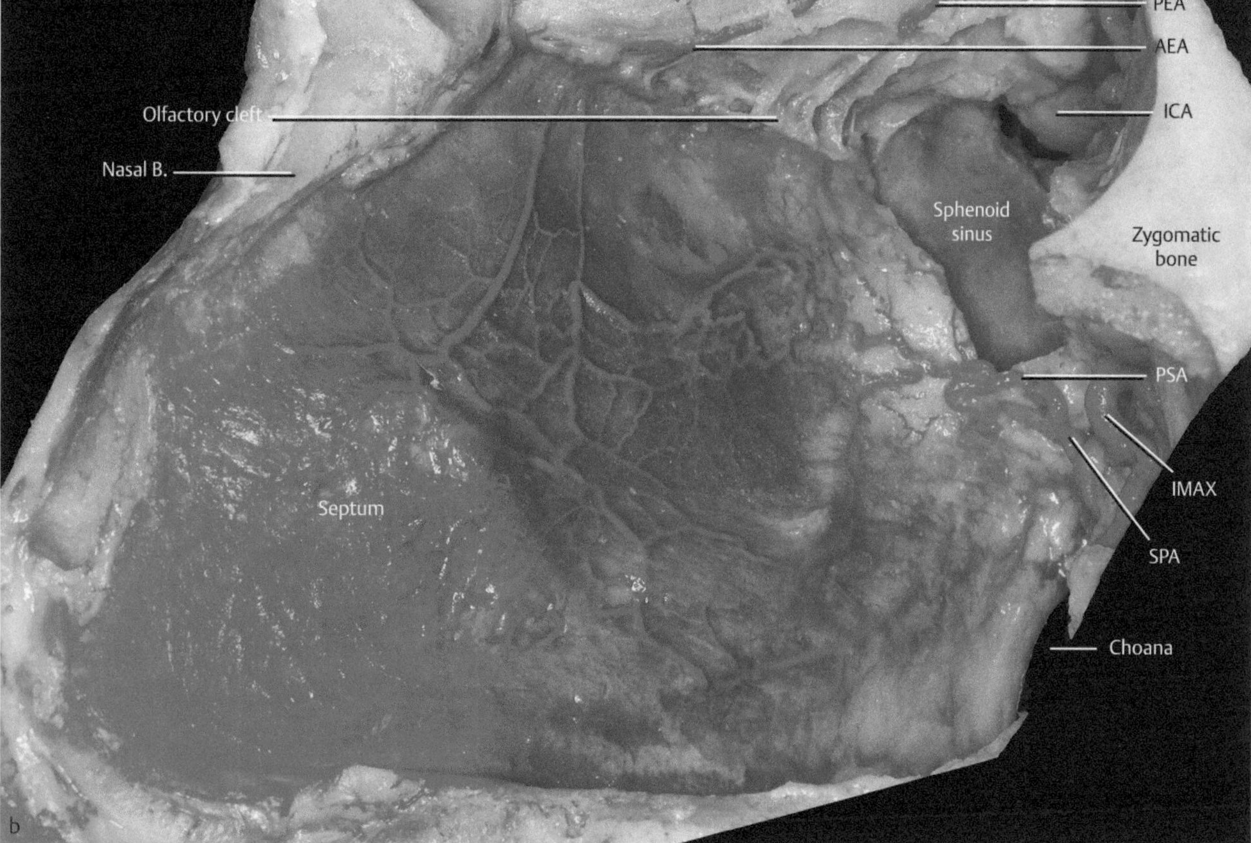

Fig. 3.1 Anatomical dissection of a sagittal hemisectioned cadaveric head to show the components of the nasal septum. (**a**) Components of the septum, the mucosa has been removed. (**b**) Vascular supply of the septum.
AEA, anterior ethmoidal artery; B., bone; ICA, internal carotid artery; IMAX, internal maxillary artery; PEA, posterior ethmoidal artery; PSA, posterior septal artery; SPA, sphenopalatine artery.

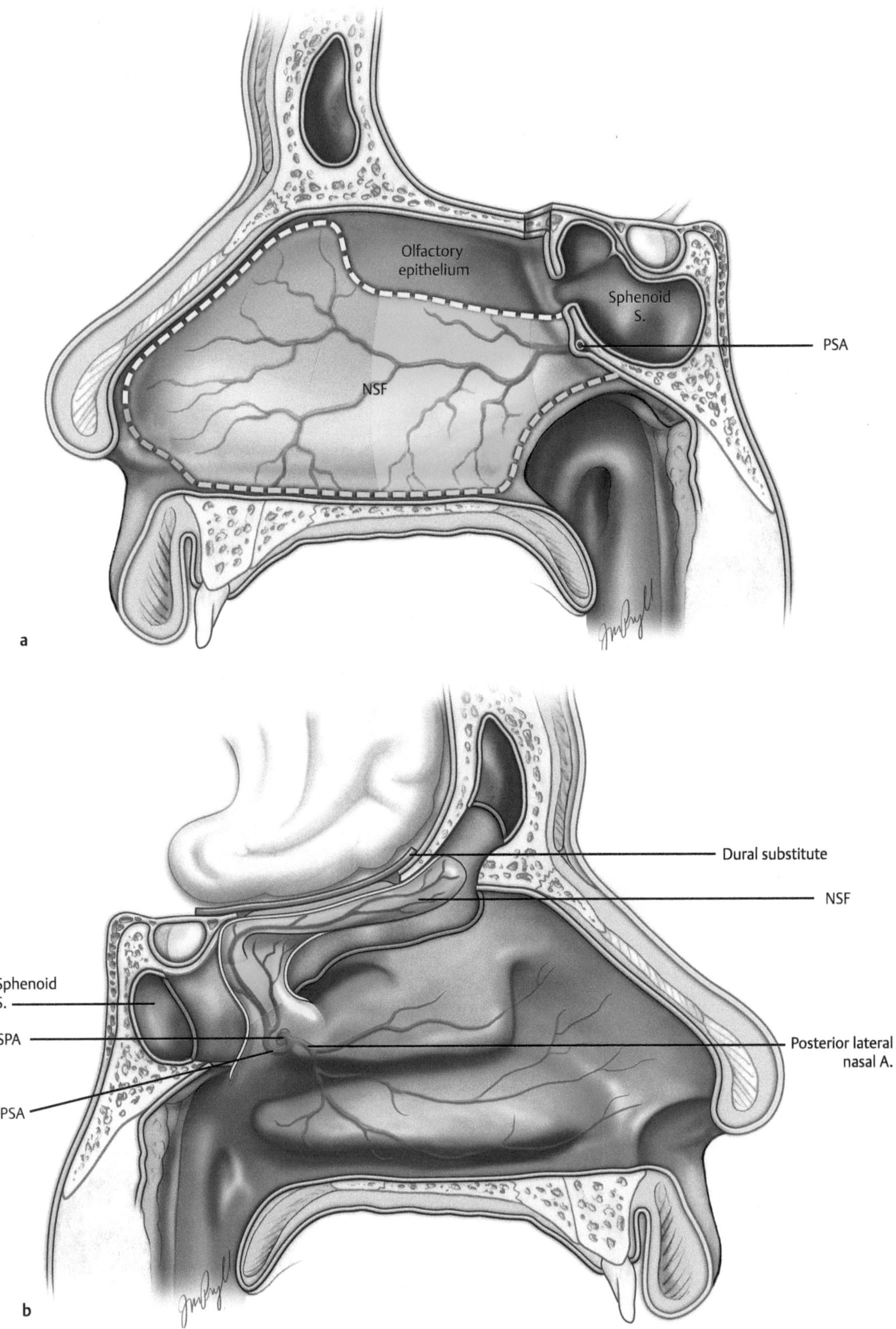

Fig. 3.2 Illustration of the left nasal cavity sagittal view. **(a)** Nasal septum and the anatomofunctional divisions of the flap: mucoperichondrium/reconstructive area (*blue*), mucoperiosteum/bridging area (*green*), and vascular pedicle (*yellow*). The three incisions to harvest the nasoseptal flap (NSF) are highlighted: inferior (*green dashed line*), anterior (*blue dashed line*), and superior (*yellow dashed line*). **(b)** Inset of the NSF to cover the anterior cranial base. The inlay dural substitute is placed first followed by the onlay flap. Observe that the pedicle is positioned along the orbital wall. A, artery; PSA, posterior septal artery; S, sinus; SPA, sphenopalatine artery.

3.3 Indications

- The wide arch of rotation allows the NSF to reach defects in all areas of the ventral cranial base: anterior, middle, or posterior fossae.
- The flap is indicated for reconstruction of a variety of skull base defects including transcribriform, transsellar, suprasellar, transclival, craniovertebral junction, transorbital, infratemporal, middle fossa approaches, etc.
- It can be used in sinonasal malignancies if negative septal margins are confirmed in frozen pathology. It is important to send an oriented single, long strip of mucosa of the entire margin.
- In the pediatric population, the harvest of the NSF has shown no obvious impact in facial growth. Regular sized endonasal instruments and endoscopes can be used in children as young as 2-year old.[6]
- The flap can be reused in revision surgery. Comprehensive inspection of the flap is important to rule out involvement with the recurrent disease.
- Elevating the flap from the skull base during reoperations requires careful dissection. Important neurovascular structures may have been exposed during the approach and the flap healed over. Sharp careful dissection with endoscopic microscissors may be required to safely release the adhesions of the flap in those areas, such as internal carotid arteries and optic nerves.

3.4 Limitations

- The anterior edge of a large anterior cranial base defect is often a concern, and modifications in the standard NSF might be required to accomplish adequate coverage.[3,7]
- Large inferior clivus defects toward the foramen magnum and craniovertebral junction commonly require modifications in the NSF and use of fat graft to fill the deep space of the clivus.[8]
- Bilateral NSFs should be avoided to prevent devascularization of the septal cartilage and potential nasal deformities as saddle nose.
- Septal perforation is not an absolute contraindication to the use of a NSF; however, it will impact the size of the flap. In such situations, the flap is designed excluding the perforation.
- History of prior septoplasty is not a contraindication for the harvest; however, it will make it more challenging and will increase the risk of mucosal lacerations. Sharp dissection with endoscopic microscissors can be used to separate the adhesions between the two septal submucosal surfaces.
- Cicatricial contraction and memory of its position assumed along the cranial base can limit the reuse of the flap during reoperations, particularly if the cranial base defect has to be enlarged during the revision surgery. In such cases, autologous or synthetic grafts can be used as well as a different flap.
- On the other hand, for sellar and suprasellar defects, the relative small size of the defect usually does not jeopardize the reconstruction with a reused flap. In those cases, the common "C"-shaped memory acquired by the flap inside the sphenoid sinus may help its repositioning.
- The NSF is a very effective option for separation and sealing of the intracranial cavity from the nose. However, it does not offer a rigid reconstruction of the bone defect. If a rigid or semirigid reconstruction is desired in selected cases, composite flaps can be used.

3.5 Surgical Technique (*Videos 3.1 and 3.2*)

3.5.1 Harvest

- Mucosal vasoconstriction is achieved with topical oxymetazoline followed by submucosal infiltration of 0.5% xylocaine with 1:2,00,000 epinephrine.
- A 0-degree endoscope is used for visualization.
- The inferior and middle turbinates are lateralized to improve space and expose the sphenoethmoidal recess.
- The vascular pedicle between the sphenoid ostium and the superior border of the arch of the choana is identified.
- A needle-tip extended monopolar electrocautery device (Bovie Medical Corporation) is used on a low setting (10 W) to make three mucosal incisions (inferior, anterior, and superior) (▶ Fig. 3.2a).
- The inferior incision starts at the superior border of the choana and is extended medially along the posterior margin of the vomer toward the nasal floor. It is continued anteriorly along the transition between the septum and nasal floor toward the caudal border of the septum.
- The incisive foramen artery is located in the transition between the nasal floor and septum about 1 cm posterior to the anterior nasal spine. The inferior incision of the flap is performed just superior to the foramen to avoid injury to the incisive foramen artery and nerves that innervate the central incisors.
- The anterior incision is performed along the caudal border of the septum at the mucocutaneous junction.
- The superior incision starts at the sphenoid ostium and is carried anteriorly and parallel to the floor of the nasal cavity approximately 1 cm inferior to the nasal vault (olfactory sulcus). When the incision reaches the level of the anterior attachment of the middle turbinate, it is directed superiorly toward the nasal dorsum to incorporate the most anterior-superior area of the septal mucosa. The incision progresses anteriorly next to the nasal dorsum mucosa to the caudal border of the septum and is connected to the anterior incision (▶ Fig. 3.3).
- The NSF is elevated from anterior to posterior from a subperichondrial plane to a subperiosteal plane until the sphenoid rostrum is widely exposed.
- After the flap is completely elevated, it is placed in the nasopharynx for later reconstruction.
- If the nasopharynx is in the route of the approach (like in transclival approaches), the flap can be placed in the maxillary sinus after performing a wide maxillary antrostomy. A large antrostomy is necessary to prevent ischemic compression of the flap.
- Another option for lower clivus and craniovertebral junction approaches is to place the flap in the sphenoid sinus after a wide sphenoidotomy.

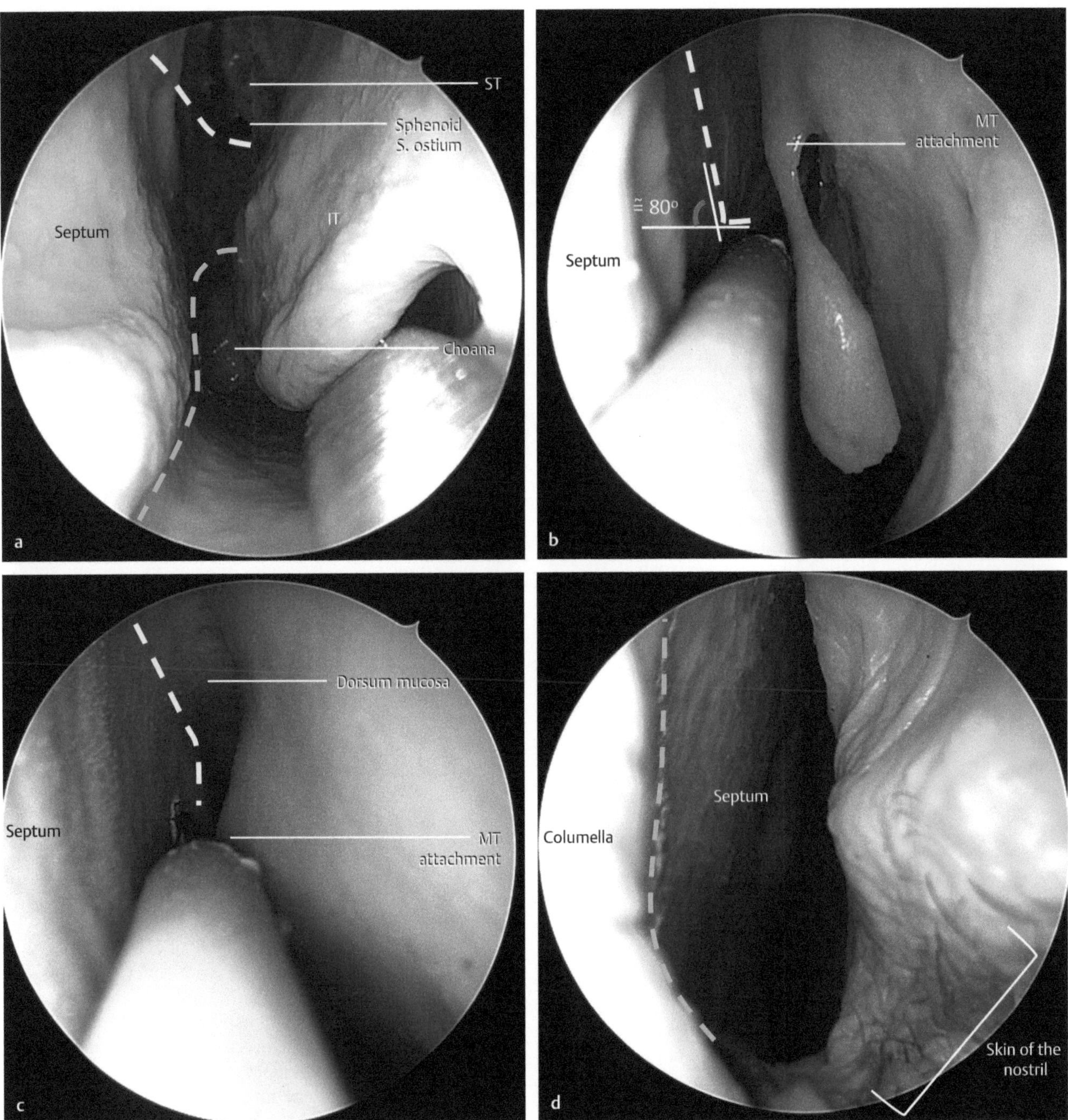

Fig. 3.3 Pictures obtained with a 0-degree endoscope during anatomical dissection of the left nasal cavity. **(a)** Inferior incision (*green dashed line*) and superior incision (*yellow dashed line*) to harvest the nasoseptal flap (NSF). **(b)** The superior incision is turned superiorly toward the nasal dorsum mucosa in an approximate 80-degree angle at the level of the middle turbinate (MT) attachment. This step allows the inclusion of the septal mucosa next to the nasal dorsum. **(c)** The superior incision is carried anteriorly in proximity to the nasal dorsum mucosa toward the caudal border of the septum. **(d)** Anterior incision at the caudal border of the septum (*blue dashed line*). IT, inferior turbinate; S, sinus; ST, superior turbinate.

3.5.2 Reconstruction

- Prior to the reconstruction, the mucosa surrounding the skull base defect should be removed and the underlying bone exposed. This includes mucosa where the pedicle of the flap will lay over as well.
- Two-layer repair is recommended: intradural (inlay) synthetic dural substitute and the extradural (onlay) NSF (▶ Fig. 3.2b).
- Autologous fascia lata graft can be used for inlay reconstruction, especially for high-flow intraoperative CSF leak with opening of suprasellar cisterns. For those cases, an inlay–onlay "button" fascia lata graft is preferred[9] (Chapter 18).
- After the inlay reconstruction, the NSF is rotated to cover the cranial base defect.
- It is important to manipulate the flap carefully to avoid trauma to the vascular pedicle or tearing of the flap.
- The nonmucosal surface of the flap should be in contact only with the inlay graft, surrounding dura, and bone. No sealant or hemostatic materials should be interposed between the flap and the defect. The nonmucosal surface of the flap should be always in contact with a structure such as an orbit or sphenoid walls. It should never be exposed to the air in order to prevent contracture due to healing by secondary intention.
- If mucosa is trapped underneath the flap, mucocele can occur.
- Special attention should be paid to the lateral recesses of the sphenoid sinus. In cases of well-pneumatized recesses, it is recommended to avoid removal of the mucosa of the recess and leave a communication with the nasal cavity during the placement of the flap.
- In cases of shallow sphenoid lateral recess, it is preferable to remove its mucosa and make sure there is adequate contact of the flap to the bone along the recess.
- When the flap is too long, the optimal placement of the reconstructive area of the flap toward the defect is achieved by folding the mucoperiosteal area. Avoiding exposure of the subperiosteum surface to the air is crucial to prevent contraction due to healing by secondary intention.
- The orientation of the flap is key to the success of the reconstruction. For sellar/planum defects, the critical area is usually the inferior edge of the defect where it is under a higher CSF pressure due to gravity. The placement of the bridging area of flap (mucoperiosteum) along the sphenoid sinus floor and clival recess would allow a natural placement of the reconstructive area (mucoperichondrium) covering the sellar/planum. This method of flap inset also allows the formation of a strong barrier against the CSF pressure inferiorly (▶ Fig. 3.4a).
- In cases of deep clival recess, the flap may not be long enough to completely cover the sellar/planum defects. Fat can be used to fill the clivus or the flap can be positioned along the lateral wall of the sphenoid with its reconstructive area covering the sella/planum (▶ Fig. 3.4b).
- If the flap is positioned along the lateral wall of the sphenoid, it is important to make sure the inferolateral recess of the sphenoid is not blocked by the flap or all the mucosa of the recess is removed. This method of flap inset may carry a higher risk of CSF leak along the inferior border of the defect since it lacks the barrier provided by the flap when positioned along the sphenoid floor and clival recess.
- For transcribriform defects, usually the flap will not cover it completely if it follows the contour of the clival recess. In such cases, the mucoperiosteal part of the flap should be placed along the medial wall of the orbit, and modifications to the flap may be necessary to optimize the reconstruction (▶ Fig. 3.5).
- Meticulous attention should be paid to the placement of the flap. This is the step where most of the errors occur, resulting in postoperative CSF leaks.
- If the defect is larger than anticipated, a second intranasal flap can be harvested. It is recommended to use a different flap than the contralateral septal mucosa in order to decrease the risk of septal deformities. Autologous or synthetic grafts can also be used.
- After the flap is positioned, it needs to be supported intranasally to counteract the intracranial pressure.
- 1 × 1 inch pieces of oxidized cellulose are placed around the periphery of the flap to improve adherence and prevent flap migration.
- Few pieces of absorbable gelatin sponge can be placed over some recessed areas of the flap to achieve a flushed surface. This would keep the pressure from the packing uniform along the flap and no dead space between the packing and the flap.
- A common area where absorbable gelatin sponges can be used is over the flap in the clival recess.
- Then a dural sealant is applied sparingly to cover the entire reconstruction.
- Finally, absorbable packing is used for all kinds of cranial base defects. It provides excellent support to the reconstruction with no need for packing removal.
- For sellar and suprasellar approaches, the packing is used only in the sphenoid sinus and sphenoethmoidal recesses, leaving the inferior nasal passages free.
- For large clival defects or extensive anterior cranial base resections, the nasal cavity is fully packed to support the reconstruction. Nonabsorbable packing is usually placed after the absorbable packing to improve the support.
- Silastic septal splints are placed bilaterally and secured anteriorly with a 2:0 Prolene. The splints help prevent synechiae and are removed in 1 week.

3.6 Postoperative Care

- The exposed septal cartilage predisposes to crust formation during the postoperative period and requires several visits to the clinic for nasal debridements.
- During the first week, saline sprays are recommended and no oxymetazoline sprays.
- Large-volume irrigation is not recommended during the first week after the surgery.
- During the first postoperative visit, besides the nasal splints removal, a limited debridement is performed to clean the nasal passages and improve the nasal breathing.
- No debridement close to the flap is performed in the first postoperative visit.
- The patient is instructed to start large-volume saline rinses once a day.
- In cases of very large cranial base defects, large-volume saline irrigation is initiated in the second or third week postoperative. Saline sprays are used until then.

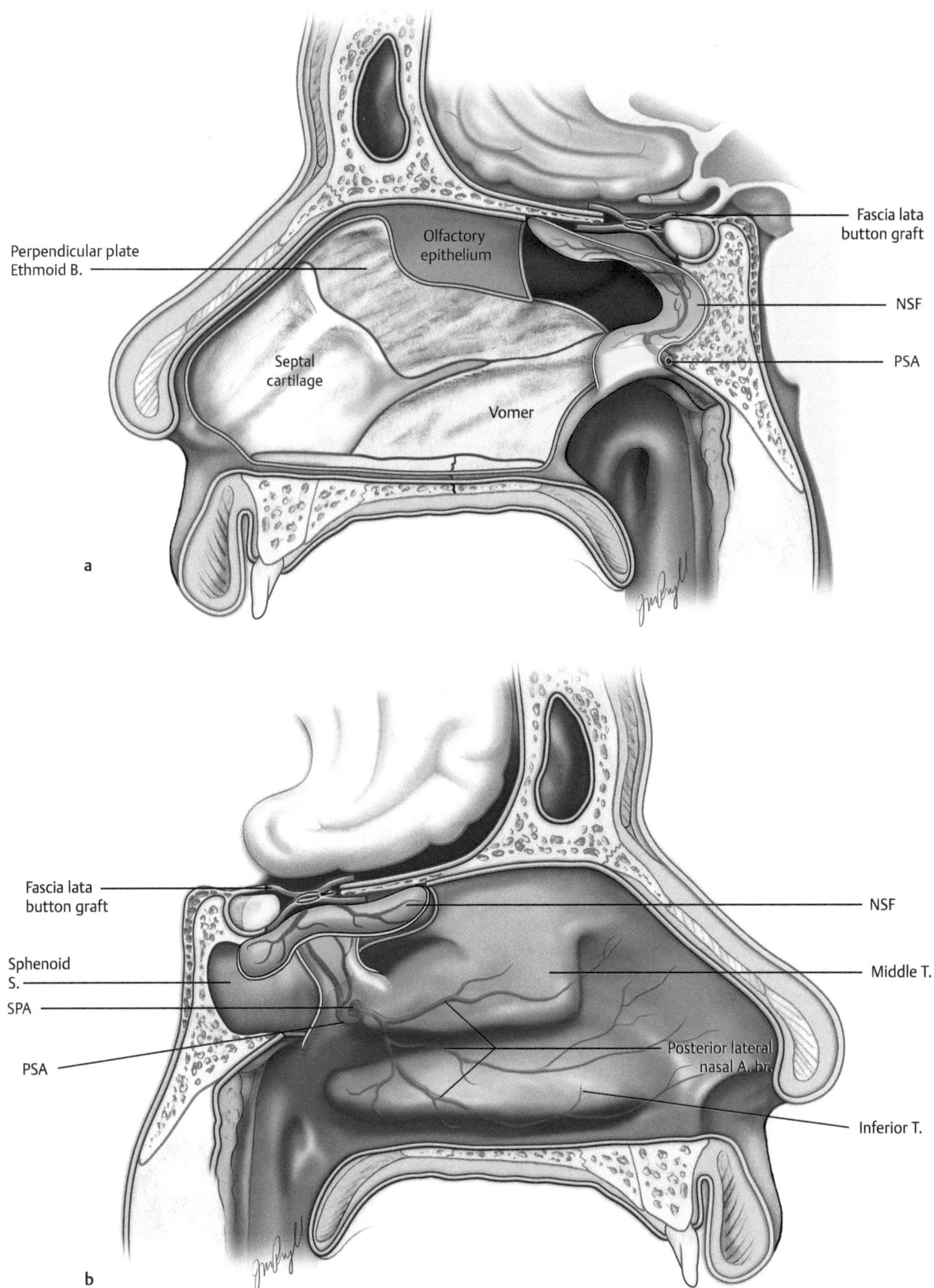

Fig. 3.4 Illustration of the left nasal cavity sagittal view to demonstrate the reconstruction of a planum sphenoidale defect with a nasoseptal flap (NSF) depending on the degree of pneumatization of the sphenoid sinus. **(a)** The presellar type of pneumatization of the sphenoid sinus usually allows the NSF inset along the sphenoid sinus floor, clivus, and anterior wall of the sella before reaching the defect. This creates a reliable closure along the inferior edge of the defect, which may be more susceptible to CSF pressure from gravity. **(b)** The sellar type of pneumatization of the sphenoid sinus is usually reconstructed positioning the NSF along the orbital wall/lateral wall of the sphenoid. The deep clival recess in such cases may prevent adequate coverage of the planum since the flap should be in contact to the sphenoid sinus floor, clival recess, sellar floor, and anterior wall of the sella before reaching the planum sphenoidale. A, artery; B, bone; br., branch; PSA, posterior septal artery; S, sinus; SPA, sphenopalatine artery; T, turbinate.

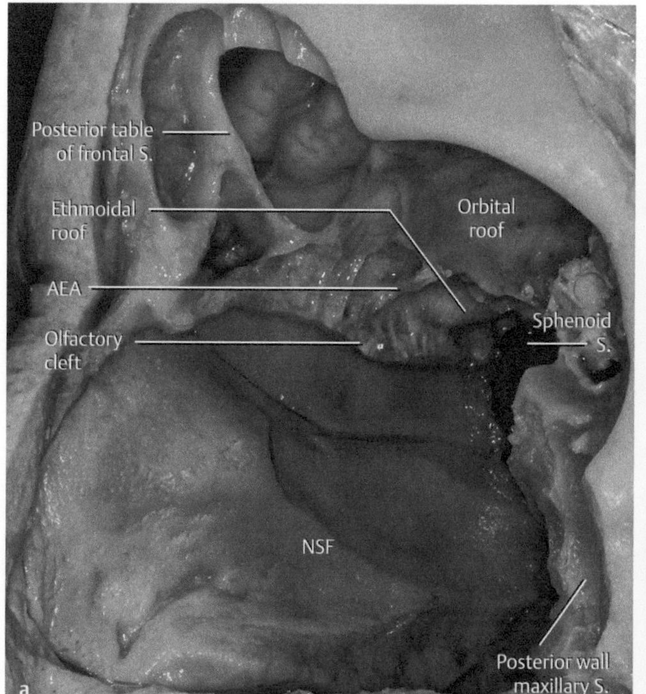

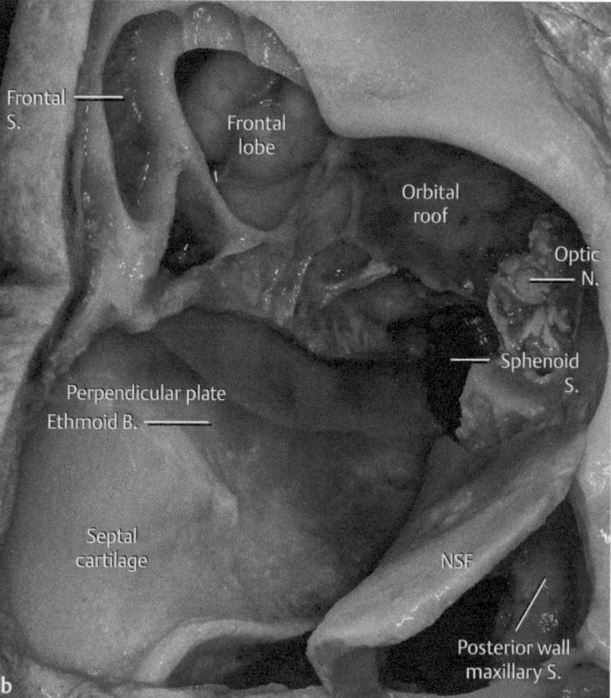

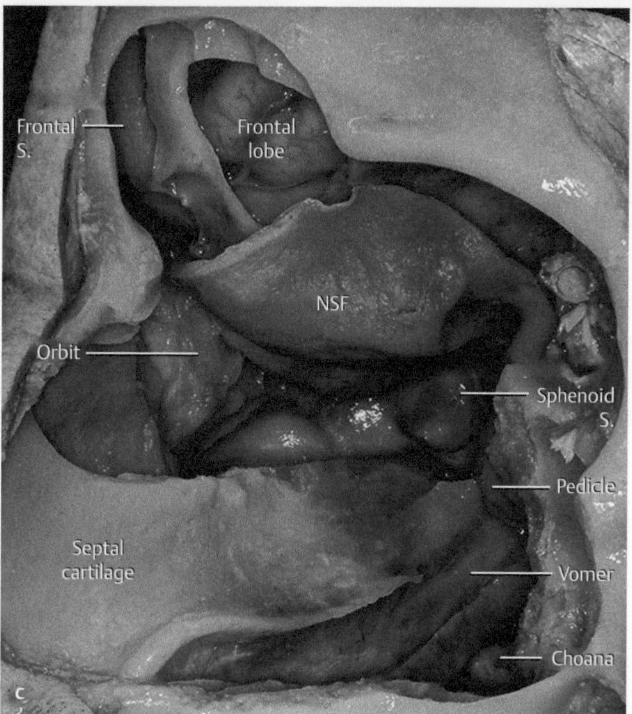

Fig. 3.5 Anatomical dissection after removal of the left hemiface and exposure of the nasal septum. **(a)** Nasoseptal flap (NSF) after the incisions were completed. **(b)** Elevation of the NSF in a subperichondrial and subperiosteal planes. **(c)** Flap inset along the anterior cranial base. Observe the pedicle is placed along the orbit to allow a better anterior reach of the flap. The dissection illustrates a defect of the posterior table of the frontal sinus. Modifications of the flap, particularly the extended dissection toward the pterygopalatine fossa, are necessary to allow its mobilization and coverage of such anterior defect. AEA, anterior ethmoidal artery; N, nerve; S, sinus.

- The second postoperative visit is 1 month after the first visit. Extensive debridement is performed with great visualization of the flap.
- The patient returns to the clinic every 3 months for further debridement until the septum is completely healed.
- It can take several months for complete mucosalization of the exposed cartilage and even when completely mucosalized, crust may still build up along the septum. This is because of impairment of the mucociliary clearance of the new septal mucosa, which can be permanent.
- The septum donor site healing process can be accelerated with placement of a free mucosal graft or mucosal flap to cover the exposed cartilage. Nasal debridement over the septum should be avoided until the graft or flap is completely healed to the septal cartilage. Early debridement in the area can cause avulsion of the graft or flap.
- It is important to assess the patency of the sinuses and make sure there is no evidence of CSF leak in follow-up nasal endoscopies. The transmission of brain pulsation to the flap is usually noticeable and has no clinical repercussion (▶ Fig. 3.6).

3.7 Managing Complications

- Patients with history of prior septoplasty or transseptal transsphenoidal surgery are at greater risk of laceration of the flap during the dissection.
- If a laceration of the flap happens during the harvesting, try to orient the flap in a way that the tear does not match with the cranial base defect.
- If the laceration coincides with the cranial base defect, the laceration can be sutured or a small plug of fat graft can be placed through the hole.
- If the laceration on the flap is large and the contralateral NSF is available, consider the harvest of a contralateral flap. The flap with the laceration is positioned back and sutured anteriorly.
- If the contralateral NSF is not available, consider the harvest of another flap: lateral nasal wall flap, pericranial flap, temporoparietal fascia flap, etc.
- Injury to the pedicle is not common. The pedicle should be protected during drilling or when using a microdebrider.
- Excessive electrocautery in proximity to the pedicle should be avoided.
- One common reason of failure of the reconstruction is a short/small flap.
- Incorporate the upper septal mucosa below the nasal bones and superior lateral cartilages to maximize the flap size. The mucosa of the nasal floor and inferior meatus can also be included.
- In order to avoid tension and extend the reach of the flap, the pedicle can be carefully mobilized and dissected laterally toward the maxillary artery within the pterygopalatine and infratemporal fossae.
- Saddle nose can occur several months after surgery. In some cases, the deformity is severe enough causing nasal obstruction and requiring septorhinoplasty. Performing the superior incision of the NSF along the nasal dorsum mucosa with microscissors instead of electrocautery decreases the thermal energy next to the upper lateral cartilages and may decrease the risk of scarring and saddle nose (Video 3.3).
- Septal cartilage necrosis and septal perforation can occur, especially if both sides of the septal mucosa are harvested.
- Anosmia or hyposmia can happen. Preservation of the superior and middle turbinates and 1 cm of the nasal septum olfactory mucosa are important to preserve the olfaction.
- Some degree of brain sagging, particularly in large anterior cranial base defects, is often a finding of no clinical relevance. If brain sagging is an anticipated concern, the use of composite flaps may help to achieve a more rigid reconstruction.

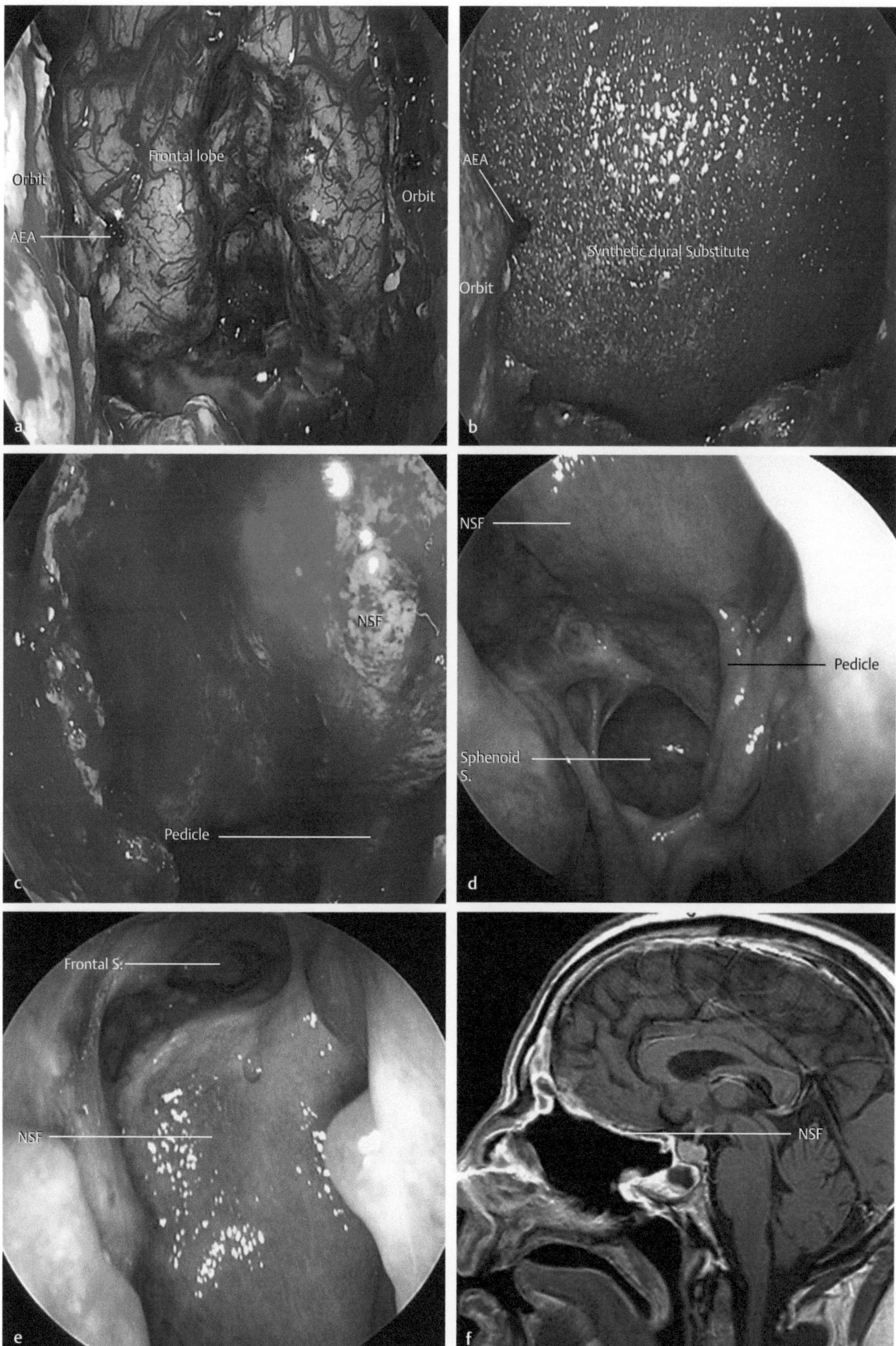

Fig. 3.6 Clinical case of a patient who had endoscopic endonasal anterior cranial base resection for esthesioneuroblastoma. **(a–c)** Intraoperative pictures obtained with a 0-degree endoscope. **(a)** Anterior cranial base defect after the resection. **(b)** Placement of the inlay synthetic dural graft. **(c)** Nasoseptal flap (NSF) inset after the superior margin of the flap was confirmed to be negative in frozen pathology. **(d, e)** Nasal endoscopy performed in clinic 12 months after the surgery with a flexible endoscope. **(d)** Observe the position of the pedicle along the left orbital wall. **(e)** Frontal sinuses outflow patent. **(f)** MRI sagittal view T1 with contrast showing the flap enhancing with contrast 12 months after the surgery. AEA, anterior ethmoidal artery; S, sinus.

References

[1] Hadad G, Bassagasteguy L, Carrau RL, et al. A novel reconstructive technique after endoscopic expanded endonasal approaches: vascular pedicle nasoseptal flap. Laryngoscope. 2006; 116(10):1882–1886

[2] Babin E, Moreau S, de Rugy MG, Delmas P, Valdazo A, Bequignon A. Anatomic variations of the arteries of the nasal fossa. Otolaryngol Head Neck Surg. 2003; 128(2):236–239

[3] Pinheiro-Neto CD, Ramos HF, Peris-Celda M, et al. Study of the nasoseptal flap for endoscopic anterior cranial base reconstruction. Laryngoscope. 2011; 121 (12):2514–2520

[4] Pinheiro-Neto CD, Carrau RL, Prevedello DM, et al. Use of acoustic Doppler sonography to ascertain the feasibility of the pedicled nasoseptal flap after prior bilateral sphenoidotomy. Laryngoscope. 2010; 120(9):1798–1801

[5] Kerr EE, Jamshidi A, Carrau RL, et al. Indocyanine green fluorescence to evaluate nasoseptal flap viability in endoscopic endonasal cranial base surgery. J Neurol Surg B Skull Base. 2017; 78(5):408–412

[6] Shah RN, Surowitz JB, Patel MR, et al. Endoscopic pedicled nasoseptal flap reconstruction for pediatric skull base defects. Laryngoscope. 2009; 119 (6):1067–1075

[7] Pinheiro-Neto CD, Prevedello DM, Carrau RL, et al. Improving the design of the pedicled nasoseptal flap for skull base reconstruction: a radioanatomic study. Laryngoscope. 2007; 117(9):1560–1569

[8] Peris-Celda M, Pinheiro-Neto CD, Funaki T, et al. The extended nasoseptal flap for skull base reconstruction of the clival region: an anatomical and radiological study. J Neurol Surg B Skull Base. 2013; 74(6):369–385

[9] Luginbuhl AJ, Campbell PG, Evans J, Rosen M. Endoscopic repair of high-flow cranial base defects using a bilayer button. Laryngoscope. 2010; 120(5): 876–880

4 Rescue Nasoseptal Flap

Carlos D. Pinheiro-Neto, Luciano C. P. C. Leonel, and Maria Peris-Celda

4.1 Fundamentals

- The rescue flap technique is not a flap; it is a technique of preservation of the pedicle (posterior septal artery) during an endoscopic endonasal approach for a possible harvest of the nasoseptal flap later in the surgery if needed.
- The main goal is to maintain intact vascular supply to the nasal septum (posterior septal artery) along the anterior wall of the sphenoid sinus during endoscopic cranial base procedures.[1] The average distance between the sphenoid ostium and the septal artery is 9.3 mm[2] (▶ Fig. 4.1).
- This technique involves the removal of the sphenoid rostrum and drilling of the sphenoid sinus floor with preservation of the pedicle.
- The preservation of the pedicle can be done in one side or both sides, depending on the degree of exposure needed. Bilateral pedicle preservation should always be attempted if possible.
- The rescue flap incision should also preserve the olfactory epithelium of the nasal septum.

4.2 Indications

- In cases where the need for vascularized reconstruction is not anticipated.
- Perform it on both sides when possible. The preservation of the vascular pedicle is important as a backup plan and for future surgeries.
- In staged procedures, when the first stage does not include intradural dissection. The pedicle can be preserved during the first stage, and the flap is harvested on the second stage.

4.3 Limitations

- The vascular pedicle crossing the anterior wall of the sphenoid limits the inferior reach toward the clival recess and laterally during transpterygoid approaches.
- Because the flap is not elevated upfront, increased attention should be taken to avoid septal mucosal lacerations or injury to the pedicle during the surgery.

4.4 Surgical Technique (*Video 4.1*)

- The middle and superior turbinates are lateralized and the natural ostium of the sphenoid sinus is identified. The natural ostium of the sphenoid sinus is medial to the superior turbinate in more than 80% of the cases.[3]
- The incision starts at the inferior aspect of the sphenoid sinus ostium and progresses anteriorly and parallel to the floor of the nasal cavity for about 1 cm (▶ Fig. 4.2a).
- The septal mucosa is gently elevated from anterior to posterior following an inferior direction to expose the bone of the sphenoid rostrum (▶ Fig. 4.2b).
- The pedicle is carefully mobilized inferiorly, and the dissection progresses posteriorly toward the roof of the nasopharynx.
- A Frazier tip suction can be placed deep in this "submucosal pocket" created toward the roof of the nasopharynx between the mucosa and the bone. The suction tip allows retraction of the pedicle inferiorly improving exposure of the bone and protecting the pedicle during the drilling (▶ Fig. 4.3).
- After wide exposure of the bone of the sphenoid rostrum, drilling can be performed with preservation of the vascular pedicle.
- If drilling of the sphenoid sinus floor is required, an additional inferior incision can be performed along the superior border of the arch of the choana. This allows mobilization of the pedicle superiorly. A Frazier tip suction can be used for retraction and protection of the pedicle during the drilling.
- Extended pedicle dissection toward the pterygopalatine fossa with removal of the osseous boundaries of the sphenopalatine foramen also improves the inferior mobilization of the rescue flap pedicle.
- If the nasoseptal flap is necessary during the surgery, the rescue flap incision is prolonged anteriorly as the superior incision for the standard nasoseptal flap. The remaining flap incisions are performed as usual.

4.5 Postoperative Care

- If the nasoseptal flap is not harvested, less crust will form in the postoperative period.
- Postoperative visits are scheduled 1 week, 1 month, and 4 months after surgery for nasal debridement.
- Saline nasal irrigation is used until the nasal mucosa is completely healed.

4.6 Complications

- The presence of the pedicle across the anterior wall of the sphenoid sinus during the surgery increases the risk of pedicle injury from the insertion of instruments. Special care should be taken, especially in the nostril with no direct endoscopic visualization.
- Be careful while resting the drill on the pedicle because of the risk of thermal injury.
- Excessive inferior retraction of the pedicle can lead to compromise of the blood supply or venous drainage.
- The inferior retraction of the pedicle can lead to a laceration next to the sphenopalatine foramen or laceration along the septal mucosa compromising the flap.

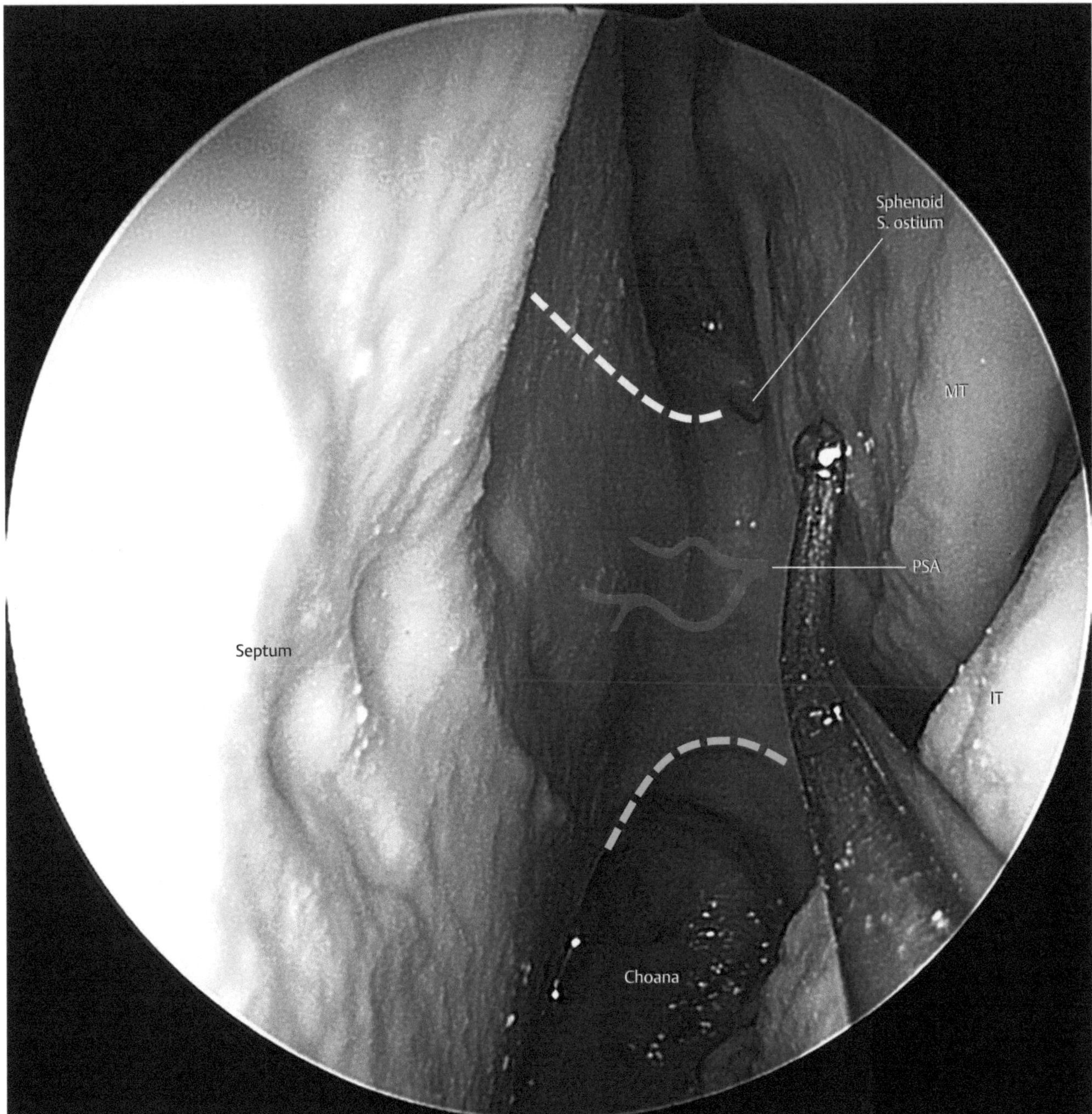

Fig. 4.1 Anatomical dissection picture obtained with a 0-degree endoscope of the left nasal cavity. The posterior septal artery (PSA) crosses the anterior sphenoid sinus wall about 9 mm below the sphenoid ostium. Often two branches of the artery are present at that level. *Yellow dashed line* represents the rescue flap incision. *Green dashed line* represents an additional incision that can be done along the superior border of the choana if drilling of the sphenoid sinus floor is needed. IT, inferior turbinate; MT, middle turbinate; S, sinus.

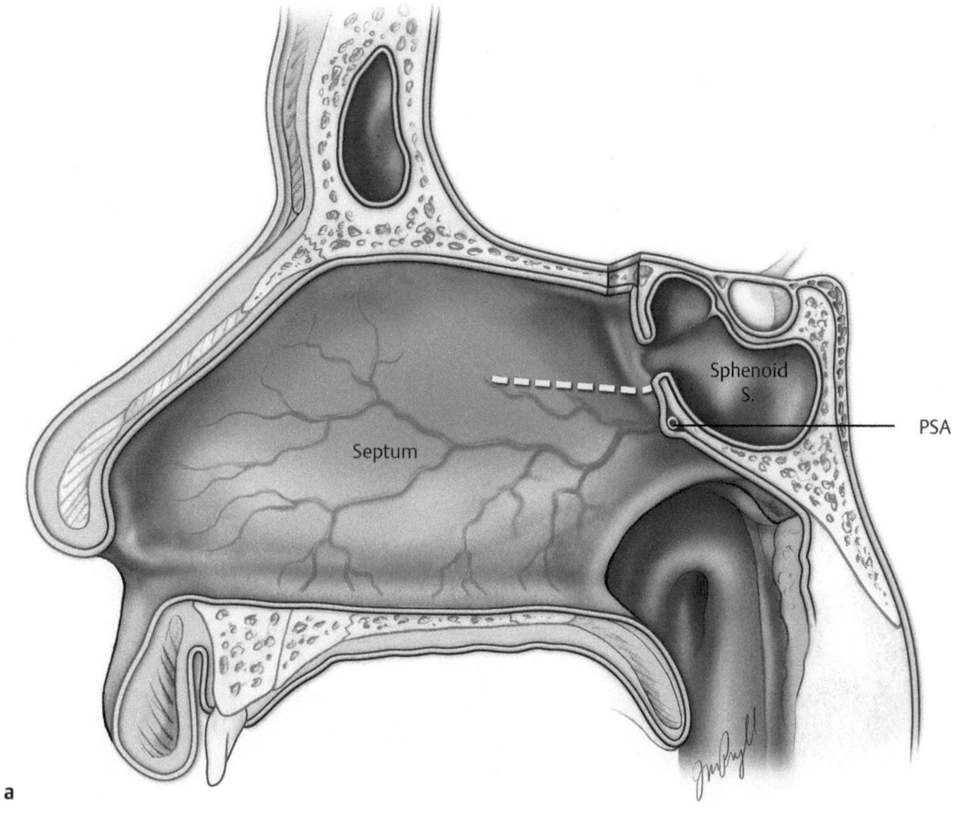

Sphenoid S.
PSA
Septum
a

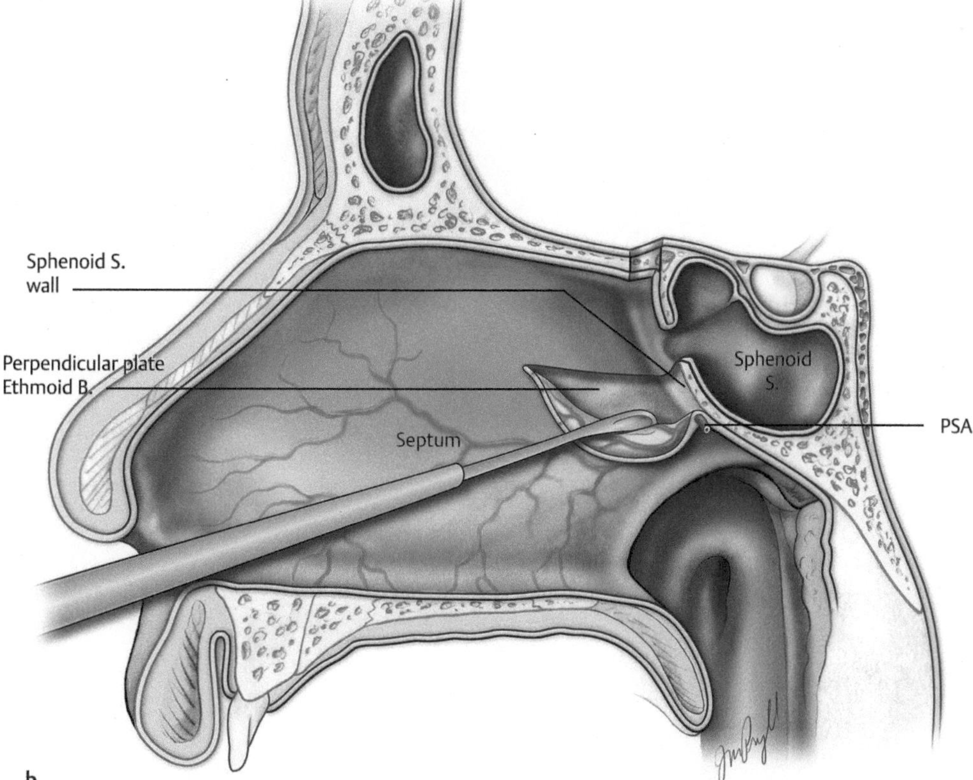

Fig. 4.2 Illustration of the rescue flap technique on the left side. **(a)** *Yellow dashed line* demonstrates the incision along the anterior sphenoid sinus wall and nasal septum. **(b)** Inferior retraction of the pedicle. B, bone; PSA, posterior septal artery; S, sinus.

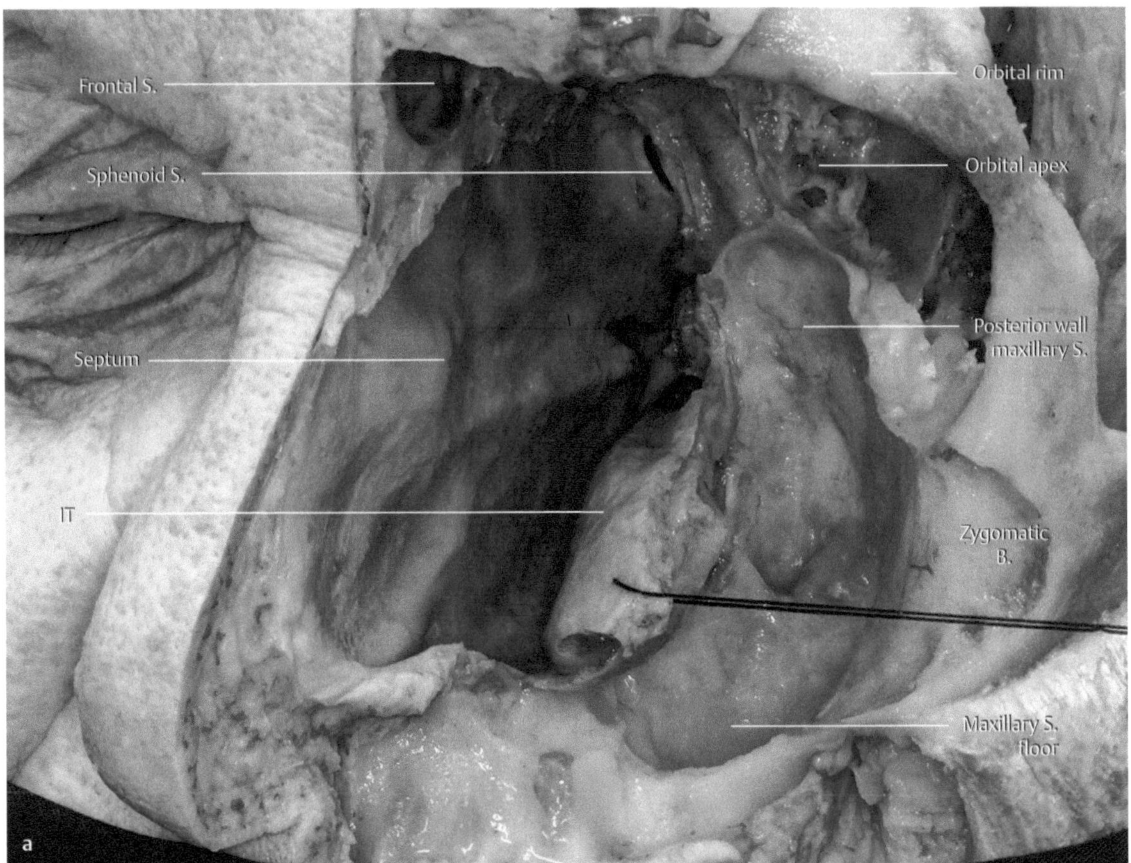

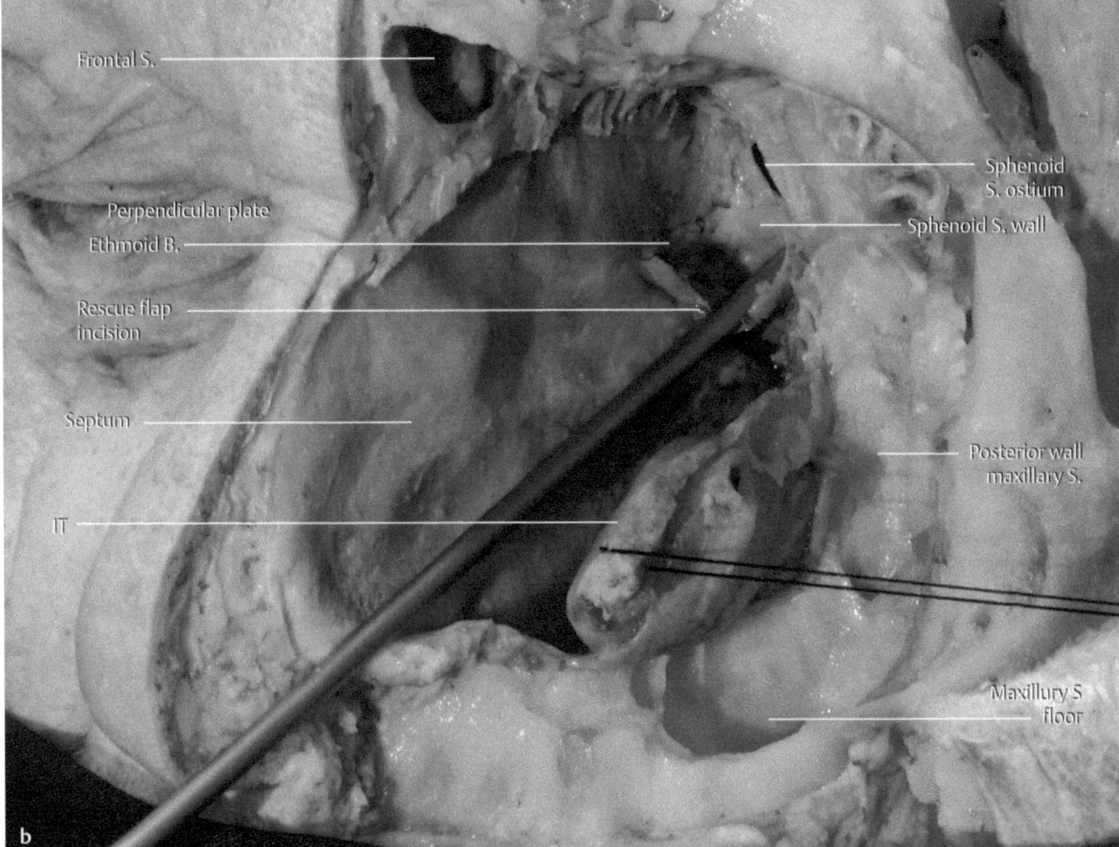

Fig. 4.3 Anatomical dissection showing the "submucosal pocket" created toward the roof of the nasopharynx and retracted inferiorly with a Frazier tip suction. This allows drilling of the anterior sphenoid sinus wall and protection of the vascular pedicle to the nasal septum. B, bone; IT, inferior turbinate; S, sinus.

References

[1] Rivera-Serrano CM, Snyderman CH, Gardner P, et al. Nasoseptal "rescue" flap: a novel modification of the nasoseptal flap technique for pituitary surgery. Laryngoscope. 2011; 121(5):990–993

[2] Pinheiro-Neto CD, Ramos HF, Peris-Celda M, et al. Study of the nasoseptal flap for endoscopic anterior cranial base reconstruction. Laryngoscope. 2011; 121 (12):2514–2520

[3] Filho BC, Pinheiro-Neto CD, Weber R, Voegels RL. Sphenoid sinus symmetry and differences between sexes. Rhinology. 2008; 46(3):195–199

5 Extended Nasoseptal Flap

Carlos D. Pinheiro-Neto, Luciano C. P. C. Leonel, and Maria Peris-Celda

5.1 Fundamentals

- The extended nasoseptal flap (ENSF) includes the mucosa of the nasal cavity floor and inferior meatus to increase the cross-sectional area of the standard nasoseptal flap (NSF).[1] The ENSF is not simply a standard NSF in a larger scale. The shape of the extended flap is different. The mucosal addition is located more posteriorly (▶ Fig. 5.1a).
- The inferior incision of the standard flap is replaced by a lateral incision within the inferior meatus.
- The nasolacrimal duct opens to the inferior meatus at the Hasner valve. This opening is located in the anterior part of the meatus.
- The amount of mucosa added to the flap can be tailored accordingly to the size and type of the defect.[2] The maximum mucosal inclusion is obtained when the lateral incision is performed along the attachment of the inferior turbinate to the lateral wall.
- The main axis of the flap is an imaginary line from the pedicle to the anterior edge and parallel to the nasal floor. This concept helps in understanding the rotation and orientation of the flap during the inset.
- Inferior clival defects where there is intracranial communication with the nasopharynx are challenging for reconstruction. Besides being an area of high intracranial pressure, the inferior edge of the extended flap is in contact to the nasopharyngeal tissues with lack of a buttress. When possible, the preservation of the nasopharyngeal roof during posterior fossa approaches is recommended to avoid intracranial communication toward the nasopharynx and keep a buttress for reconstruction. In such cases, the standard NSF may be enough to cover the defect.[3]

5.2 Indications

- Large posterior fossa defects with violation of the nasopharynx. In such cases, not only the nasal floor mucosa is included but also the mucosa of the inferior meatus lateral wall. The lateral incision is made along the attachment of the inferior turbinate. The flap is positioned with the main axis parallel to the sellar floor, and extra mucosa from the inferior meatus will naturally lie over inferiorly toward the craniovertebral junction. Fat graft is commonly used to fill the clival defect prior to the inset of the extended flap. This will move the contact point of the flap anteriorly, optimizing the positioning of the flap. Additionally, the fat graft creates a thicker reconstructive layer to decrease the risk of encephalocele (▶ Fig. 5.1b).
- Large anterior cranial base defects from the sella to the posterior wall of the frontal sinus.[4] The rotation of the flap is performed leaving the pedicle along the ipsilateral orbit. The main axis of the flap is oriented diagonally along the anterior skull base with the reconstructive area anteriorly and the extra mucosa from the nasal floor toward the sella (▶ Fig. 5.1c).
- The extended flap can also be used for large infratemporal fossa and middle cranial fossa defects.

5.3 Limitations

- Harder inset due to the configuration and size of the flap.
- The increase in the cross-section area of the flap is not uniform.
- The extra mucosa added to flap is located posterior and inferior to the mucoperichondrium (main reconstructive area of the standard flap).[5]

5.4 Surgical Technique (*Video 5.1*)

5.4.1 Harvest

- Zero-degree endoscope is used. ▶ Fig. 5.2 illustrates the incisions for the ENSF. The superior and anterior incisions are the same as the standard NSF, and the inferior incision is different. Usually, the inferior incision is performed first, then the anterior, and finally the superior, but this order can be changed.
- The inferior turbinate is initially outfractured laterally.
- The inferior incision starts at the superior border of the choana and is carried along the posterior border of the vomer toward the nasal cavity floor (same as the one used for the standard NSF).
- At the floor of the nasal cavity, the incision is progressed laterally toward the inferior meatus along the transition between the hard and soft palates.
- A vertical incision with endoscopic sinus scissors can be performed at the head of the inferior turbinate to improve its superior mobilization and exposure of the inferior meatus.
- In some cases, the nasal septum can be used to support the inferior turbinate in a superior position while working on the inferior meatus.
- After wide exposure of the inferior meatus, the inferior flap incision is continued laterally toward the inferior meatus lateral wall. The amount of extra mucosa included is tailored according to the defect.
- The inferior flap incision can be extended toward the attachment of the inferior turbinate. Then it is carried anteriorly along the inferior turbinate attachment toward the head of the inferior turbinate. Care should be taken with the Hasner valve (▶ Fig. 5.3).
- At the head of the inferior turbinate, the incision is turned toward the septum and carried along the inferior border of the piriform aperture.
- After the anterior and superior incisions of the flap are completed, the ENSF is elevated in three steps:
  1. Septum:
     - The inferior turbinate is moved back to its natural position.
     - The flap is elevated from the septal cartilage in the subperichondrial plane.

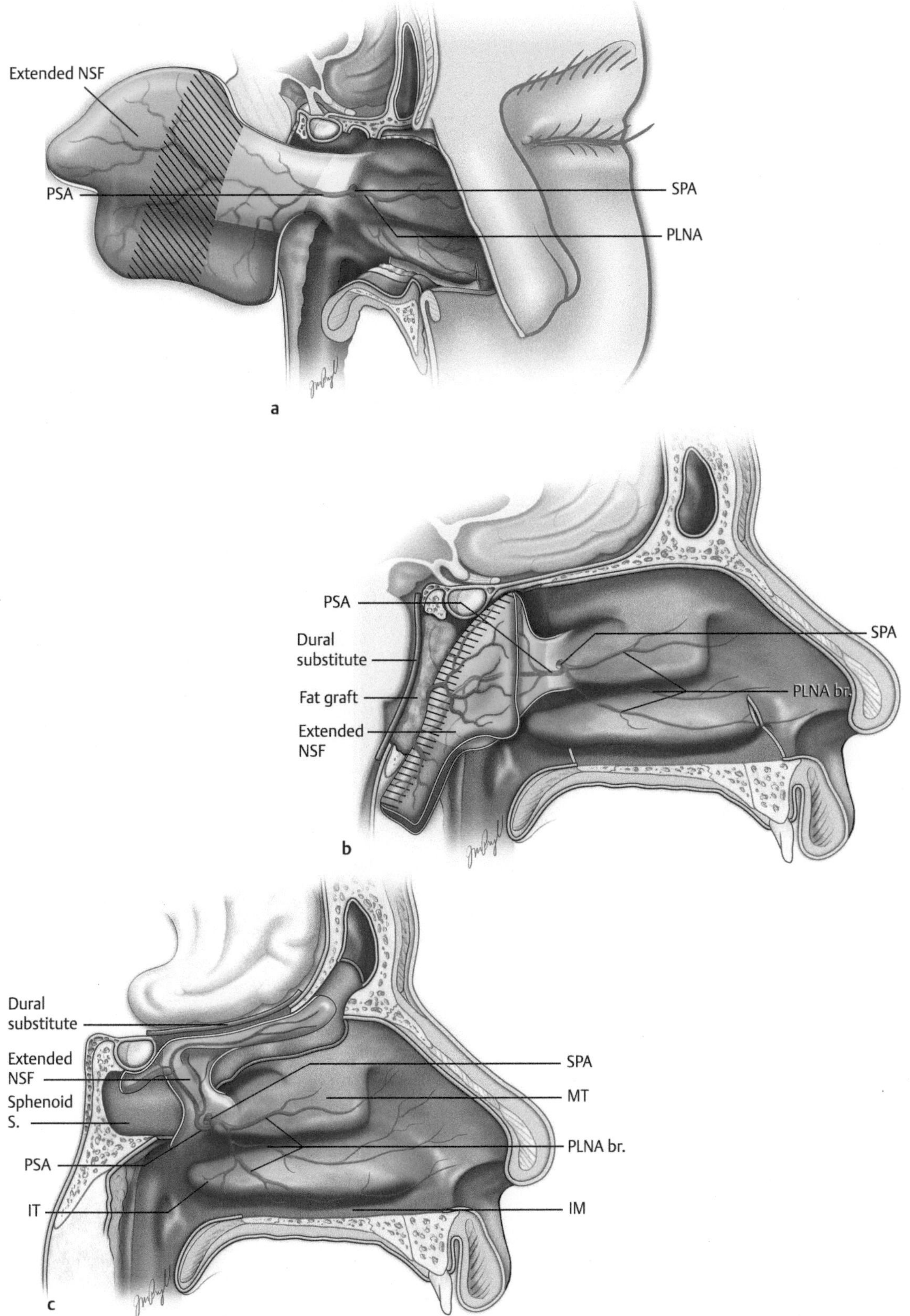

Fig. 5.1 Illustration of a hemisectioned head to show the anatomofunctional divisions of the extended nasoseptal flap (ENSF). **(a)** Note that the ENSF is not a standard nasoseptal flap (NSF) in a larger scale. The incorporation of the extra mucosa (*red*) from the nasal floor and inferior meatus (IM) does not evenly augment the reconstructive area (*blue*) of the standard flap. Half of the extra mucosa added is actually related to the bridging area (*green*) of the standard flap. *Yellow* represents the pedicle area. Because of this unequal augmentation, when the extended flap is used to cover a large clival defect, its reconstructive area (hatched zone) is different from the reconstructive area (*blue*) of the standard flap. **(b)** Inset of the ENSF to cover a large clival defect. Observe the layers of reconstruction: Inlay dural substitute, fat graft filling the clival defect, and onlay ENSF. Note hatched zone working as the reconstructive area of the extended flap. **(c)** Inset of the extended flap to reconstruct a large anterior cranial base defect. Note the extra mucosa (*red*) from the nasal floor/IM positioned toward the planum sphenoidale. br., branch; IT, inferior turbinate; MT, middle turbinate; PLNA, posterior lateral nasal artery; PSA, posterior septal artery; S, sinus; SPA, sphenopalatine artery.

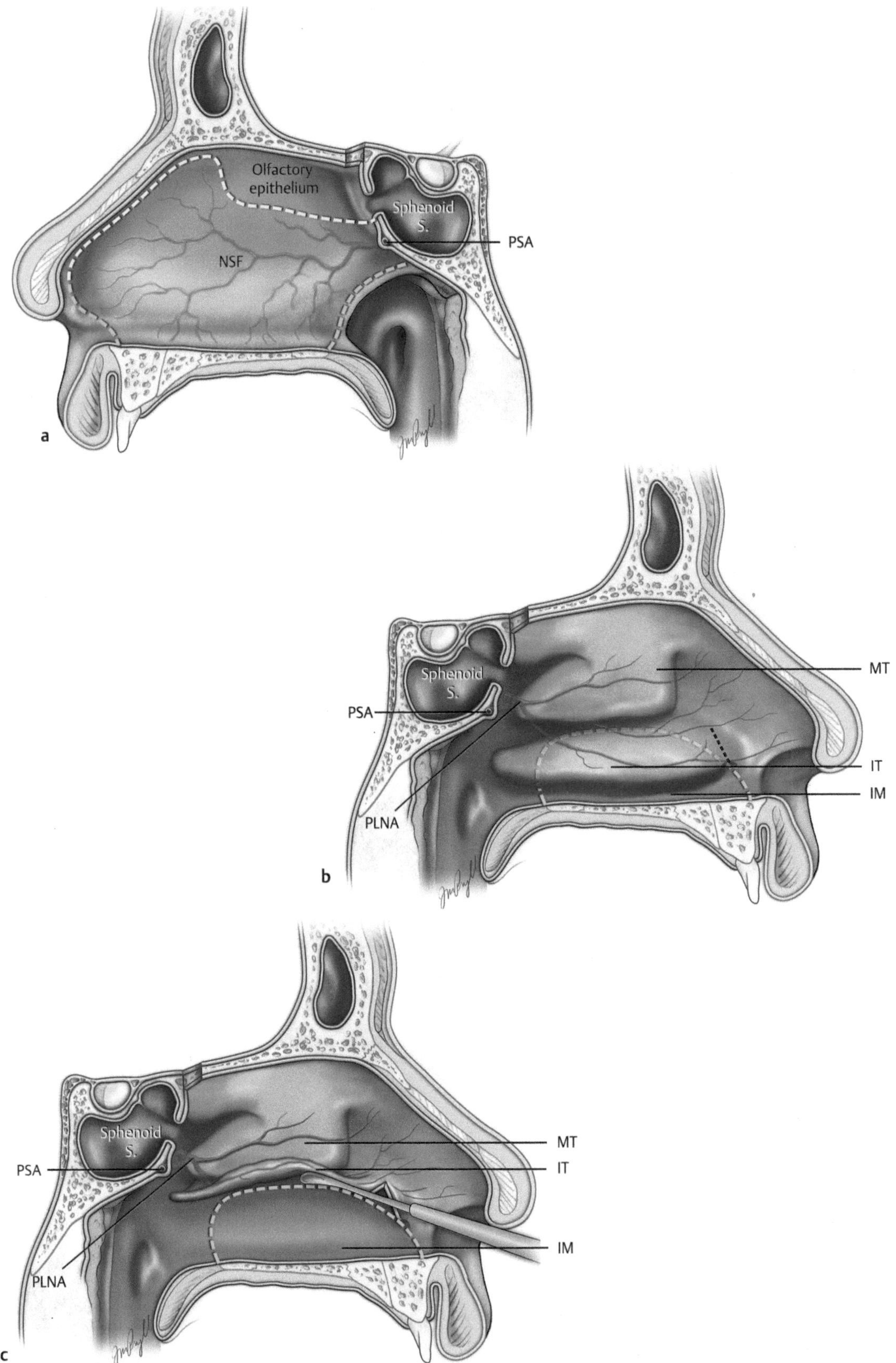

Fig. 5.2 Sagittal view of the left nasal cavity to demonstrate the incisions for the extended nasoseptal flap (ENSF). **(a)** Superior incision (*yellow dashed line*), anterior incision (*blue dashed line*), and inferior incision along the posterior border of the vomer (*green dashed line*). Observe that the inferior incision is not progressed anteriorly along the transition between the septum and the nasal floor as done for the standard nasoseptal flap (NSF). **(b)** Left lateral nasal wall. *Green dashed line* represents the extension of the inferior incision laterally toward the inferior meatus (IM). *Black dashed line* shows the incision that can be performed at the head of the inferior turbinate (IT). This allows the superior mobilization of the turbinate and great exposure of the IM. **(c)** Lateral incision along the attachment of the IT within the IM after superior mobilization of the IT. MT, middle turbinate; PLNA, posterior lateral nasal artery; PSA, posterior septal artery; S, sinus.

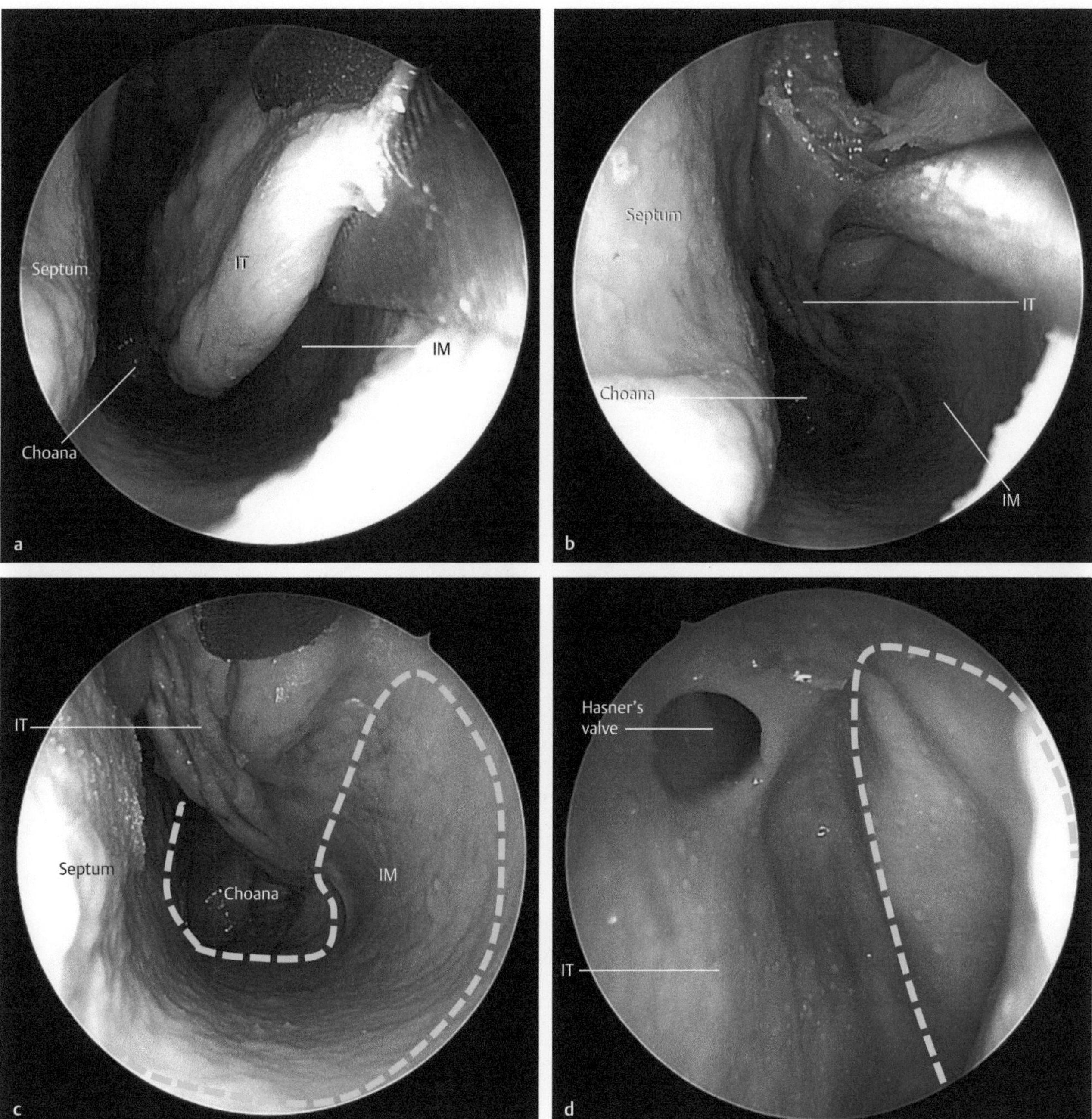

Fig. 5.3 Pictures obtained with a 0-degree **(a–c)** and 45-degree **(d)** endoscopes during anatomical dissection of the left nasal cavity. **(a)** Incision at the head of the inferior turbinate (IT). **(b)** Superior mobilization of the turbinate to expose the inferior meatus (IM). **(c)** *Green dashed line* shows the incisions along the nasal floor and IM. **(d)** Close-up view of the nasolacrimal duct opening (Hasner valve) and its relation with the lateral incision of the flap.

   - The mucosa is elevated from the perpendicular plate of the ethmoid and vomer in the subperiosteal plane.
2. Floor and inferior meatus:
   - The inferior turbinate is mobilized again superiorly to expose the inferior meatus.
   - The mucosa of the nasal cavity floor and inferior meatus lateral wall is elevated in the subperiosteal plane.
   - It is easier to elevate the inferior meatus lateral wall mucosa starting from the incision site toward the nasal floor.
   - 30- or 45-degree endoscopes may be useful in some cases for the anterior part of the elevation due to anatomical variations of the piriform aperture.
3. Transition septum/nasal cavity floor:
   - After those two steps, the flap is attached only to the transition area between the septum and nasal floor.
   - The mucosa is gently elevated from anterior to posterior until the incisive (nasopalatine) foramen and its neurovascular bundle are identified. The incisive foramina, one on each side of the septum are located 8 to 10 mm posterior to the anterior nasal spine. This is an area of neurovascular anastomosis (nasopalatine nerve with greater palatine nerve; and posterior septal artery with descending palatine artery).
   - A ball probe can be used to elevate the mucosa posterior to the nasopalatine bundle. Once the bundle is completely isolated in a 360-degree circumference, a needle tip Bovie is used to transect it and free the flap.

- ► Fig. 5.4a–e shows an anatomical dissection of the ENSF harvest and inset to reconstruct the clival region.

5.4.2 Reconstruction

- Prior to the flap inset, preparation of the recipient site should be done as described for the standard NSF (Chapter 3).
- Because of its configuration, the ENSF fits well for reconstruction of the clivus and craniovertebral junction.
- The main axis of the flap should be positioned horizontally, and the extended mucosa of the inferior meatus will lie inferiorly. ► Fig. 5.4f illustrates a surgical example of reconstruction of a clival defect with an ENSF.
- Fat graft can be used to fill the clival defect prior to the inset of the extended flap.
- Lumbar drain is recommended in the postoperative period for 3 to 5 days for posterior fossa defects.
- For large anterior cranial base defects from the sella to the posterior table of the frontal sinus, the ENSF is usually harvested, including the nasal floor mucosa and possibly the mucosa of the lateral wall of the inferior meatus. The pedicle is placed along the orbital wall vertically toward the cranial base. Then the reconstructive area of the flap is placed anteriorly with the main axis of the flap oriented diagonally along the defect. The extra mucosa of the flap is positioned posteriorly to cover the planum sphenoidale, tuberculum of the sella, and the upper part of the sellar region.
- In cases of large anterior cranial base meningiomas or other tumors with mass effect in the frontal lobes, the tumor resection leaves a large empty space intracranially. The inlay reconstruction is challenging in such situations and the NSF tends to displace intracranially with the brain pulsation. To minimize these issues, it is recommended to partially fill the intracranial space with pieces of absorbable gelatin sponge and/or fat graft, especially along the anterior edge of the defect, prior to the placement of the inlay dural substitute (synthetic or fascia lata). This will allow some pressure on the inlay dural substitute layer against the defect and minimize gaps. It will also help to prevent intracranial displacement of the flap and consequent cerebrospinal fluid leak. It is important to avoid placement of too much fat to prevent mass effect from the fat graft.
- Lumbar drain is usually not necessary for anterior cranial base defects.

5.5 Postoperative Care

- The nasal floor and inferior meatus mucosalization is faster than the nasal septum.

5.5.1 One-Week Postoperative Visit

- Nasal splints are removed and limited nasal debridement is performed to clean the nasal passages and improve the nasal breathing.
- In cases of very large defects, the patients are instructed to start large-volume saline irrigation once a day after 2 or 3 weeks from the surgery.
- No need for debridement within the inferior meatus.
- Do not remove the fibrin that covers the nasal cavity floor.
- Do not remove the crust over the septum donor site.

5.5.2 One-Month Postoperative Visit

- At this point, the nasal floor should mostly be covered with new mucosa and granulation tissue.
- The septal cartilage is still mostly exposed, and only partial removal of crusting from the septum is recommended.
- Careful debridement next to the flap and pedicle is performed.

5.5.3 Four-Month Postoperative Visit

- The nasal floor should be totally mucosalized, and septum donor site should be mostly mucosalized.
- Not uncommonly, crusting still forms along the septum despite good mucosalization. This could be related to changes in the mucus quality and mucociliary movements from the secondary intention healing process.
- Follow-up visits are scheduled accordingly to the severity of nasal crusting.

5.6 Complications

- Higher risk of flap laceration anteriorly at the transition between the septum and the nasal floor.
- Numbness of the upper central incisors due to the transection of the incisive foramen (nasopalantine) neurovascular bundle, which can be permanent.

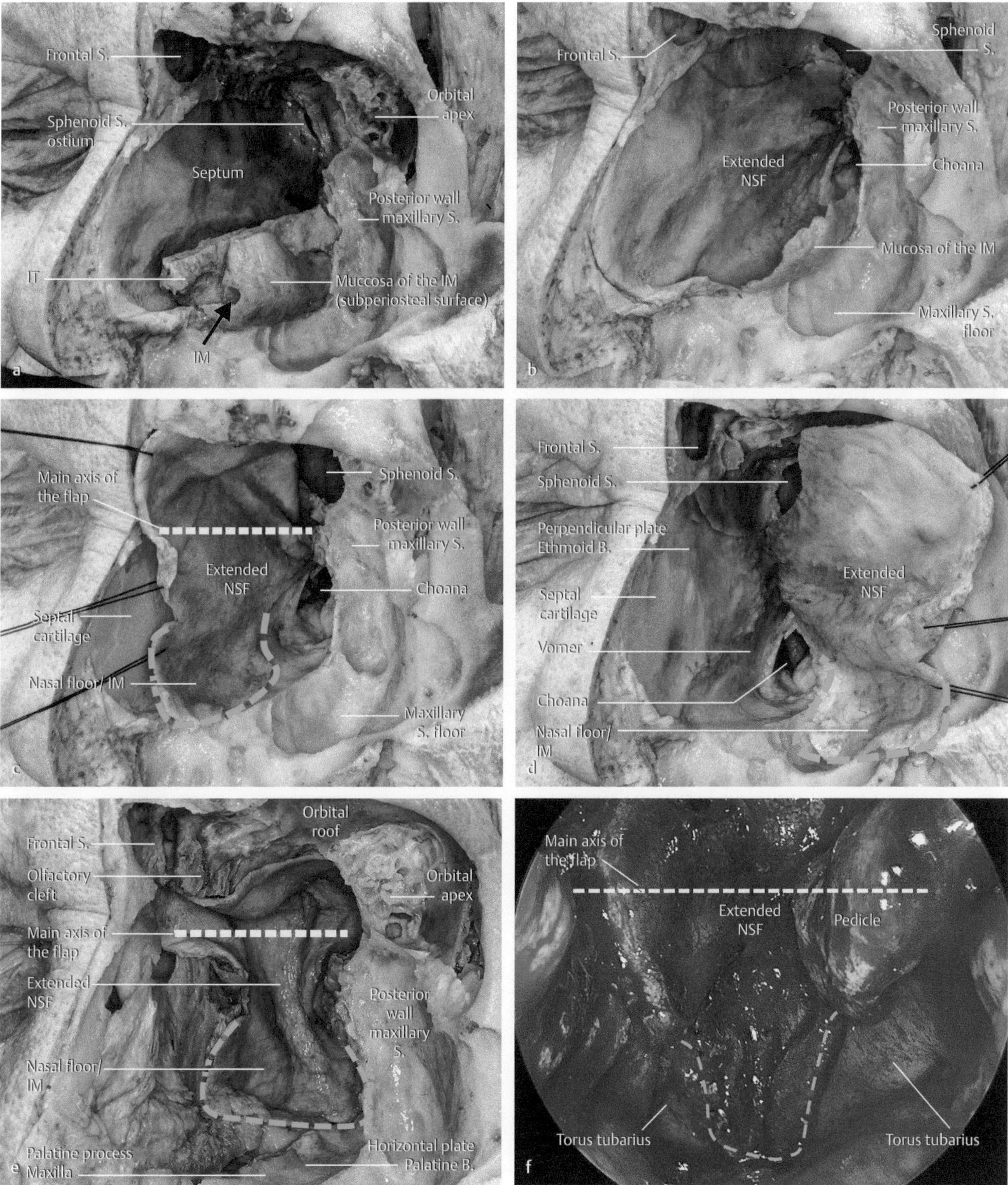

Fig. 5.4 Anatomical dissection after removal of the left hemiface and exposure of the nasal cavity. **(a)** Relation between the nasal septum, inferior turbinate (IT), and inferior meatus (IM). Note that the bone of the medial maxillary sinus wall was removed. **(b)** After completion of the incisions for the extended nasoseptal flap (ENSF), the IT was removed to improve the view. **(c)** The flap was elevated in three steps: Septal mucosa; nasal floor, and IM mucosa; and transection of the neurovascular bundle at the incisive foramen. *Green dashed line* shows the added mucosa from the nasal floor and IM to the nasoseptal flap (NSF). *Yellow dashed line* shows the main axis of the flap which helps in understanding the rotation of the extended flap to cover the clival region. **(d)** Subperichondrial and subperiosteal view of the extended flap. **(e)** Inset of the flap to cover the clival defect after near total septectomy and clivectomy. Observe the extra mucosa lying toward the inferior edge of the defect. **(f)** Clinical case of a patient who had endoscopic endonasal transclival approach for resection of a posterior fossa meningioma. Intraoperative picture obtained with a 0-degree endoscope. Note the mucosa from the nasal floor and IM covering the inferior edge of the defect (*green dashed line*). B, bone; S, sinus.

- Risk of perforation in the flap at the area of the nasopalatine neurovascular bundle transection.
- Penetration into the maxillary sinus during the elevation of the inferior meatus mucosa. This can lead to a permanent communication between the sinus and the inferior meatus causing potential issues such as recirculation of mucus and chronic sinusitis.
- Injury to the nasolacrimal duct opening may lead to obstruction and epiphora (rare complication).
- The descending palatine artery and greater palatine nerve passes through the greater palatine canal which is formed between a groove in the vertical plate of the palatine bone and the maxilla. Inadvertent injury to the descending palatine nerve can cause palatal numbness. This may occur during the dissection within the inferior meatus next to the tail of the inferior turbinate.
- Care must be taken with the posterior incision between the soft and hard palates to avoid injury to the muscles of the soft palate.
- Asymptomatic brainstem prolapse toward the clival defect has been described. The use of fat graft to fill the clival defect may help to prevent the prolapse.

References

[1] Peris-Celda M, Pinheiro-Neto CD, Funaki T, et al. The extended nasoseptal flap for skull base reconstruction of the clival region: an anatomical and radiological study. J Neurol Surg B Skull Base. 2013; 74(6):369–385

[2] Pinheiro-Neto CD, Snyderman CH. Nasoseptal flap. Adv Otorhinolaryngol. 2013; 74:42–55

[3] Pinheiro-Neto CD, Salgado-Lopez L, Leonel LCPC, Aydin SO, Peris-Celda M. Endoscopic Endonasal Approaches to the Clivus with no Violation of the Nasopharynx: Surgical Anatomy and Clinical Illustration. J Neurol Surg B Skull Base DOI:10.1055/s-0041-1729905

[4] Pinheiro-Neto CD, Ramos HF, Peris-Celda M, et al. Study of the nasoseptal flap for endoscopic anterior cranial base reconstruction. Laryngoscope. 2011; 121 (12):2514–2520

[5] Pinheiro-Neto CD, Prevedello DM, Carrau RL, et al. Improving the design of the pedicled nasoseptal flap for skull base reconstruction: a radioanatomic study. Laryngoscope. 2007; 117(9):1560–1569

6 Nasoseptal Flap Pedicle Release

Carlos D. Pinheiro-Neto, Luciano C. P. C. Leonel, and Maria Peris-Celda

6.1 Anatomy

- In order to perform the release of the pedicle of the nasoseptal flap (NSF) into the pterygopalatine fossa (PPF), it is essential to understand the anatomy of the sphenopalatine foramen and PPF.
- The sphenopalatine foramen is a notch in the palatine bone between the orbital process anteriorly and the sphenoid process posteriorly (▶ Fig. 6.1).
- Besides the sphenopalatine artery (SPA), veins that drain the nasal cavity mucosa also pass through the sphenopalatine foramen to drain into the pterygoid venous plexus.
- The PPF is a narrow pyramidal shape space with the apex pointing inferiorly. This space is formed by the palatine bone medially, maxillary bone anteriorly, pterygoid base/plates posteriorly, orbit superiorly, and infratemporal fossa laterally. Inferiorly, the PPF ends at the articulation between the maxilla and the pterygoid plates.
- The neurovascular contents within the PPF include the pterygopalatine ganglion, vidian nerve, and branches of the maxillary division of the trigeminal nerve (V2); maxillary artery (MA) and its branches. The vascular structures are located anterior to the nerves (▶ Fig. 6.2).
- A periosteal layer covers adipose tissue and neurovascular structures within the PPF.
- At the level of the SPA foramen, the artery is very attached to the periosteum. However, within the PPF, the MA is free and surrounded by adipose tissue.
- The PPF has seven different openings where important neurovascular structures pass and communicate with different areas within the cranial base (▶ Table 6.1).
- The greater palatine canal is formed by a groove in the medial wall of the maxillary bone and a groove in the perpendicular plate of the palatine bone.

6.2 Fundamentals

- The lateral release of the NSF pedicle involves the opening of the maxillary sinus and its posterior wall to expose the periosteum of the PPF.
- The lateral dissection of the NSF pedicle can be used for two main reasons: ipsilateral transpterygoid approach and improvement of the flap reach and reconstructive area.
- When a transpterygoid approach is required on the same side of the flap, the pedicle release allows great lateral mobilization of the flap and safe drilling of the pterygoid base.[1]
- In some cases, the vidian nerve needs to be sacrificed to improve the lateral mobilization of the flap and exposure of the pterygoid base.
- The lateral pedicle dissection not only improves the reach of the flap but also increases its effective reconstructive surface. With more freedom after the pedicle release, the posterior part of the flap (mucoperiosteal surface/bridging area) can be successfully used for reconstruction.[2]
- Two steps of pedicle release are involved: removal of the osseous boundaries of the sphenopalatine foramen (osseous release) and 360-degree periosteal incision around the SPA (periosteal release).
- The descending palatine artery can be transected to increase the pedicle release and reach of the flap.
- The osseous release increases the reach of the flap about 0.6 cm and the periosteal release 3 cm.[3]

6.3 Indications

- Ipsilateral transpterygoid approaches (osseous release).
- Posterior table of the frontal sinus defect.
- Clival/craniovertebral junction defect. The pedicle release allows the inset of the flap with its main axis in a more craniocaudal orientation. Note that this is different to what is normally performed with the extended NSF where the main axis of the flap is parallel to the floor of the sella.
- Upper cervical spine/posterior pharyngeal wall (periosteal release). Orientation of the main axis of the flap is in a craniocaudal direction.
- The extended pedicle dissection into the PPF virtually allows the flap to reach any area of the ventral cranial base. This technique allows the flap to be used in other areas of head–neck reconstruction such as oropharyngeal defects after transoral robotic surgery and reconstruction of the external nose after rhinectomy.[4,5]

Table 6.1 Communication between the PPF and different regions within the cranial base

Opening	To	Structures passing through
Pterygomaxillary fissure	Infratemporal fossa	MA
Inferior orbital fissure	Orbit	Infraorbital nerve and artery
Sphenopalatine foramen	Nasal cavity	SPA and veins, posterior superior lateral nasal nerve, and the nasopalatine nerve
Palate	Greater palatine canal	Descending palatine artery and greater and lesser palatine nerves
Intracranial space	Foramen rotundum	V2
Intracranial space/foramen lacerum	Vidian canal	Vidian nerve and artery
Nasopharynx	Palatovaginal (palatosphenoidal) canal	Pharyngeal nerve from the pterygopalatine ganglion and the pharyngeal branch of the MA

Abbreviations: MA, maxillary artery; PPF, pterygopalatine fossa; SPA, sphenopalatine artery.

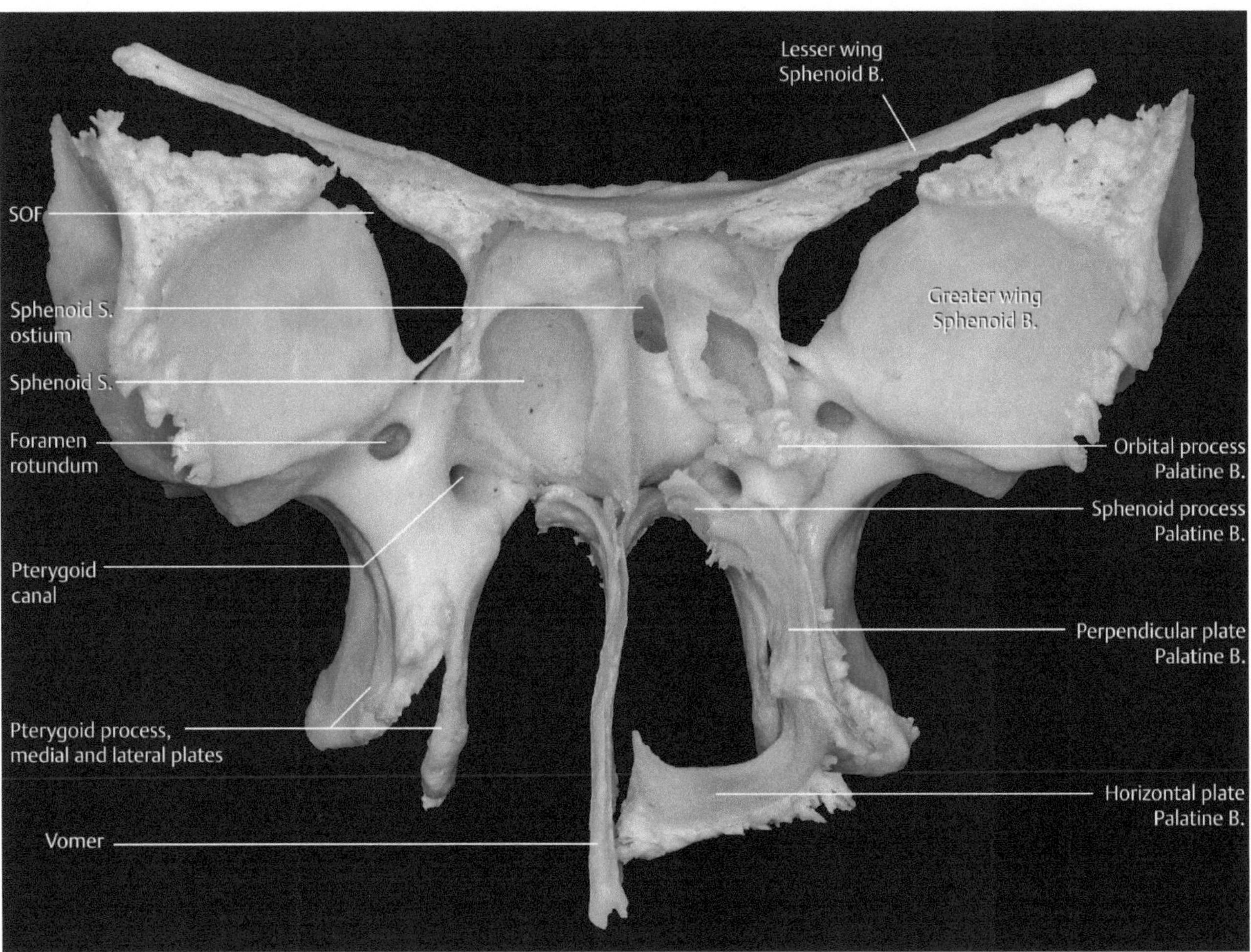

Fig. 6.1 Dry sphenoid bone articulating with the left palatine bone. Important step for the nasoseptal flap (NSF) pedicle release is the removal of the orbital process and the sphenoid process of the palatine bone. B, bone; S, sinus; SOF, superior orbital fissure.

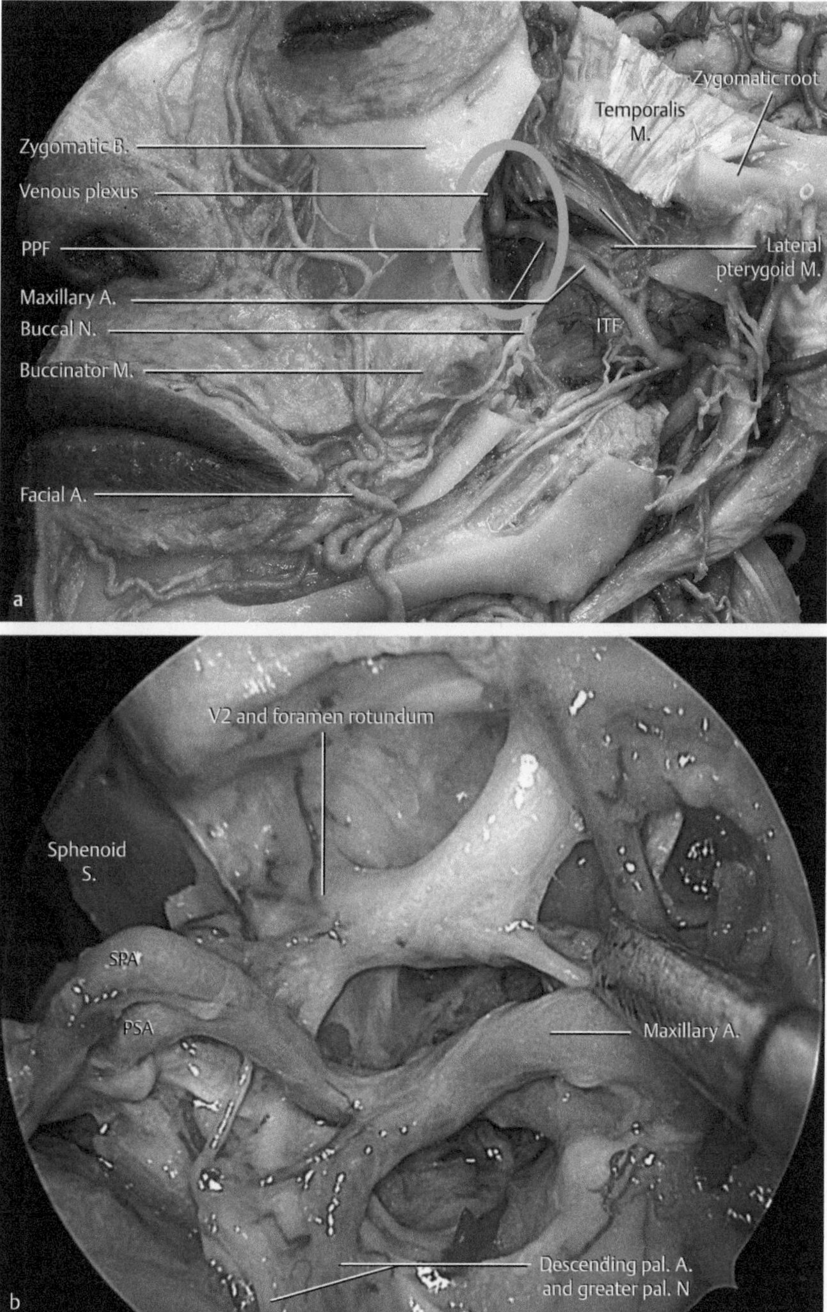

Fig. 6.2 (a) Anatomical dissection of the left infratemporal fossa (ITF) to demonstrate the vascularization of the region. *Blue circle* shows the maxillary artery (MA) entering the pterygopalatine fossa (PPF) through the pterygomaxillary fissure surrounded by a venous plexus. **(b)** Picture obtained with a 0-degree endoscope during anatomical dissection of the left nasal cavity. Neurovascular structures within the PPF. Note the arterial branches anterior to the neural structures. (Reproduced with permission from Pinheiro-Neto et al 2019.[2]) A, artery; B, bone; M, muscle; N, nerve; Pal, palantine; PSA, posterior septal artery; S, sinus; SPA, sphenopalatine artery.

6.4 Limitations

- Narrow vascular pedicle.
- MA exposed to the nasal cavity has to be covered with autologous or synthetic graft.
- Technically challenging dissection with risk of injury of the vascular pedicle or neural structures within the PPF.

6.5 Surgical Technique (*Videos 6.1 and 6.2*)

- Total ethmoidectomy, middle turbinectomy, maxillary antrostomy, and sphenoidotomy are performed with preservation of the nasoseptal pedicle. Resection of the horizontal portion of the middle turbinate can be performed instead of its total resection, with preservation of the vertical attachment of the middle turbinate to the cranial base.
- Harvest of the NSF and placement in the nasopharynx.
- Just posterior to the maxillary antrostomy, the mucosa is elevated from the palatine bone until exposure of the ethmoidal crest and the SPA is identified.

6.5.1 360-Degree Bone Removal around the SPA Foramen (Osseous Release)

- The orbital process of the palatine bone is removed with a Kerrison rongeur. This step should be done carefully to avoid injury of the SPA. The blade of the Kerrison is placed inside the SPA foramen just anterior to the artery. The bone removal is carried laterally toward the posterior wall of the maxillary sinus to expose the periosteum of the PPF. High-speed drill with a 3 mm diamond burr can be used to thin the bone prior to its removal with the rongeur.
- The bone superior to the SPA foramen is removed toward the inferior orbital fissure.
- Part of the perpendicular plate of the palatine bone underneath the SPA foramen is removed with exposure of the medial aspect of the PPF. The greater palatine canal can be opened with exposure of its contents enclosed in a periosteal layer (descending palatine artery and greater palatine nerve).
- The flap is placed inside the maxillary sinus or superiorly in the ethmoid/sphenoid region. This allows exposure of the arch to the choana. The inferior flap incision along the arch of the choana is extended laterally and anteriorly toward the maxillary antrostomy. This incision should be passing inferior to the SPA.
- The mucosa is elevated posteriorly to the SPA and the sphenoid process of the palatine bone is identified. The sphenoid process of the palatine bone is drilled with exposure of the palatovaginal (or palatosphenoidal) canal and its contents (pharyngeal branch of the MA and nerve filaments).
- At this point, the entire osseous boundaries of the sphenopalatine foramen have been removed.
- The osseous release provides a great mobilization of the pedicle, allowing dissection of tumor behind it as well as drilling of the pterygoid base for ipsilateral transpterygoid approaches. If further pedicle release is needed, a 360-degree periosteal incision should be performed (▶ Fig. 6.3).

6.5.2 Ipsilateral Transpterygoid Approach

- The palatovaginal (or palatosphenoidal) canal contents are transected, and the PPF encased in its periosteum is lateralized to allow the identification of the vidian nerve.[6]
- At this point, the transpterygoid approach can be carried out by drilling the pterygoid base medially, superiorly, and inferiorly to the vidian nerve. This drilling can be progressed posteriorly to the lacerum portion of the internal carotid artery, with preservation of the vascular pedicle of the NSF.[7]
- If exposure lateral to the vidian nerve is needed, the nerve can be transected, allowing further lateral mobilization of the PPF contents and wide exposure of the lateral part of the pterygoid base. The drilling can be extended with exposure of the maxillary (V2) and the mandibular (V3) divisions of the trigeminal nerve and dura of the middle fossa with preservation of the vascular pedicle of the NSF.

6.5.3 360-Degree Circumferential Incision in the Periosteum of the PPF around the SPA (Periosteal Release)

- Once the osseous boundaries of the SPA foramen are removed with exposure of the underlying periosteum, the 360-degree periosteal incision around the SPA is performed (▶ Fig. 6.4).
- A sickle knife or microscissors are used to make the first periosteal incision and open the anterior aspect of the PPF inferior to the SPA/MA and exposing the PPF fat.
- A ball probe (seeker probe) is used to carefully elevate the periosteum from PPF contents, allowing a safer incision around the SPA.
- The periosteal incision is carried laterally toward the infratemporal fossa since the periosteum is adherent to the artery at the level of the SPA foramen.
- At that point, the incision is turned superiorly toward the inferior orbital fissure and then medially from the inferior orbital fissure toward the vidian and palatovaginal canals.
- Then, the medial cut is performed just inferior to the SPA toward the palatovaginal canal. Attention should be paid to the descending palatine artery and greater palatine nerve during this inferior incision.
- Similar to what is performed for ipsilateral transpterygoid approaches, the pharyngeal branch of the MA that passes through the palatovaginal (palatosphenoidal) canal from the PPF to the nasopharynx is cauterized and transected.
- Once the 360-degree incision around the SPA is completed, the artery is carefully mobilized with a ball probe anteriorly and is completely freed from the PPF periosteum. This allows full freedom of the pedicle of the NSF, which remains attached to the MA (▶ Fig. 6.5).
- Keep fat from the PPF around the MA to avoid disruption of the periarterial venous drainage.

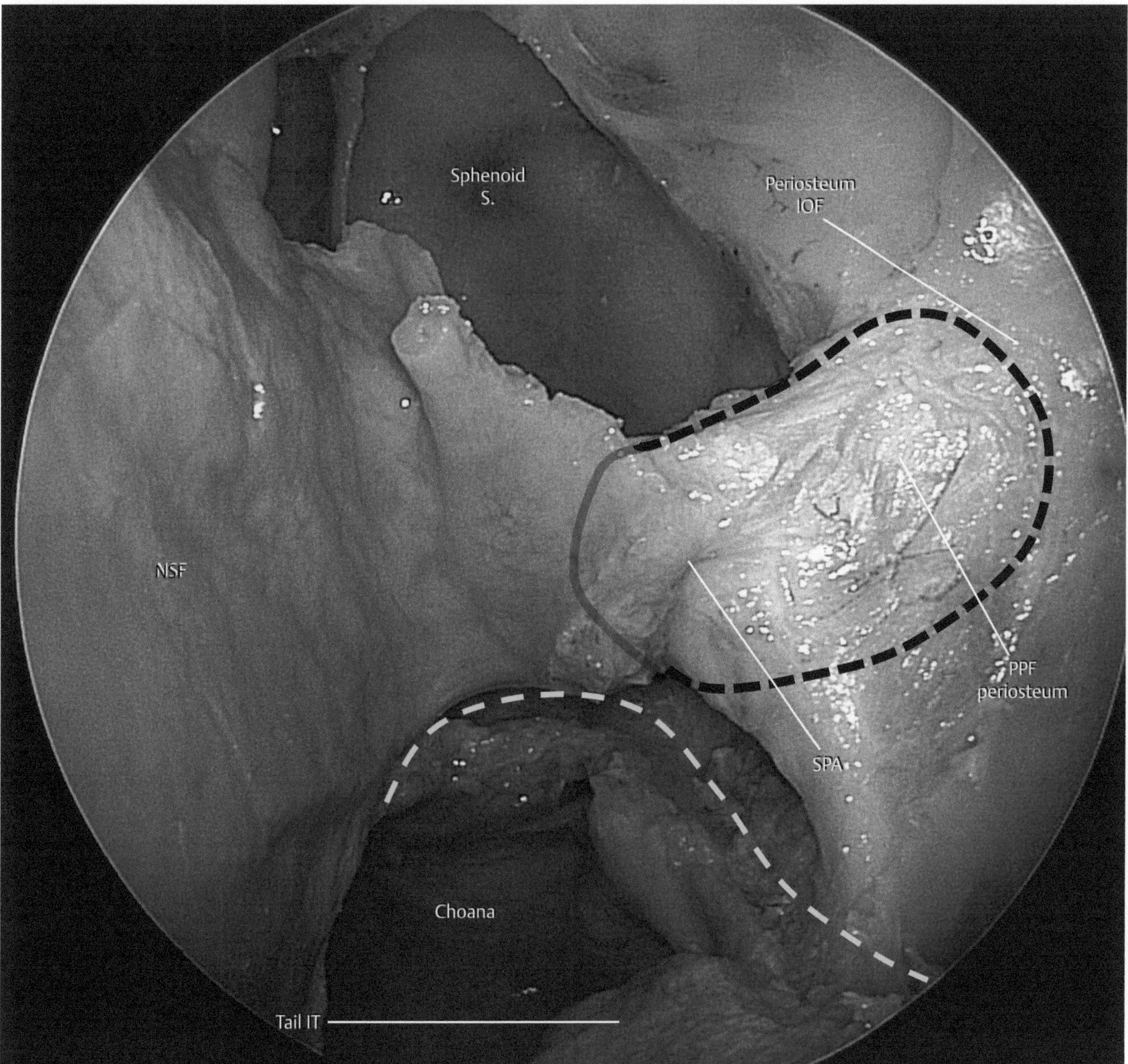

Fig. 6.3 Picture obtained with a 0-degree endoscope during anatomical dissection of the left nasal cavity after the osseous release around the sphenopalatine foramen. Observe the pedicle of the flap in continuity with the periosteum of the pterygopalatine fossa (PPF). This picture also illustrates the pterygoid base drilled behind the PPF (ipsilateral transpterygoid approach). *Green dashed line* represents the extension of the inferior incision of the nasoseptal flap (NSF) from the arch of the choana to the maxillary antrostomy. *Black dashed line* shows the anterior periosteal incision that can be done for further release of the pedicle. *Continuous back shaded line* illustrates the posterior periosteal incision needed to complete a 360-degree circumferential periosteal release of the pedicle. (Reproduced with permission from Pinheiro-Neto et al 2019[2].) IOF, inferior orbital fissure; IT, inferior turbinate; S, sinus; SPA, sphenopalatine artery.

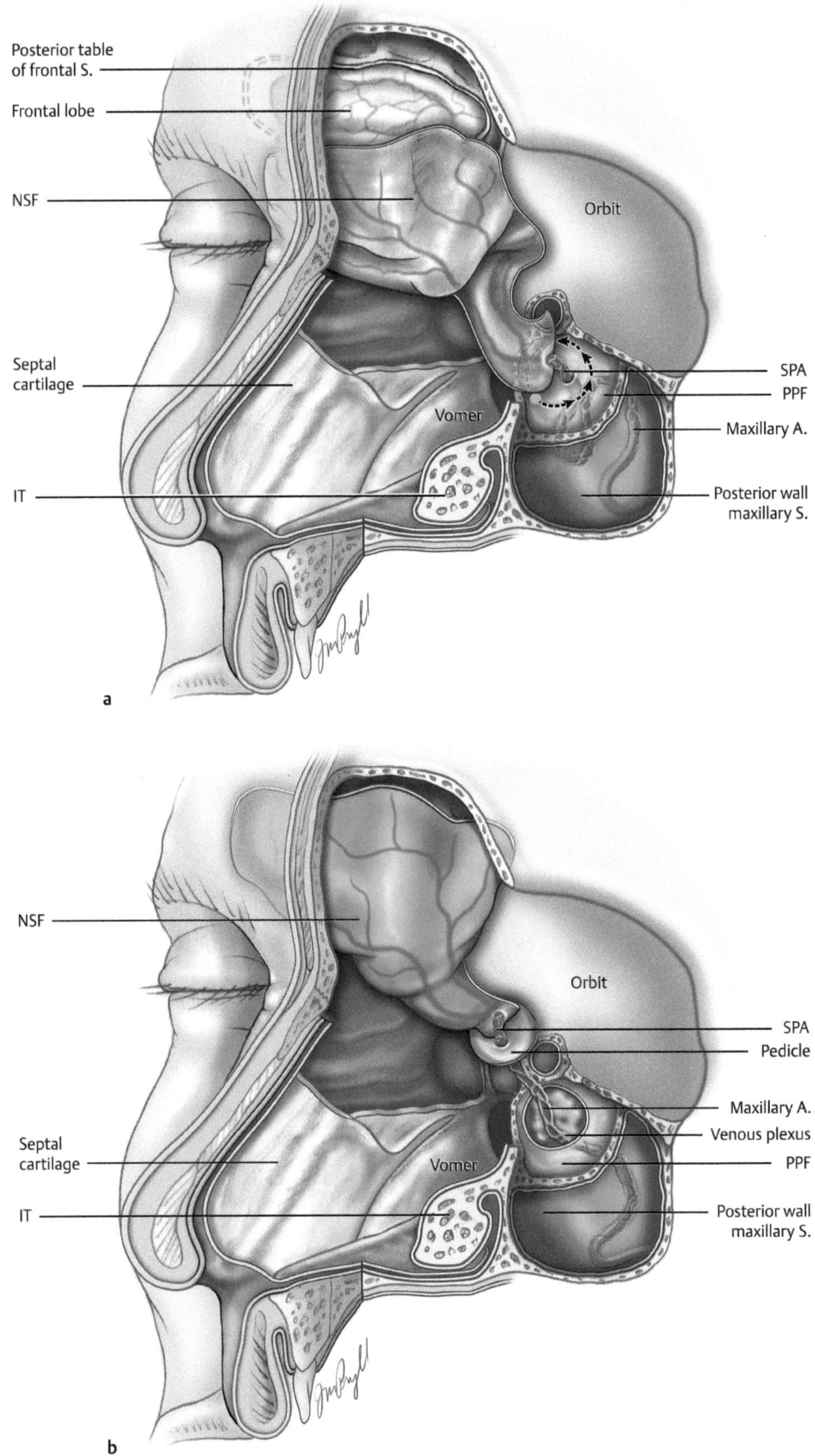

Fig. 6.4 Illustration of the nasal cavity after removal of the left hemiface and orbital contents. **(a)** Nasoseptal flap (NSF) after the osseous release of the pedicle. Note that this release is not sufficient for the flap to cover the entire skull base defect involving the posterior table of the frontal sinus. *Black arrowed line* shows the anterior periosteal incision. *Blue arrowed line* illustrates the posterior periosteal incision behind the sphenopalatine artery (SPA). **(b)** Improved anterior reach of the NSF is achieved after the 360-degree circumferential periosteal incision and release of the maxillary artery (MA). A, artery; IT, inferior turbinate; PPF, pterygopalatine fossa; S, sinus.

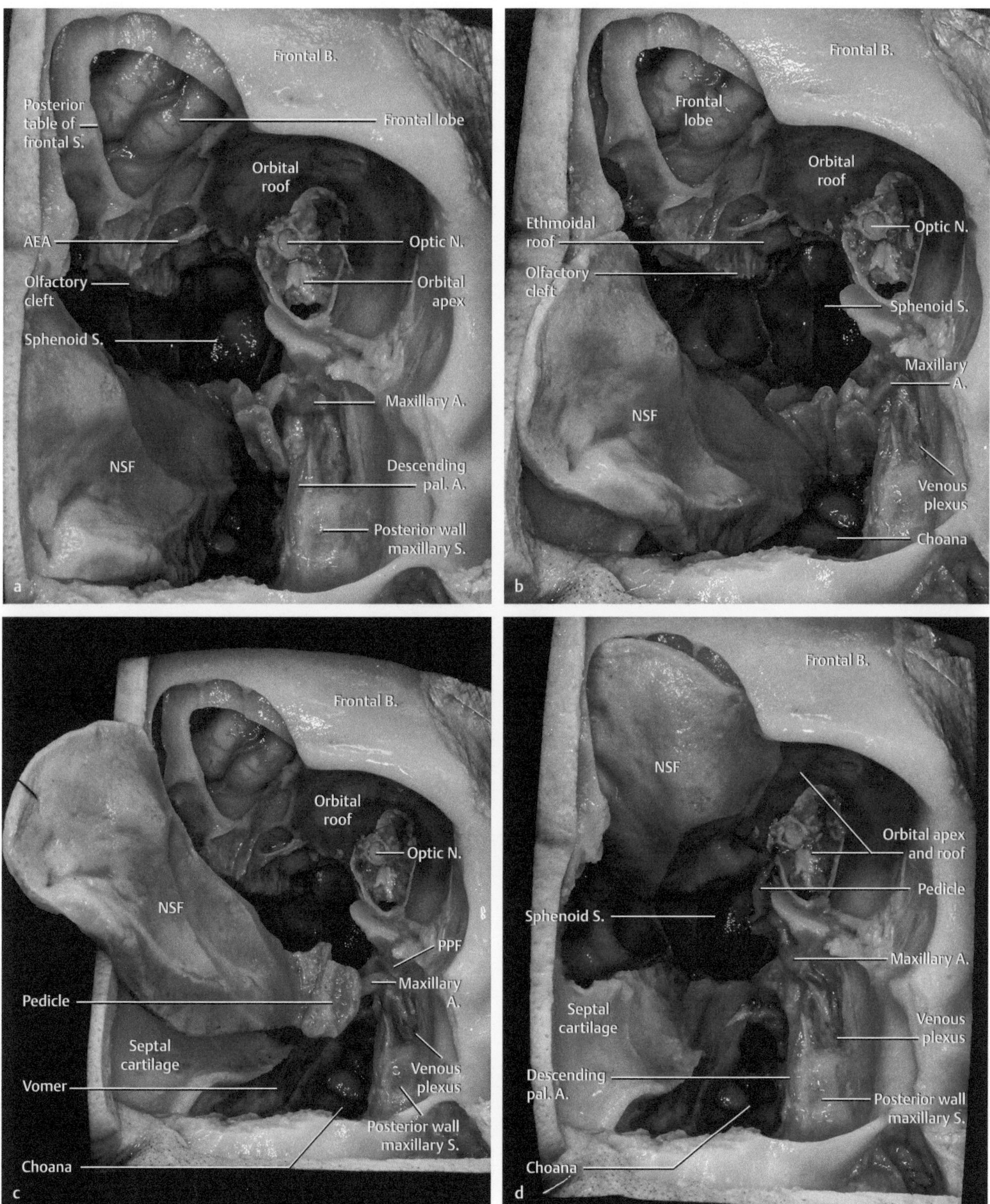

Fig. 6.5 Anatomical dissection after removal of the left hemiface and orbital contents with exposure of the nasal cavity. **(a)** Dissection of the pterygopalatine fossa (PPF) and exposure of the maxillary artery (MA). **(b)** Elevation of the flap. **(c)** The MA release allows an average of 3 cm increase in the flap reach, expanding the application of this flap.[3] **(d)** Reconstruction of a defect of the posterior table of the frontal sinus. Note that the flap inset follows the same principles of the nonreleased nasoseptal flap (NSF). It is important to place the pedicle along a structure (e.g., orbit) to minimize contraction during the healing process. The PPF and MA should be covered with an autologous or synthetic graft. A, artery; AEA, anterior ethmoidal artery; B, bone; N, nerve; pal., palatine; S, sinus.

- The descending palatine artery may be transected to increase the freedom of the pedicle and improve the flap reach.
- After the inset of the flap, the MA should be covered with a free mucosal graft and/or pieces of oxidized cellulose.
  Fat or muscle graft or other synthetic graft may also be used instead.
- ▶ Fig. 6.6 illustrates a surgical example of pedicle release with MA dissection.

6.6 Postoperative Care

6.6.1 One-Week Postoperative Visit

- Limited nasal debridement to clean the nasal passages and improve the nasal breathing.
- No debridement close to the flap pedicle or posterior wall of the maxillary sinus should be performed.
- Instruction of the patient to start large-volume saline rinses once a day.

6.6.2 One-Month Postoperative Visit

- Careful debridement inside the maxillary sinus.
- Meticulous debridement along the NSF pedicle.
- Pay attention to the area below the SPA where part of the greater palatine nerve may be exposed. Severe dental pain may be elicited during the debridement.
- Do not force the removal of firm and attached crusts due to the risk of neurovascular injury within the PPF

6.7 Complications

- Potential complications of this technique are related to neurovascular injury within the PPF:
  - Palate/dental numbness (greater palatine nerve).
  - Dry eye (vidian nerve).
  - Numbness on the cheek (V2/infraorbital nerve).
  - Severe intraoperative bleeding (MA) and flap compromise.
- Flap congestion due to narrow pedicle and flap necrosis.
- Severe postoperative bleeding from the MA.

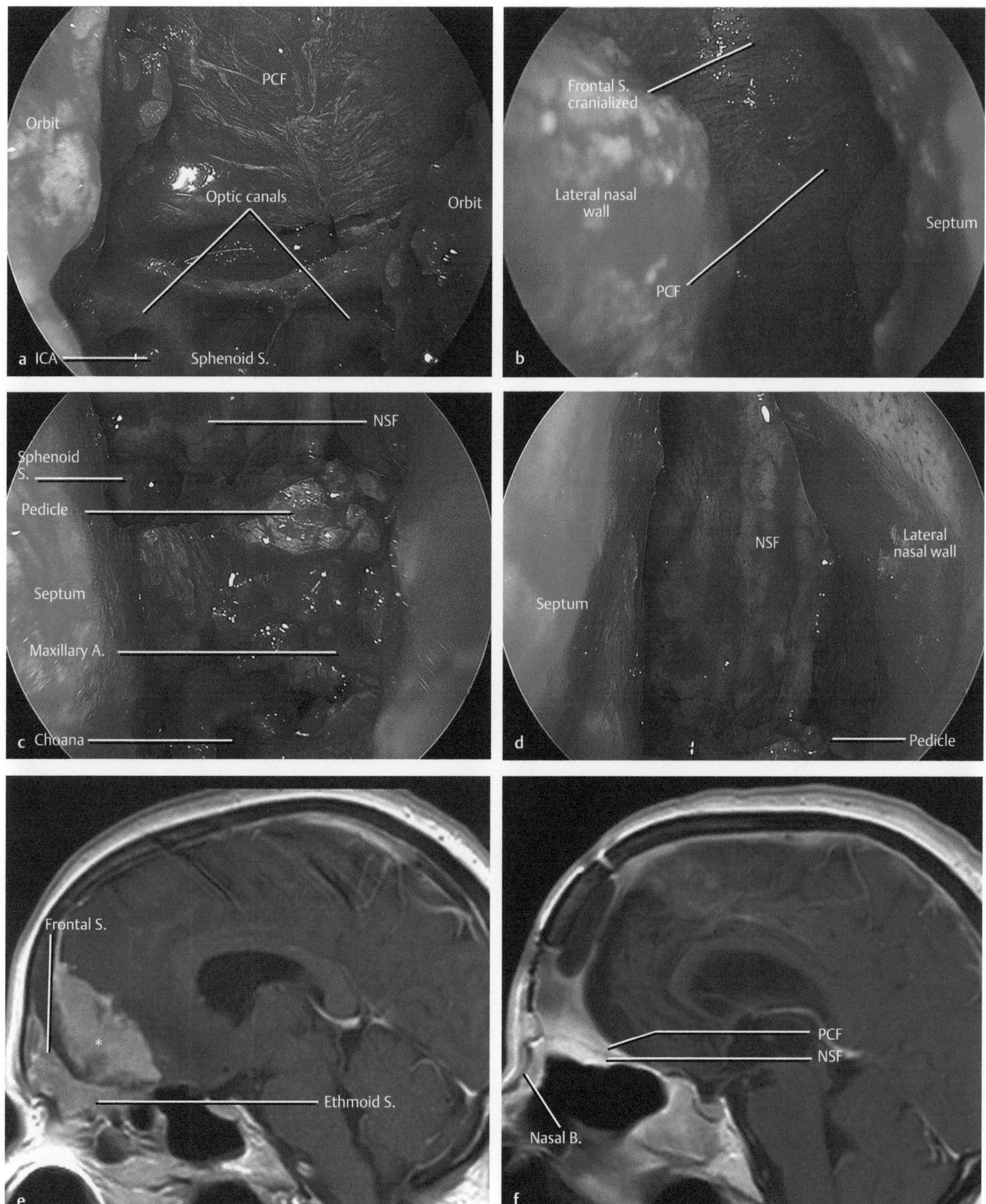

Fig. 6.6 Clinical case of a patient who presented with an anterior cranial base meningioma and underwent combined open and endoscopic endonasal approaches for resection. **(a–c)** Intraoperative pictures obtained with a 0-degree endoscope. **(a)** Endonasal view after the tumor was resected. The inlay dural reconstruction was performed with a pericranial flap (PCF) inset through the craniotomy. **(b)** Right nasal cavity showing that the frontal sinus was cranialized. The consequent skull base defect was very large from the planum sphenoidale to the anterior table of the frontal sinus. **(c)** A periosteal release of the flap pedicle providing freedom of the maxillary artery (MA) was necessary. **(d)** An extended nasoseptal flap (NSF) was harvested with inclusion of the nasal floor mucosa. With the pedicle release, both areas of the flap (mucoperichondrium and mucoperiosteum) worked as reconstructive surface and the flap covered the entire defect. **(e)** Preoperative magnetic resonance imaging (MRI) T1 with contrast sagittal view. Observe that the tumor (*asterisk*) was extremely anterior involving the frontal and ethmoid sinuses and required a combined approach. **(f)** Postoperative MRI T1 with contrast sagittal view 4 months after the surgery. Note the NSF enhancing with contrast and covering the anterior cranial base defect all the way to the nasal bones. Besides reinforcing the reconstruction, the coverage of the endonasal surface of the PCF with an intranasal mucosal flap minimizes the crust formation along the pericranium and reduces the time of mucosalization of the PCF. A, artery; B, bone; ICA, internal carotid artery; S, sinus.

References

[1] Pinheiro-Neto CD, Paluzzi A, Fernandez-Miranda JC, et al. Extended dissection of the septal flap pedicle for ipsilateral endoscopic transpterygoid approaches. Laryngoscope. 2014; 124(2):391–396

[2] Pinheiro-Neto CD, Peris-Celda M, Kenning T. Extrapolating the limits of the nasoseptal flap with pedicle dissection to the internal maxillary artery. Oper Neurosurg (Hagerstown). 2019; 16(1):37–44

[3] Shastri KS, Leonel LCPC, Patel V, et al. Lengthening the nasoseptal flap pedicle with extended dissection into the pterygopalatine fossa. Laryngoscope. 2020; 130(1):18–24

[4] Pinheiro-Neto CD, Galati LT. Nasoseptal flap for reconstruction after robotic radical tonsillectomy. Head Neck. 2016; 38(9):E2495–E2498

[5] Shastri KS, Lin Y, Scordino J, Pinheiro-Neto CD. Composite cartilage-osseous-mucosal nasoseptal flap for reconstruction after near total rhinectomy. Ann Otol Rhinol Laryngol. 2021; 130(1):98–103

[6] Pinheiro-Neto CD, Fernandez-Miranda JC, Rivera-Serrano CM, et al. Endoscopic anatomy of the palatovaginal canal (palatosphenoidal canal): a landmark for dissection of the vidian nerve during endonasal transpterygoid approaches. Laryngoscope. 2012; 122(1):6–12

[7] Prevedello DM, Pinheiro-Neto CD, Fernandez-Miranda JC, et al. Vidian nerve transposition for endoscopic endonasal middle fossa approaches. Neurosurgery. 2010; 67(2) Suppl Operative:478–484

7 Composite Cartilagomucosal Nasoseptal Flap

Carlos D. Pinheiro-Neto, Luciano C. P. C. Leonel, and Maria Peris-Celda

7.1 Fundamentals

- The mucosal reconstruction of skull base defects provided by the nasoseptal flap is sufficient to effectively separate the intracranial cavity from the nose and has excellent clinical outcomes. However, in selected cases, it may be beneficial to add some degree of rigidness to the reconstruction.
- The composite cartilagomucosal nasoseptal flap consists of the nasoseptal flap with part of the septal cartilage attached to the flap.
- The cartilage with the attached mucosa works as a single unit and is placed onlay to cover the skull base defect.
- The size of the cartilage harvested should be smaller than the mucosal component of the flap. This allows appropriate contact of the subperichondrial layer to the bony edges of the defect. Usually leaving 5 mm of mucosa around the cartilage is sufficient to ensure good mucosal contact with the borders of the defect.
- The harvest technique of the cartilage is similar to what is performed in septoplasties, leaving an L-shaped strut to support the nose. The remaining septal cartilage is left attached to the mucosal flap.
- The vomer can be left attached to the flap if a larger rigid reconstruction is required. In such cases, the composite flap becomes an osteocartilagomucosal nasoseptal flap (▶ Fig. 7.1).
- If needed, lateral pedicle dissection (osseous release or periosteal release) can be performed to facilitate the inset (Chapter 6).

7.2 Indications

- Transplanum/transtuberculum defects.[1]
- Meningoencephalocele, particularly in obese patients with severe high intracranial pressure.
- Ventral cranial base defects in patients with severe obstructive sleep apnea with the need for elevated pressure while using continuous positive airway pressure (CPAP) or bilevel positive airway pressure (BiPAP).
- Clival defects to reinforce the reconstruction and decrease the risk of catastrophic injuries consequent to nasal intrusions such as nasogastric tubes.
- After partial rhinectomy, the composite flap allows reconstruction of the endonasal lining and framework with a single flap.[2]
- Reconstruction of medial orbital wall or orbital floor defects.[3]

7.3 Limitations

- The maximum size of the septal cartilage that can be harvested is limited due to the need to leave an "L" strut to support the nose.
- History of septal perforations or prior septoplasty due to the absence of enough cartilage.
- Severe septal deviation due to a nonlinear configuration of the cartilage.
- History of septal fracture or septal hematoma/abscess.

7.4 Surgical Technique (*Video 7.1*)

7.4.1 Flap Harvest

- The mucosal incisions are the same as for the standard nasoseptal flap.
- The inferior incision may be performed along the nasal floor mucosa about 5 mm lateral to the nasal septum. This modification increases the distance from the mucosal edge of the flap to the cartilage in that area, which helps the mucosal contact of the flap to the borders of the defect. If needed, an extended composite nasoseptal flap can be harvested, where this mucosal incision is performed further laterally within the inferior meatus.
- The mucosal elevation starts at the caudal border of the septum and the mucosa is elevated from the underlying cartilage about 1 cm posteriorly. It is important to stop the elevation at this level because the cartilage beyond that should be left attached to the mucosa.
- Then the mucosa next to the nasal dorsum incision is elevated from cartilage about 1 cm from the nasal dorsum. The dissection is progressed posteriorly and superiorly parallel to the nasal dorsum until identification of the perpendicular plate of the ethmoid bone.
- Along the inferior mucosal incision of the flap, the mucosa is elevated from the nasal floor medially toward the septum until the attachment of the septal cartilage to the maxillary crest is identified.
- Next, an L-shaped cartilaginous incision is made similar to what is performed for septoplasty.
- Using a "D" knife, the cartilaginous incision starts 1 cm from and parallel to the caudal border of the septum, right next to where the septal mucosa was left attached to the cartilage.
- Along the nasal dorsum, a similar incision is performed respecting 1 cm of cartilage from the nasal dorsum and parallel to it. Once these two cartilaginous incisions are completed, a 1 cm, L-shaped septal strut is preserved and all cartilage posteriorly can be elevated with the flap.[4]
- A Cottle dissector is used through the cartilaginous incisions to carefully elevate a contralateral subperichondrial plane and separate the cartilage from the contralateral mucosa. This step leaves the piece of cartilage attached to the nasoseptal flap.
- The dissection in the contralateral subperichondrial plane is carried posteriorly and inferiorly until the perpendicular plate of the ethmoid, vomer, and maxillary crest are identified.
- At this point, the piece of cartilage is gently disarticulated from the perpendicular plate of the ethmoid, vomer, and maxillary crest, and it remains only attached to the nasoseptal flap.

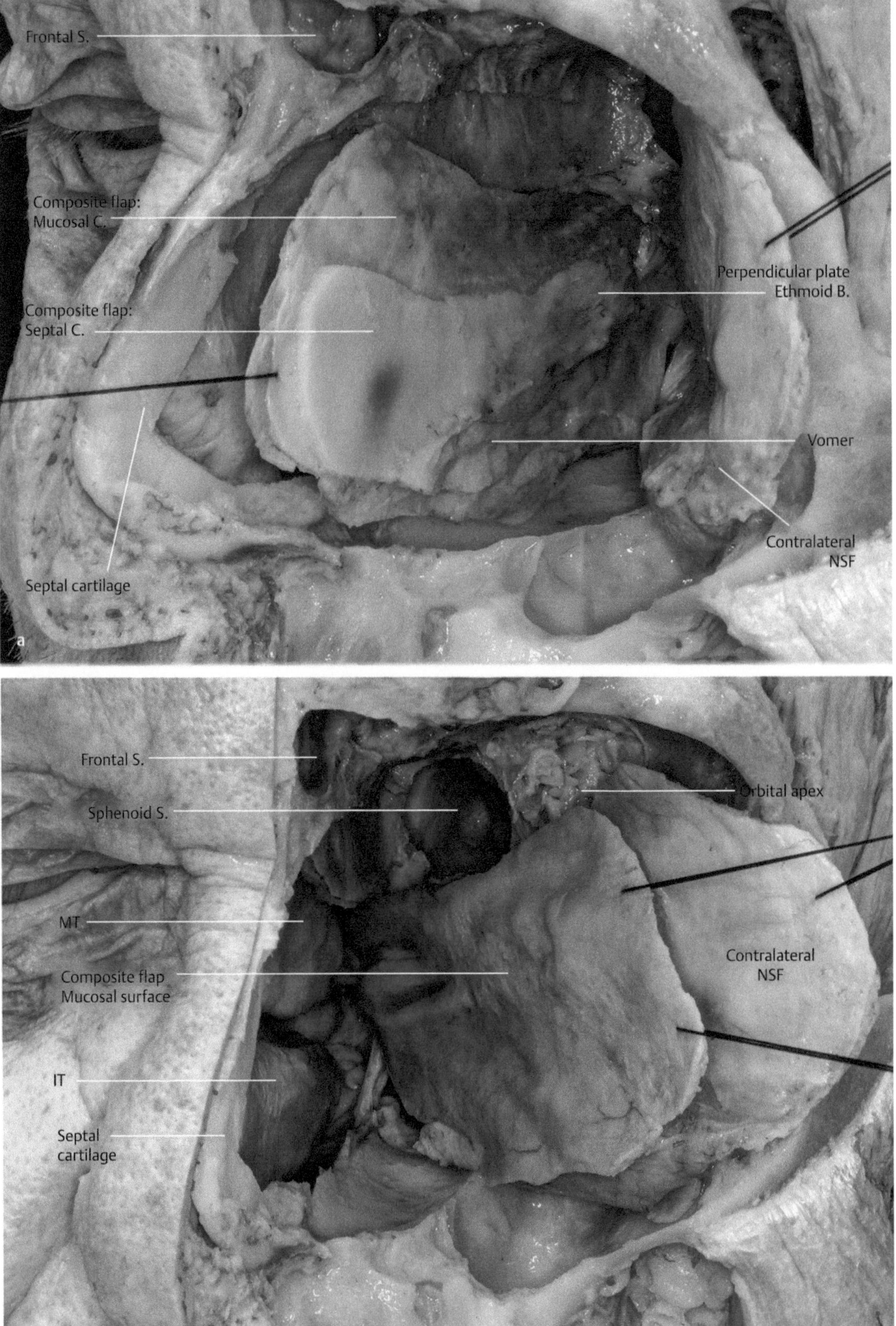

Fig. 7.1 Anatomical dissection after removal of the left hemiface, orbital contents, and exposure of the nasal cavity. **(a)** A standard NSF was harvested on the left side and a composite osteocartilagomucosal nasoseptal flap (NSF) on the right side. Note the L-shaped strut of septal cartilage preserved to provide support to the external nose. **(b)** Mucosal surface of the composite flap. B, bone; C, component; IT, inferior turbinate; MT, middle turbinate; S, sinus.

- The dissection continues ipsilaterally with elevation of the flap posteriorly as usual toward the choana.
- The composite flap is carefully placed in the nasopharynx. If the piece of cartilage is too large, the flap can be placed back along the septum and temporarily sutured anteriorly during the surgery (▶ Fig. 7.2a).

7.4.2 Reconstruction

- The reconstruction is performed similarly to other nasoseptal flaps.
- The cartilaginous part of the flap faces the defect.
- It is important to make sure that the mucosal edges of the flap are in good contact with the borders of the defect.
- After the inlay reconstruction is completed, the composite flap is inset onlay.
- Both mucosal and cartilaginous components of the flap stay onlay.
- The presence of the cartilage maintains the flap unfolded and facilitates the flap inset (▶ Fig. 7.2b).
- ▶ Fig. 7.3 illustrates a surgical case of a patient who had skull base reconstruction with a composite cartilagomucosal nasoseptal flap.
- ▶ Fig. 7.4 demonstrates a surgical example of a patient who had nasal reconstruction with composite osteocartilagomucosal nasoseptal flap after pedicle release along the maxillary artery.

7.5 Postoperative Care

- Postoperative visits 1 week, 1 month, and 4 months for nasal debridement (see Chapter 3).
- During postoperative nasal endoscopies, the classical pulsations of the nasoseptal flap due to transmission of the brain pulsations are not usually noticeable. The presence of the cartilaginous component of the flap seems to improve stability and strength of the reconstruction against intracranial pressure.

7.6 Complications

- Saddle nose if too much septal cartilage is resected.
- Septal perforation.
- Numbness in the upper central incisors due to dissection at the incisive foramen.
- Cartilage compression of neurovascular structures. Gentle packing with absorbable material is important to avoid any neurovascular trauma.

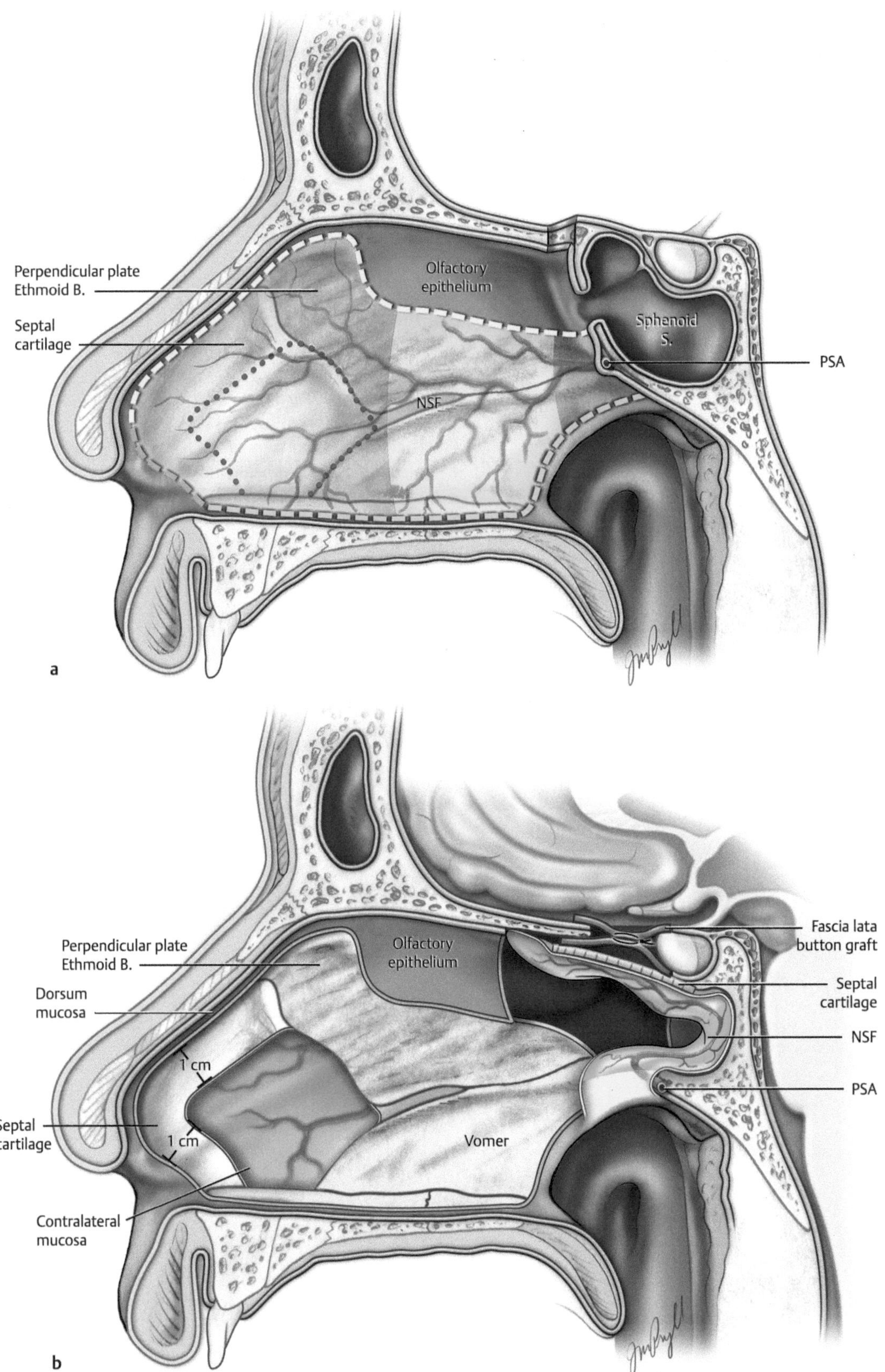

Fig. 7.2 Sagittal illustration of the left nasal septum. **(a)** The mucosal incisions for the composite cartilagomucosal nasoseptal flap (NSF) are the same ones used for the standard NSF. *Yellow dashed line*—superior incision. *Light blue dashed line*—anterior incision along the caudal border of the septum. *Green dashed line*—inferior incision. The inferior incision may be performed 5 mm lateral to the nasal septum along the nasal floor to incorporate mucosa of the floor and increase the rim of mucosa around the cartilaginous part of the flap. *Dotted dark blue lines*—cartilaginous incisions. Observe that the anatomofunctional divisions of the composite cartilagomucosal flap are similar to the standard flap. The mucoperichondrium with the attached cartilage is the main reconstructive area (*blue shade*). *Green shade*—mucoperiosteum (bridging area). *Yellow shade*—pedicle area. **(b)** Flap inset. Note the cartilaginous component placed onlay to reconstruct a suprasellar defect. The inlay reconstruction is performed with an inlay–onlay fascia lata button graft. Observe the preservation of 1 cm, L-shaped strut of the septal cartilage. B, bone; PSA, posterior septal artery; S, sinus.

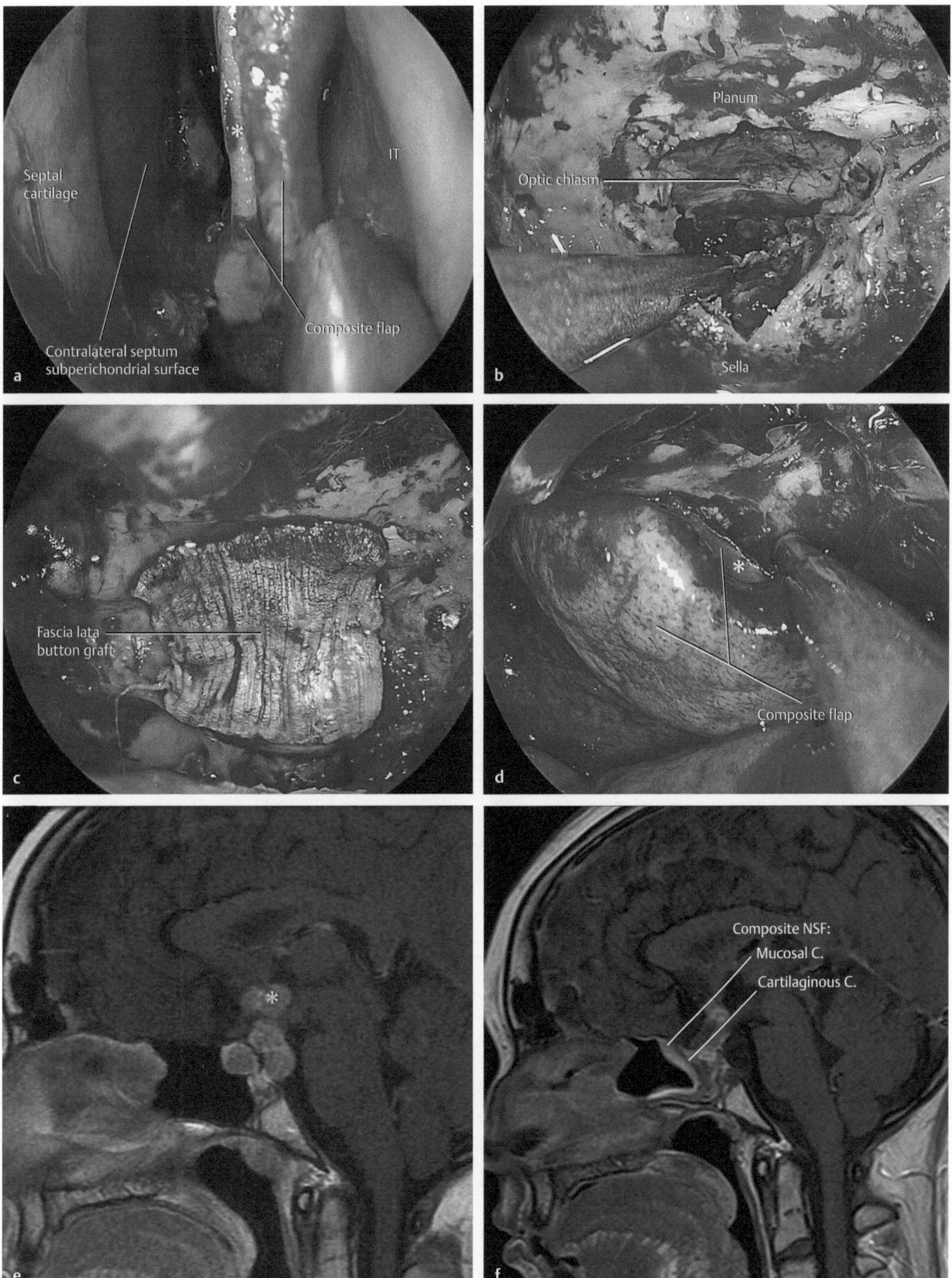

Fig. 7.3 Surgical case of a 17-year-old female who had an endoscopic endonasal resection of a suprasellar mass. Reconstruction was performed with a cartilagomucosal nasoseptal flap (NSF) to add a stronger reconstructive layer and improve long-term skull base protection for this young patient. **(a, c, d, and e)** Intraoperative pictures obtained with a 0-degree endoscope. **(a)** Harvest of a left-sided composite flap. Elevation of the cartilage (*yellow asterisk*) from the contralateral mucosa, leaving it attached to the ipsilateral NSF. **(b)** Suprasellar defect. **(c)** Outer layer of the fascia lata inlay–onlay button graft. **(d)** Composite flap inset. Note the cartilaginous component of the flap (*yellow asterisk*). **(e)** Preoperative magnetic resonance imaging (MRI) T1 with contrast sagittal view showing the suprasellar tumor (*green asterisk*). **(f)** Postoperative MRI T1 with contrast sagittal view 4 months after the surgery. Note the NSF enhancing with contrast and the cartilage protecting the suprasellar space. C, component; IT, inferior turbinate.

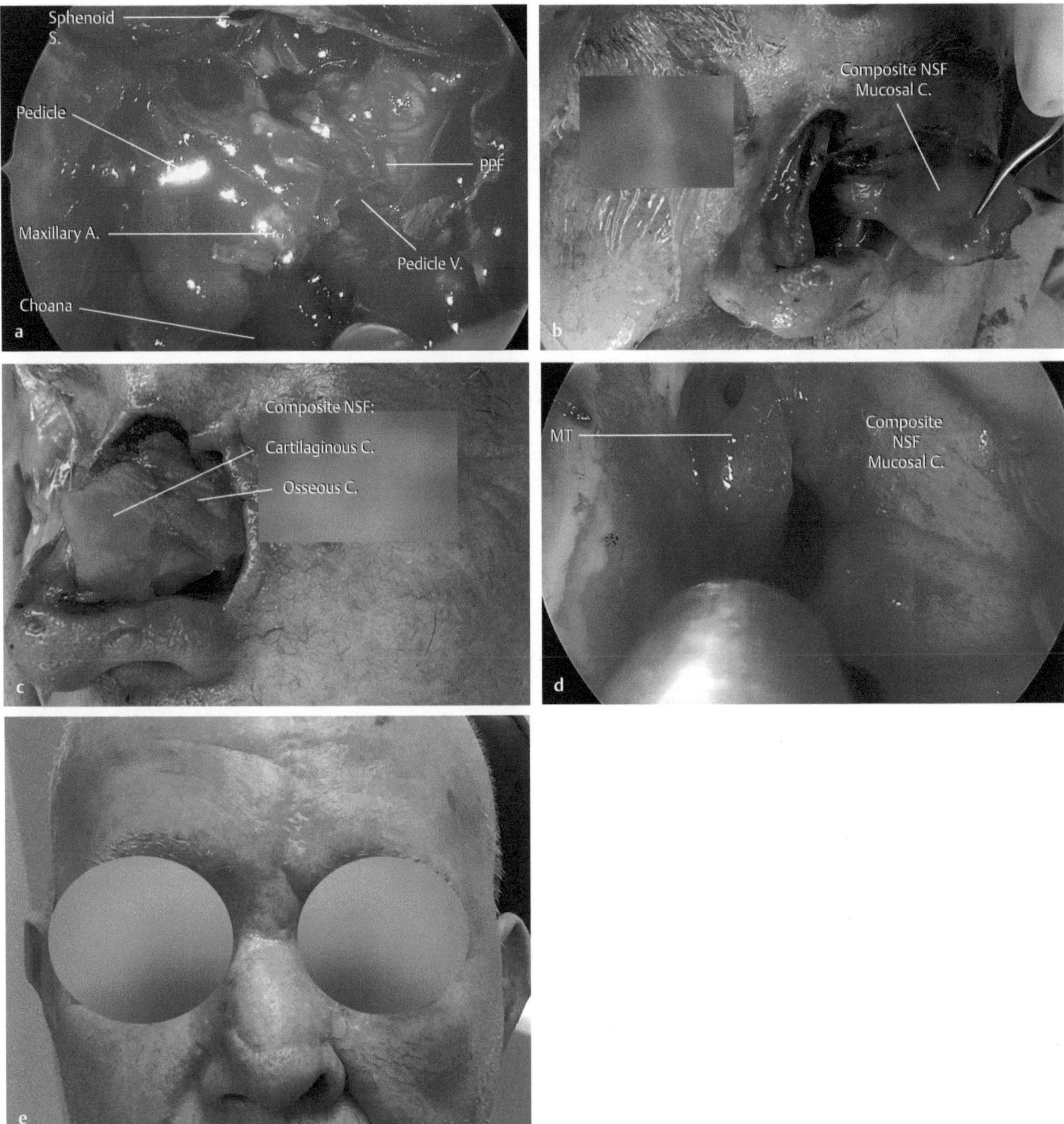

Fig. 7.4 Surgical case of a 68-year-old male with a cutaneous nasal melanoma with extensive cartilaginous and bone invasion. He underwent partial rhinectomy and reconstruction with a left-sided composite osteocartilagomucosal nasoseptal flap (NSF) to provide endonasal lining and framework with a single pedicled flap. Paramedian forehead flap was used for skin coverage. In order to mobilize the composite flap for the reconstruction, a pedicle release along the maxillary artery (MA) was performed. **(a)** Intraoperative picture obtained with a 0-degree endoscope showing the left pterygopalatine fossa (PPF) opened and the pedicle/MA release after maxillary antrostomy. **(b)** The flap was rotated and mobilized anteriorly after the pedicle release. **(c)** Flap inset. **(d)** Endoscopic view of the left nasal cavity during the division of the paramedian forehead flap 1 month after the surgery. Observe the mucosalization of the subperichondrial surface of the contralateral septum (*blue asterisk*). **(e)** Patient after 12 months from the reconstruction. A, artery; C, component; MT, middle turbinate; S, sinus; V, vein.

References

[1] Ramsey T, Shastri K, Curran K, Debiase C, Peris-Celda M, Pinheiro-Neto CD. Composite Chondromucosal Nasoseptal Flap for Reconstruction of Suprasellar Defects. World Neurosurg. 2021 May;149:11–14. doi: 10.1016/j.wneu.2021.01.137. Epub 2021 Feb 5. PMID: 33556598

[2] Shastri KS, Lin Y, Scordino J, Pinheiro-Neto CD. Composite cartilage-osseous-mucosal nasoseptal flap for reconstruction after near total rhinectomy. Ann Otol Rhinol Laryngol. 2021; 130(1):98–103

[3] Kalyoussef E, Schmidt RF, Liu JK, Eloy JA. Structural pedicled mucochondral-osteal nasoseptal flap: a novel method for orbital floor reconstruction after sinonasal and skull base tumor resection. Int Forum Allergy Rhinol. 2014; 4 (7):577–582

[4] Kim DW, Gurney T. Management of naso-septal L-strut deformities. Facial Plast Surg. 2006; 22(1):9–27

8 Resurface of the Septum Donor Site

Carlos D. Pinheiro-Neto and Maria Peris-Celda

8.1 Fundamentals

- There are two main vascularized flaps for mucosal resurface of the septum donor site after nasoseptal flap (NSF) harvest:
  - Reverse contralateral NSF.[1]
  - Inferior meatal mucosal flap.[2]
- The reverse flap is based on a broad pedicle with the blood supply from the anterior nasal septum circulation.
- The posterior septal artery does not contribute to the reverse NSF. This branch is actually transected to allow the anterior rotation of the flap.
- The inferior meatal flap is based on the greater palatine artery at the incisive (nasopalatine) foramen.
- The exposed cartilage and bone after harvesting the NSF heal by secondary intention.
- The mucosalization of the denuded septum can last for more than 3 months.[3]
- Nasal crust formation on the septum donor site has an important negative impact on patients' quality of life.
- Even after total mucosalization of the septum donor site, nasal crusting can still happen. This could be possibly related to inefficiency of the mucociliary clearance of the new epithelium.
- The denuded septal cartilage, particularly the area next to the nasal dorsum, is at increased risk of scar contraction and consequent saddle nose.[4]
- Patients who undergo concurrent septoplasty seem to be at increased risk of saddle nose due to loss of support associated with the cartilage resection.
- Nasal blockage, sleep difficulties, nasal pain/pressure, foul smell, and hyposmia are common symptoms related to nasal crusting.
- The exposed cartilage anteriorly seems to form more crusting than the exposed bone posteriorly.
- Techniques to resurface the septum donor site with mucosa are important to minimize areas of healing by secondary intention, nasal crusting, and possibly risk of saddle nose.
- Those surgical techniques may have a positive impact on patients' quality of life.

8.2 Indications

- To cover exposed septal cartilage at the donor site after NSF harvest.

8.3 Limitations

8.3.1 Reverse Contralateral NSF

- The reverse flap requires a large posterior septectomy, with impact on nasal airflow and crust formation at the sphenoid rostrum.
- The reverse flap carries increased risk to the olfactory area since both sides of the septal mucosa near the cribriform plate are incised.
- The mucosa rotated corresponds mostly to the mucoperiosteum (bridging area) of the nasal septum, which is smaller than the exposed septal cartilage, limiting the coverage of the cartilage next to the nasal dorsum.
- Harvesting a reverse flap precludes the use of the contralateral NSF in future reconstructions if needed.

8.3.2 Inferior Meatal Flap

- The inferior meatal flap is not available if the nasal floor/inferior meatus mucosa is added to an extended NSF.
- Since there is no septectomy required for this flap, the rotation of the mucosa covers the cartilage anteriorly, but the vomer is left uncovered.
- The bone of the nasal floor is left exposed and its mucosalization happens by secondary intention. Interestingly, the nasal floor is an area that heals rapidly with no major issues with crusting or negative impact in postoperative quality of life.[5] Maybe the less intense airflow in this region helps with less crust formation.

8.4 Surgical Technique

8.4.1 Reverse Contralateral NSF

- The reverse NSF consists of the anterior rotation of the contralateral posterior septal mucosa to resurface the septal cartilage exposed after the harvest of the NSF.
- After harvesting the NSF and working through the same nostril, the vomer and the inferior part of the perpendicular plate of the ethmoid are removed with exposure of the subperiosteal surface of the contralateral septal mucosa.
- Then through the contralateral nasal cavity, a needle tip bovie is used to perform the mucosal incisions for the reverse flap.
- The inferior incision starts as the standard NSF harvest at the superior border of the choana and is carried along the posterior border of the vomer, and transition between the nasal floor and septum. The difference is that this incision ends next to the anterior edge of the middle turbinate.
- The superior incision starts the same as for the standard NSF. At the level of the sphenoid sinus ostium, the incision is carried anteriorly and parallel to the palate up to the level of the anterior edge of the middle turbinate.
- Finally, a posterior incision is performed to connect the inferior and superior incisions along the anterior wall of the sphenoid. This posterior incision transects the septal artery, which should be coagulated. The blood supply to the flap is guaranteed by the broad pedicle anteriorly and the anterior septum vascularization.
- The reverse flap incisions can also be performed from the side where the NSF was harvested in the subperiosteal surface, if preferred.
- Once those incisions are concluded, the contralateral flap is rotated anteriorly to cover the septal cartilage exposed.

- Finally, the mucosa is sutured anteriorly with absorbable sutures similar to what is performed to suture the septal mucosa after a septoplasty (▶ Fig. 8.1).
- If needed, the posterior edge of the septal cartilage can be partially removed in order to facilitate the anterior reach of the reverse flap.

8.4.2 Inferior Meatal Flap (*Video 8.1*)

- Four incisions are made to harvest the inferior meatal flap.
- The posterior incision is performed from the septum to the tail of the inferior turbinate at the transition between the nasal surface of the soft palate and the nasal floor.
- The lateral incision is carried along the attachment of the inferior turbinate.
- The anterior incision is made along the nostril at the mucocutaneous junction from the inferior turbinate head toward the anterior nasal spine.
- The medial incision was already performed along the transition between the septum and nasal floor during the harvest of the NSF.
- The flap is elevated leaving it attached to the incisive foramen neurovascular bundle (▶ Fig. 8.2a).
- After the harvest, the inferior meatal flap is rotated to cover the septal cartilage and sutured anteriorly along its caudal border (▶ Fig. 8.2b).
- ▶ Fig. 8.3 illustrates a surgical example of a patient who had inferior meatal flap to resurface the septal cartilage after harvesting a NSF.

8.5 Postoperative Care

- For both flaps, Doyle open-lumen plastic splints are used in both sides. The splints help pressuring the flap against the denuded septal cartilage.
- Nasal splints are removed 1 week after the surgery.
- Postoperative visits 1 week, 1 month, and 4 months after surgery for nasal debridement. Do not remove crusting over the septum at the 1-week postoperative visit to avoid detachment of the flap from the septal cartilage.

8.6 Complications

- Reverse flap: Risk of hyposmia/anosmia with bilateral septal incisions next to the olfactory cleft. Change in the posterior airflow within the nasal cavity due to the large posterior septectomy.
- Inferior meatal flap: Dental numbness (central incisors) due to manipulation of the neurovascular bundle of the incisive canal. Potential risk of nasolacrimal obstruction due to the lateral incision of the flap next to the nasolacrimal duct opening (Hasner valve). Bulky pedicle anteriorly due to the mucosal fold and risk of nasal obstruction. Usually during the healing process, the pedicle area contracts and there is no need for division of the pedicle postoperatively.

8.7 Free Mucosal Grafts

- Besides the use of vascularized flaps to resurface the septal cartilage after the NSF harvest, the use of free mucosal grafts (FMGs) is also described in the literature.
- The middle turbinate mucosa can be used as FMG.[3]
- Instead of removing the posterior septum and rotating the posterior septal mucosa to cover the denuded cartilage as described for the reverse flap, the contralateral posterior septal mucosa can be harvested as a FMG. This technique leaves the posterior bony septum intact in both sides to heal by secondary intention.[6]
- The contralateral nasal floor/inferior meatus mucosa can also be harvested and used as a FMG.

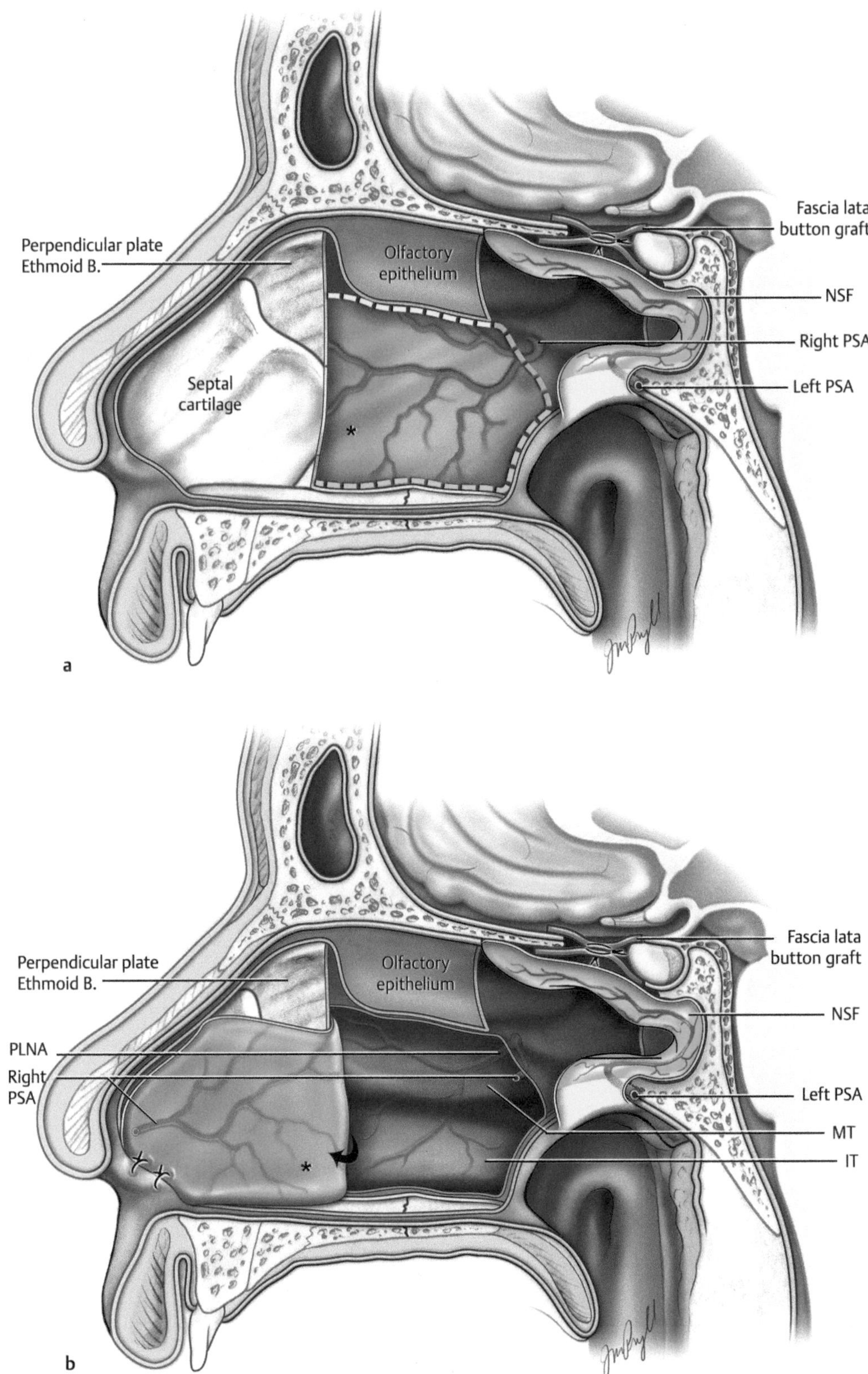

Fig. 8.1 (a) Illustration of the nasal septum sagittal view after harvesting a left-sided nasoseptal flap (NSF) for reconstruction of a planum sphenoidale defect. The vomer and part of the perpendicular plate of the ethmoid bone were removed with exposure of the underlying subperiosteal surface of the contralateral septal mucosa (*asterisk*). The harvest of the reverse contralateral NSF includes three incisions: Superior (*yellow dashed line*), inferior (*green dashed line*), and posterior (*blue dashed line*). Note the preservation of the equivalent olfactory mucosa on the contralateral side. The flap incisions can be performed on either side. **(b)** The *arrow* demonstrates the rotation of the reverse flap to cover septal cartilage. Sutures are placed anteriorly to secure the flap in place. *Asterisk* shows the right septal mucosa covering the denuded cartilage. Observe the transection of the right posterior septal artery to allow the rotation of the flap. B, bone; IT, inferior turbinate; MT, middle turbinate; PLNA, posterior lateral nasal artery; PSA, posterior septal artery.

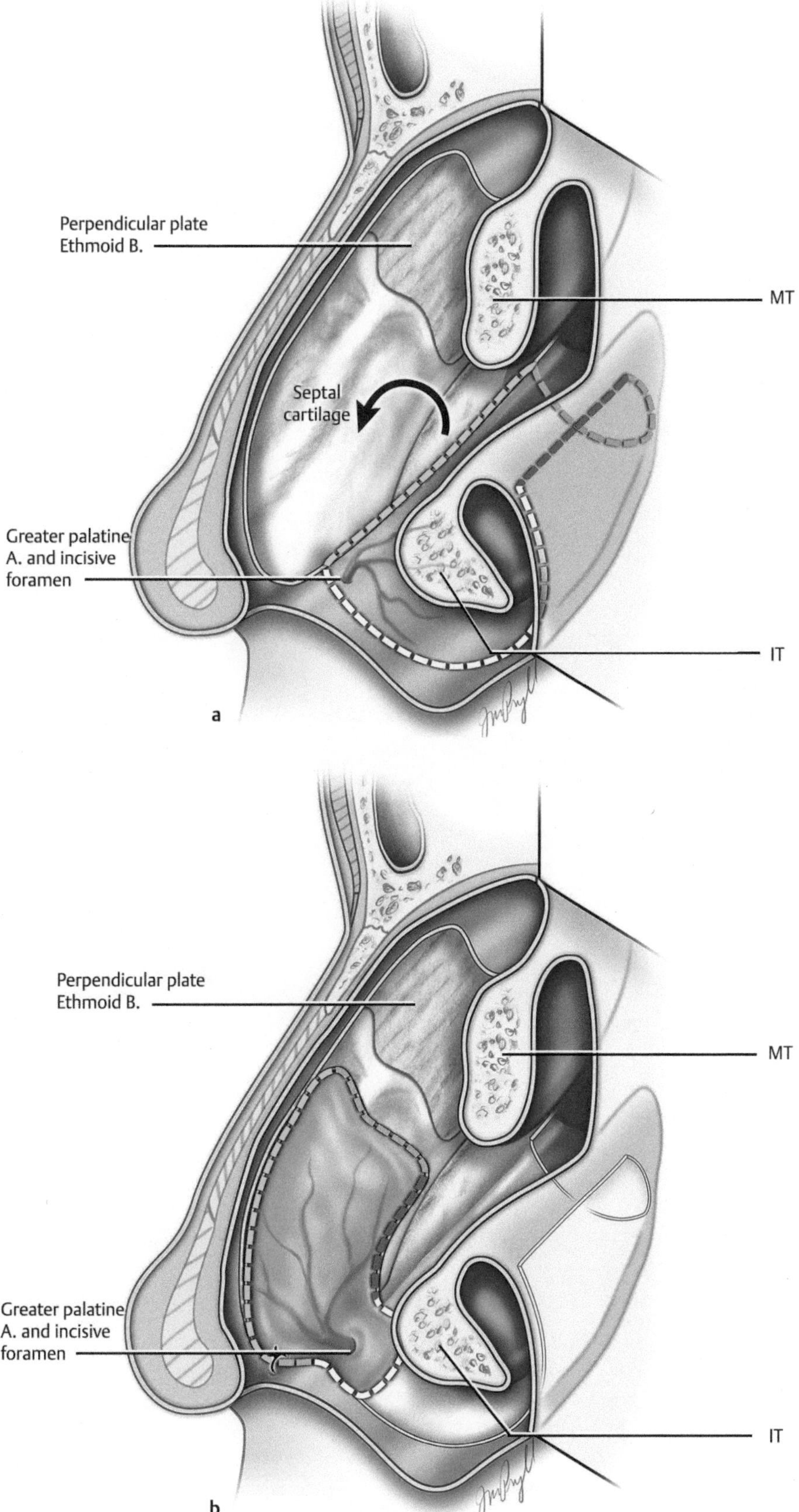

Fig. 8.2 Illustration of the left nasal cavity to demonstrate the harvest and inset of the inferior meatal flap to cover the septal cartilage after harvesting of a nasoseptal flap (NSF). **(a)** Three incisions are made since the medial one (*green dashed line*) corresponds to the same inferior incision for the NSF: Posterior incision along the transition between the hard and soft palates (*orange dashed line*); lateral incision along the attachment of the inferior turbinate (IT) within the inferior meatus (*purple dashed line*); and the anterior incision along the mucocutaneous junction of the nostril (*white dashed line*). The *arrow* demonstrates the rotation of the flap toward the septum. **(b)** Flap inset and suture placed anteriorly. A, artery; B, bone; MT, middle turbinate.

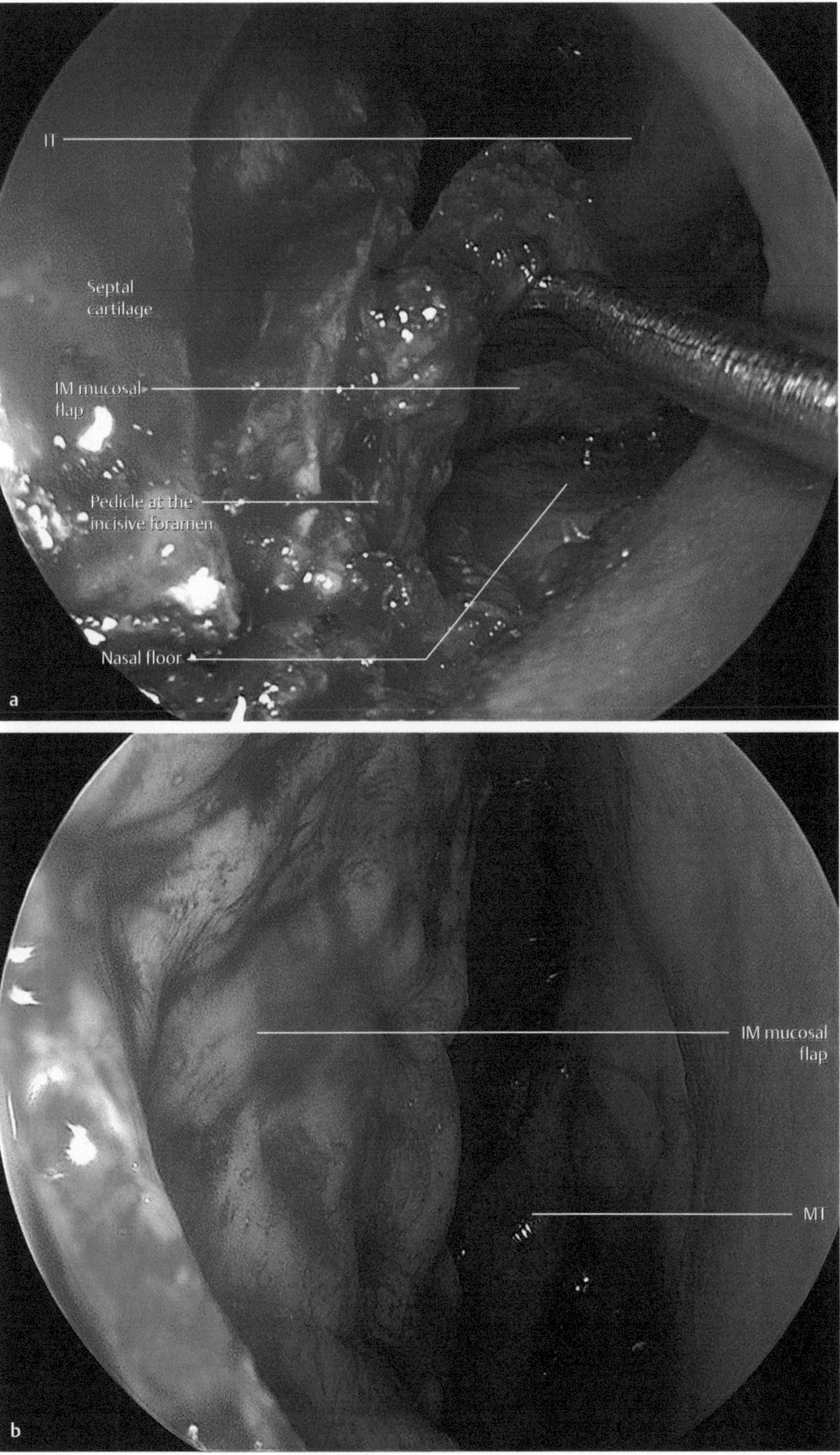

Fig. 8.3 Intraoperative pictures of the left nasal cavity obtained with a 0-degree endoscope to show the resurface of the septal cartilage after harvesting of a nasoseptal flap (NSF). **(a)** Vascular pedicle based on the neurovascular bundle at the incisive foramen (greater palatine artery). **(b)** Flap inset. IM, inferior meatus; IT, inferior turbinate; MT, middle turbinate.

References

[1] Kasemsiri P, Carrau RL, Otto BA, et al. Reconstruction of the pedicled nasoseptal flap donor site with a contralateral reverse rotation flap: technical modifications and outcomes. Laryngoscope. 2013; 123(11):2601–2604

[2] Ruffner R, Pereira MC, Patel V, Peris-Celda M, Pinheiro-Neto CD. Inferior Meatus Mucosal Flap for Septal Reconstruction and Resurfacing After Nasoseptal Flap Harvest. Laryngoscope. 2021 May;131(5):952–955

[3] Kimple AJ, Leight WD, Wheless SA, Zanation AM. Reducing nasal morbidity after skull base reconstruction with the nasoseptal flap: free middle turbinate mucosal grafts. Laryngoscope. 2012; 122(9):1920–1924

[4] Rowan NR, Wang EW, Gardner PA, Fernandez-Miranda JC, Snyderman CH. Nasal deformities following nasoseptal flap reconstruction of skull base defects. J Neurol Surg B Skull Base. 2016; 77(1):14–18

[5] Scagnelli RJ, Patel V, Peris-Celda M, Kenning TJ, Pinheiro-Neto CD. Implementation of free mucosal graft technique for sellar reconstruction after pituitary surgery: outcomes of 158 consecutive patients. World Neurosurg. 2019; 122: e506–e511

[6] Yoo F, Kuan EC, Bergsneider M, Wang MB. Free mucosal graft reconstruction of the septum after nasoseptal flap harvest: a novel technique using a posterior septal free mucosal graft. J Neurol Surg B Skull Base. 2017; 78(2): 201–206

Section III

Other Intranasal Flaps

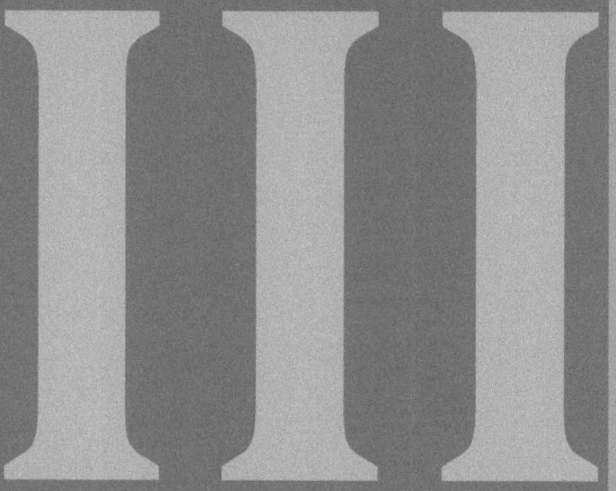

9 Middle Turbinate Flap

Carlos D. Pinheiro-Neto, Luciano C. P. C. Leonel, and Maria Peris-Celda

9.1 Anatomy

- The middle turbinate (MT) is part of the ethmoid bone.
- The middle meatus is the space between the turbinate and the nasal lateral wall where the ostiometal complex is located.
- Frontal sinus, anterior ethmoidal cells, and maxillary sinus drain through the ostiometal complex.
- The MT has three portions with different insertions (▶ Fig. 9.1a):
  - Vertical portion (anterior 1/3): Insertion in the sagittal plane to the skull base between the medial and lateral lamellas of the cribriform plate.
  - Diagonal portion (middle 1/3): Insertion in the coronal plane to the lamina papyracea. The diagonal portion is also called basal lamella and separates the anterior and posterior ethmoidal cells.
  - Horizontal portion (posterior 1/3): Insertion in the axial plane to the vertical plate of the palatine bone.
- A proximal branch of the posterior lateral nasal artery near the sphenopalatine foramen supplies the MT.[1]
- The MT artery enters the turbinate along the attachment of the horizontal portion (▶ Fig. 9.1b).
- The MT can present different degrees of pneumatization (concha bullosa) that could impact the space within the middle meatus.
- The natural curvature of the MT has a concavity in its meatal/lateral surface. The paradoxical curvature of the MT is an anatomical variation where the concavity faces the septum, and the convex part of the turbinate protrudes toward the middle meatus narrowing that space.

9.2 Fundamentals

- The MT can be used as an intranasal flap for reconstruction of the cranial base.
- The middle turbinate flap (MTF) is usually used in selected cases when the nasoseptal flap is not available or in cases where the defect is small enough and suitable for this flap.
- The MTF is a mucoperiosteal flap. The elevation of the MT mucosa is performed with the turbinate still attached to the skull base. If the turbinate is detached too early, the mucosal harvesting is more challenging due to the instability of the turbinate.
- The reconstructive area of the MT corresponds to the mucosa attached to its vertical portion and can be divided in two areas: Nasal or medial surface and meatal or lateral surface.
- The diagonal portion of the MT does not contribute to the flap and is removed during the flap harvest to improve its mobilization.
- The pedicle area of the MTF corresponds to the horizontal portion of the MT.
- The meatal and the nasal mucosa of the MTF are continuous along the inferior edge of turbinate after the bone removal (▶ Fig. 9.1c).
- The MTF can be harvested as a composite osteomucosal flap when the MT bone is left attached to the mucosa.[2]

9.3 Indications

- Anterior cranial base defects involving the cribriform plate and fovea ethmoidalis.[3]
- Sellar and suprasellar defects.
- Selected cases of oroantral fistulas to reconstruct the maxillary sinus floor (pedicle release is necessary).

9.4 Limitations

- The limited cross-sectional area restricts its reconstruction capability to smaller defects.
- Some areas of the MT mucosa are extremely thin which increases the risk of inadvertent laceration during harvesting.
- The MT bone next to the skull base is thin and may be inadvertently dettached during the harvest. The resultant instability makes the mucosal elevation more difficult.
- The different shapes of the MT with a variety of recesses make the harvest more challenging and with increased risk of mucosal lacerations.
- In cases of concha bullosa, the harvest of the flap is harder due to the narrow space within the middle meatus.
- The wide attachment of the pedicle (horizontal portion of the MT) to the lateral wall limits the flap reach. This can be optimized with careful extended dissection of the pedicle, releasing the horizontal attachment of the MT toward the sphenopalatine foramen.

9.5 Surgical Technique

9.5.1 Harvest

- The MT is gently medialized.
- An anterior ethmoidectomy can be performed to improve the space within the middle meatus. If a posterior ethmoidectomy is also performed, this step detaches the diagonal portion of the MT, separating it from the orbit.
- The MTF incision starts at the anterior face of the vertical portion of the MT from superior to inferior. A needle tip bovie set at 10 W is used (▶ Fig. 9.2a).
- The middle meatus mucosa is carefully elevated from anterior to posterior until exposure of the posterior border of the MT bone. Similar elevation is performed on the nasal surface of the MT.
- The superior incision corresponds to the separation of the vertical and diagonal attachments of the MT, leaving the turbinate attached only at its horizontal portion (pedicle of the flap).
- The MT is transected right next to the skull base (vertical attachment) with endoscopic scissors. This incision is progressed posteriorly and inferiorly along the diagonal attachment if the posterior ethmoidectomy was not performed.
- The detachment of the MT from the skull base (vertical portion) is performed in all three layers of the turbinate: meatal mucosa, MT bone, and nasal mucosa (▶ Fig. 9.2b).

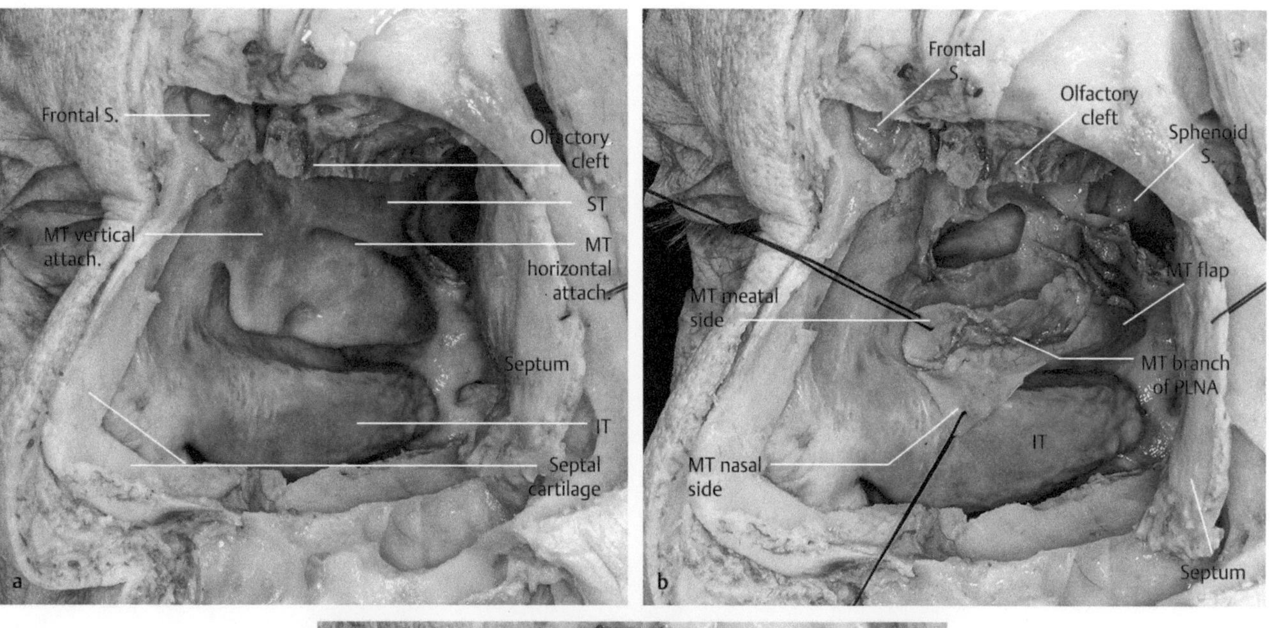

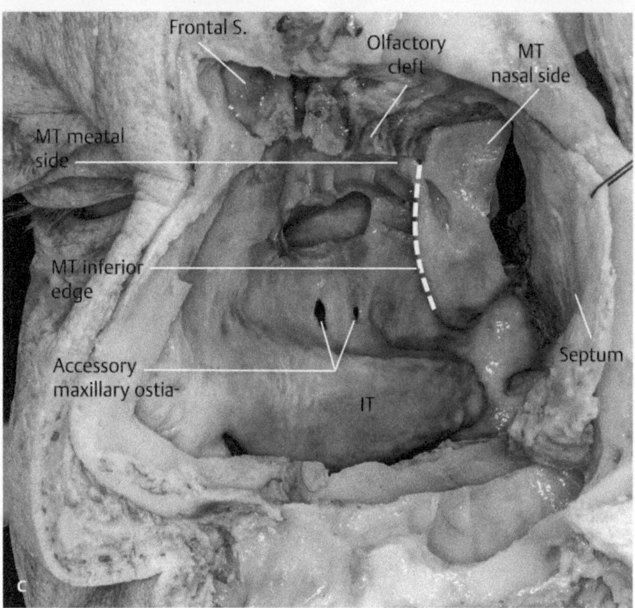

Fig. 9.1 Anatomical dissection after removal of the left hemiface, orbital contents, and exposure of the nasal cavity. **(a)** Right lateral nasal wall. **(b)** After detachment of the middle turbinate (MT) from its vertical insertion to the skull base and its diagonal attachment to the orbit. The MT bone was removed, and the turbinate was opened like a "book." Note the two surfaces of the MT: Nasal and meatal; and the MT artery arising from its horizontal portion. **(c)** Middle turbinate flap (MTF) inset. *White dashed line*—mucosa along the inferior border of the MT connecting the nasal and the meatal surfaces. attach, attachment; IT, inferior turbinate; PLNA, posterior lateral nasal artery; S, sinus; ST, superior turbinate.

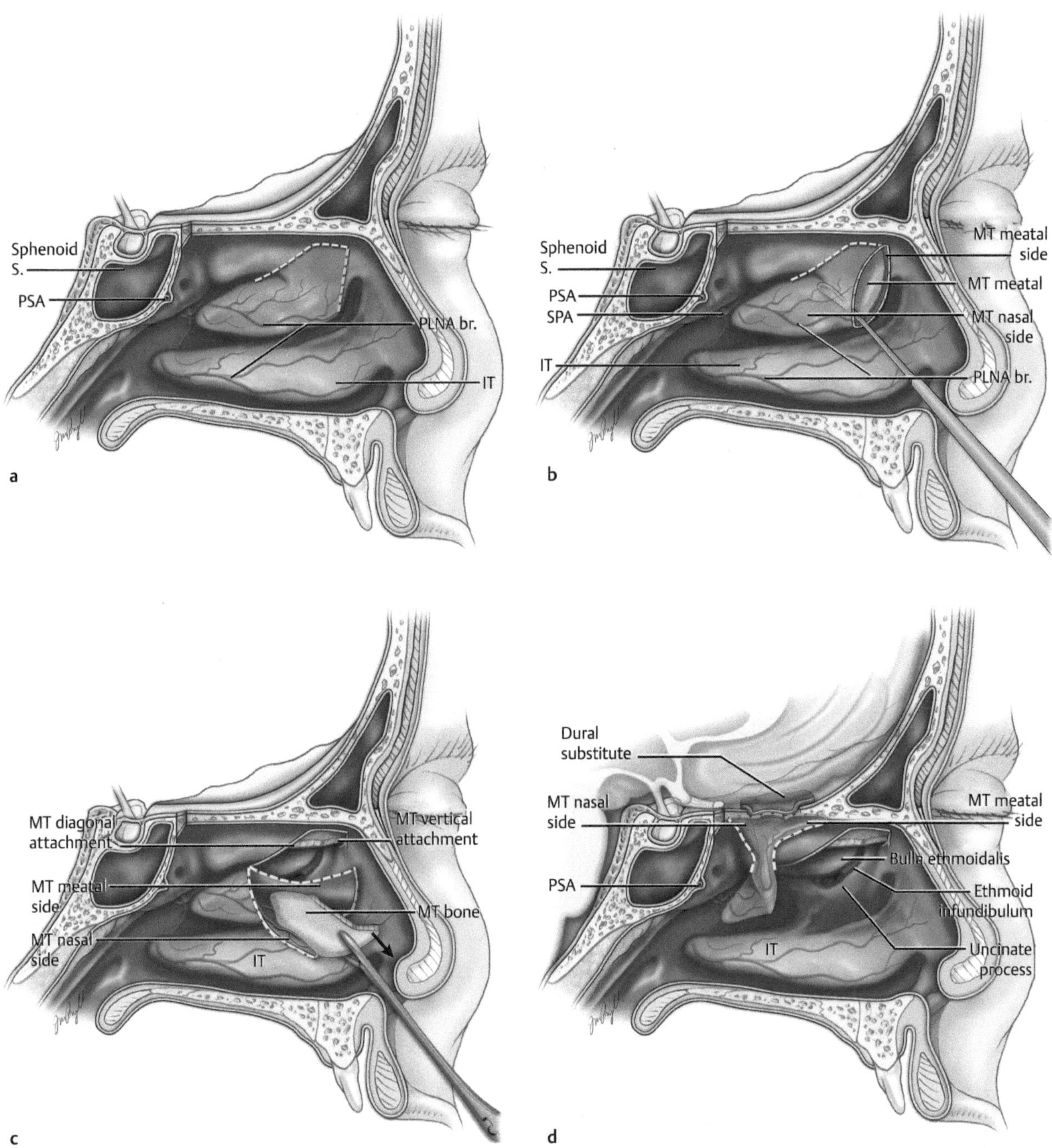

Fig. 9.2 Illustration of a sagittal view of the left lateral nasal wall to show the harvest of the middle turbinate flap (MTF). **(a)** *Blue dashed line*—anterior incision. *Yellow dashed line*—superior incision. **(b)** First, the anterior incision is performed and two subperiosteal submucosal pockets are created: One in the nasal surface and another one in the meatal surface. This exposes the middle turbinate (MT) bone. **(c)** The superior incision is performed detaching the MT from the skull base (vertical attachment) and from the orbit (diagonal attachment). The MT bone is finally dissected from the mucosa of the inferior border and removed (*arrow*). **(d)** Inset of the MTF to reconstruct an anterior cranial base defect. br., branch; IT, inferior turbinate; PLNA, posterior lateral nasal artery; PSA, posterior septal artery; S, sinus; SPA, sphenopalatine artery.

- At this point, the MT bone is attached only to the mucosa of its inferior border, which corresponds to the mucosa between the meatal surface and nasal surface of the MT.
- The MT is open like a "book" and the bone is gently removed from the mucosa of the inferior border[4] (▶ Fig. 9.2c).
- Finally, the boneless MT can be used as a flap for cranial base reconstruction.
- To increase the flap reach, a 360-degree circumferential mucosal incision around the horizontal portion of the MT can be performed. The horizontal portion of the MT is carefully elevated until the sphenopalatine artery is identified. If further release is needed, the dissection can be progressed toward the pterygopalatine fossa and maxillary artery.

9.5.2 Reconstruction

- During repair of defects of the ethmoidal roof, the flap is moved upward, leaving the periosteal surface in contact with the skull base (▶ Fig. 9.2d).
- For defects of the planum sphenoidale or sella, the flap is rotated posteriorly.
- After the placement of the MTF, pieces of oxidized cellulose are applied to the borders of the flap, followed by dural sealant and absorbable packing.
- ▶ Fig. 9.3 illustrates a surgical example of a composite MTF used for reconstruction of an oroantral fistula.

9.6 Postoperative Care

- Postoperative visits 1 week, 1 month, and 4 months for nasal debridement.
- During the first postoperative visit (1 week after surgery), the debridement is performed mostly to improve nasal breathing. The absorbable packing and crusting around the MTF are not removed.
- Large-volume saline nasal irrigation is used during the first month.
- During the second postoperative visit (1 month after the surgery), the nasal debridement is performed next to the reconstruction area and the flap is visualized.
- During the following 3 months, large-volume saline irrigation can be used as needed and the patient comes to clinic for the third postoperative visit (4 months after the surgery) for final assessment of healing. After that visit, the follow-up is scheduled according to the baseline disease or if the patient has any issues with nasal crusting or sinusitis.
- Because the MT is totally used for reconstruction, there is no donor site morbidity related to exposed cartilage or bone as seen with other intranasal flaps.

9.7 Complications

- Due to the limited flap reach, extensive elevation of the horizontal portion of the MT can lead to avulsion of the arterial blood supply of the MT. To minimize this risk, dissection around the sphenopalatine foramen is recommended.
- Fracture of the cribriform plate during the harvest and consequent cerebrospinal fluid leak.[5]
- Hyposmia or anosmia due to damage of olfactory filaments next to the cribriform plate.
- The use of the MT for reconstruction may impact the physiologic airflow through the nasal cavity.

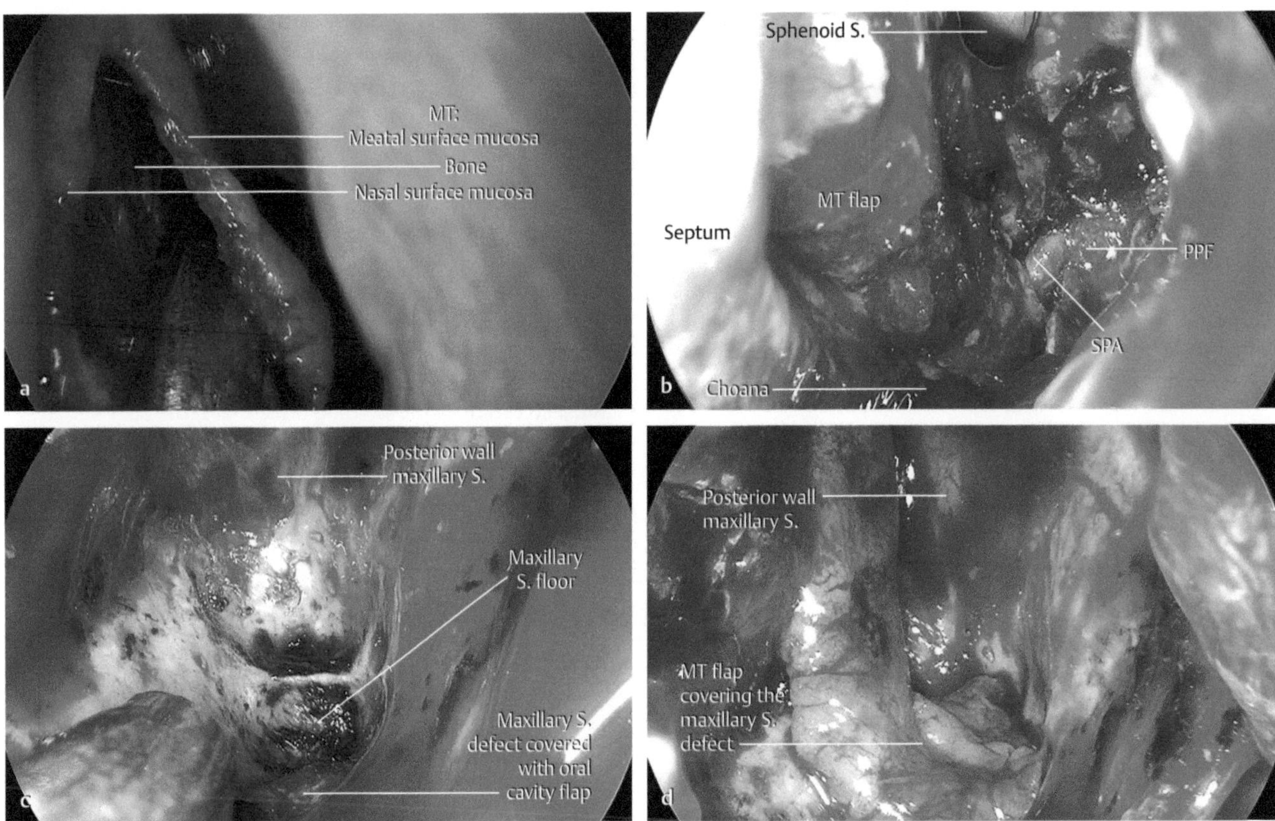

Fig. 9.3 Clinical case of a patient who had a composite middle turbinate flap (MTF) for reconstruction of the maxillary sinus surface of an oroantral fistula. Patient had seven previous surgeries, and an intranasal flap was recommended to cover the maxillary sinus defect in addition to an oral cavity flap for the oral surface of the defect. Intraoperative pictures obtained with a 0-degree endoscope. **(a)** Left nasal cavity showing the anterior incision for the MTF and elevation of the subperiosteal submucosal pocket along the meatal surface. **(b)** The middle turbinate (MT) bone was left attached to the mucosa as a composite osteomucosal flap. A 360-degree circumferential mucosal incision around the horizontal attachment of the MT was performed. The mucosa next to the sphenopalatine artery (SPA) was elevated and the artery exposed. Maxillary antrostomy and osseous release of the pedicle were performed with removal of the osseous boundaries of the sphenopalatine foramen to allow sufficient mobilization of the flap toward the maxillary sinus floor. **(c)** View through sublabial transmaxillary approach after removal of the maxillary sinus mucosa to allow appropriate healing of the flap. An intraoral flap was previously rotated to cover the oral surface of the defect. **(d)** Composite MTF covering the floor of the maxillary sinus. This inferior reach was possible due to the pedicle release. Absorbable packing was used to fill the maxillary sinus and promote gentle pressure of the flap toward the defect. PPF, pterygopalatine fossa; S, sinus.

References

[1] MacArthur FJ, McGarry GW. The arterial supply of the nasal cavity. Eur Arch Otorhinolaryngol. 2017; 274(2):809–815

[2] Amin SM, Fawzy TO, Hegazy AA. Composite vascular pedicled middle turbinate flap for reconstruction of sellar defects. Ann Otol Rhinol Laryngol. 2016; 125(9):770–774

[3] Tamura R, Toda M, Kohno M, et al. Vascularized middle turbinate flap for the endoscopic endonasal reconstruction of the anterior olfactory groove. Neurosurg Rev. 2016; 39(2):297–302, discussion 302

[4] Prevedello DM, Barges-Coll J, Fernandez-Miranda JC, et al. Middle turbinate flap for skull base reconstruction: cadaveric feasibility study. Laryngoscope. 2009; 119(11):2094–2098

[5] Chakravarthi S, Gonen L, Monroy-Sosa A, Khalili S, Kassam A. Endoscopic endonasal reconstructive methods to the anterior skull base. Semin Plast Surg. 2017; 31(4):203–213

10 Posterior-Based Lateral Nasal Wall Flaps

Carl H. Snyderman and Paul A. Gardner

10.1 Anatomy

- The posterior-based lateral nasal wall flap (posterior LNWF) is based on the vascular territory of the lateral nasal wall branch of the sphenopalatine artery which sends branches to the middle and inferior turbinates.[1] The inferior turbinate branch courses along the inferior concha with smaller branches to the inferior meatus and lateral nasal wall.[2]
- A standard flap consists of the mucosa investing the inferior concha, the mucosa of the lateral nasal wall superior to the attachment of the inferior turbinate, and the mucosa of the inferior meatus (▸ Fig. 10.1).[3]
- The vascular pedicle of the posterior LNWF is a short segment from the posterior attachment of the inferior turbinate to the sphenopalatine foramen. The pedicle is superior and anterior to the Eustachian tube.
- Extended versions of the posterior LNWF include mucosa from the nasal floor and nasal septum (▸ Fig. 10.1).[4,5] These extended flaps greatly increase the surface area and reach of the posterior LNWF.
- There is a dominant inferior branch of the lateral nasal wall artery that supplies the inferior meatus and a portion of the nasal floor.[2] Anatomical studies demonstrate anastomoses (average of three vessels) of these vessels with the inferior branch of the nasoseptal artery.[5]
- The nasolacrimal duct enters the nasal cavity through the lateral nasal wall at the anterior limit of the inferior meatus under cover of the inferior concha.

10.2 Fundamentals

- The introduction of the vascularized nasoseptal flap (NSF) in 2006 had a major impact on cerebrospinal fluid (CSF) leak rates and has become the workhorse for reconstruction of most ventral skull base defects.[6]
- Systematic reviews of the literature demonstrate that reconstruction with vascularized tissue rather than free tissue grafts is associated with fewer postoperative CSF leaks.[7]
- An NSF cannot be used in all cases due to prior surgery with sacrifice of the vascular pedicle, prior use of NSF, or tumor involvement of the vascular pedicle or nasal septum. Alternative intranasal flaps include the middle turbinate flap (MTF) and posterior LNWF.[8,9,10,11,12] The MTF has limited applications due to its small size and limited reach and is rarely used.[8,12]

10.3 Indications

- The posterior LNWF, also called an inferior turbinate flap, is most suitable for reconstruction of sellar and clival defects.[9,10,11] It is a good option for the reconstruction of clival defects when reconstruction with an NSF is not an option or other repairs have failed, such as NSF necrosis.[13]
- In our experience, posterior LNWFs were used to cover sellar and suprasellar defects in 6 out of 24 cases and posterior fossa defects in 18 out of 24 cases.[2] The posterior LNWFs were performed in revision surgery because of NSF unavailability (41.7%), for postoperative CSF leaks secondary to NSF necrosis (41.7%) and for postoperative CSF leaks that required additional vascularized tissue coverage (16.6%).
- The blood supply to a posterior LNWF is usually preserved during endoscopic transphenoidal approaches, preserving the option of a posterior LNWF in revision cases where an NSF is not an option or has been used previously.
- Extended posterior LNWFs are an option when prior surgery or tumor involvement of the sphenoid rostrum precludes use of a NSF.

10.4 Limitations

- It is difficult to dissect the inferior conchal bone, and this may result in retained bone fragments or mucosal lacerations.
- Due to its short vascular pedicle, the posterior LNWF has limited mobility and reach.
- The conchal portion of the flap retains its shape and does not conform well to the surgical site.
- With extended flaps, it is unclear if the blood supply to the septum is robust enough to support a large flap.

10.5 Surgical Technique

- Intraoperatively, the posterior LNWF is not harvested until after tumor resection as it typically lies outside of the surgical field where it is protected from instrument trauma for most sagittal plane approaches. For coronal plane approaches, early harvest and mobilization of the vascular pedicle may be necessary.

10.5.1 Standard Posterior LNWF[3] (*Videos 10.1 and 10.2*)

- A middle meatal antrostomy is first performed with removal of part of the uncinate process.
- Using an extended needle-tip electrocautery device, an incision is made from the antrostomy superiorly over the lateral nasal wall. Once the nasal dorsum is reached, the incision follows the margin of the pyriform aperture anteriorly and inferiorly to the anterior attachment of the inferior turbinate. The incision is extended to the anterior tip of the inferior concha. The vertical incision continues to follow the pyriform aperture at the anterior limit of the inferior meatus to the nasal floor. The incision then extends posteriorly along the junction of the lateral nasal wall and nasal floor to the Eustachian tube. The vascular pedicle is at the posterior attachment of the inferior concha and can be preserved by staying below this level. In order to maximize mobility of the flap, it is important to extend the incision above the Eustachian tube posterior to the vascular pedicle (▸ Fig. 10.2).
- It is preferable to dissect the mucoperiosteum from the bone of the inferior concha before detaching the bone from the lateral nasal wall. The inferior concha has an irregular surface

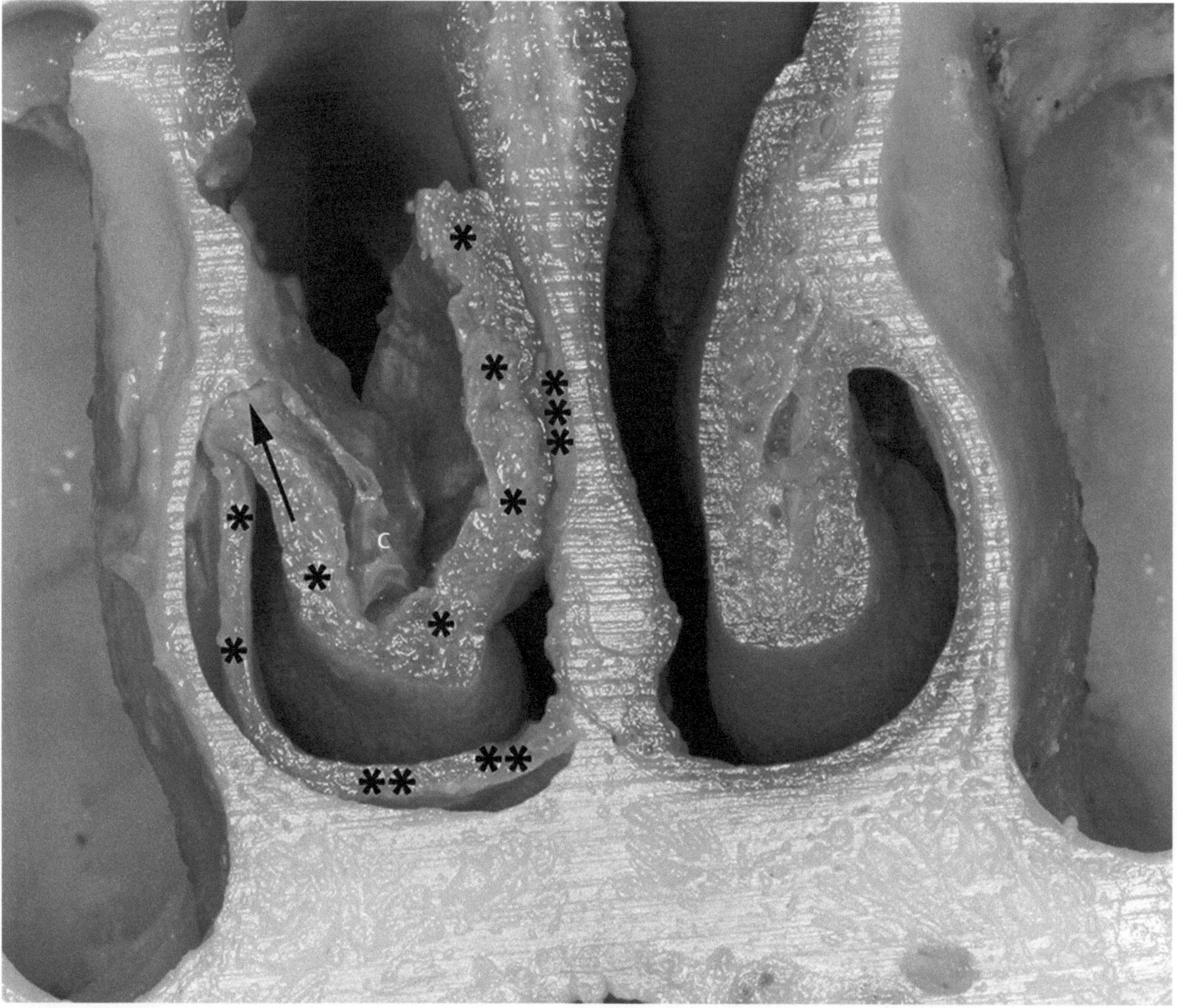

Fig. 10.1 A standard posterior-based lateral nasal wall flap (*single asterisks*) includes the mucosa of the lateral nasal wall superior to the inferior concha (C), the inferior concha itself, and the inferior meatus lateral wall. It may be extended to include the mucosa of the nasal floor (*double asterisks*) and even the nasal septum (*triple asterisks*). The nasolacrimal duct (*arrow*) is exposed and transected in the nasolacrimal canal to preserve the mucosa of the inferior meatus.

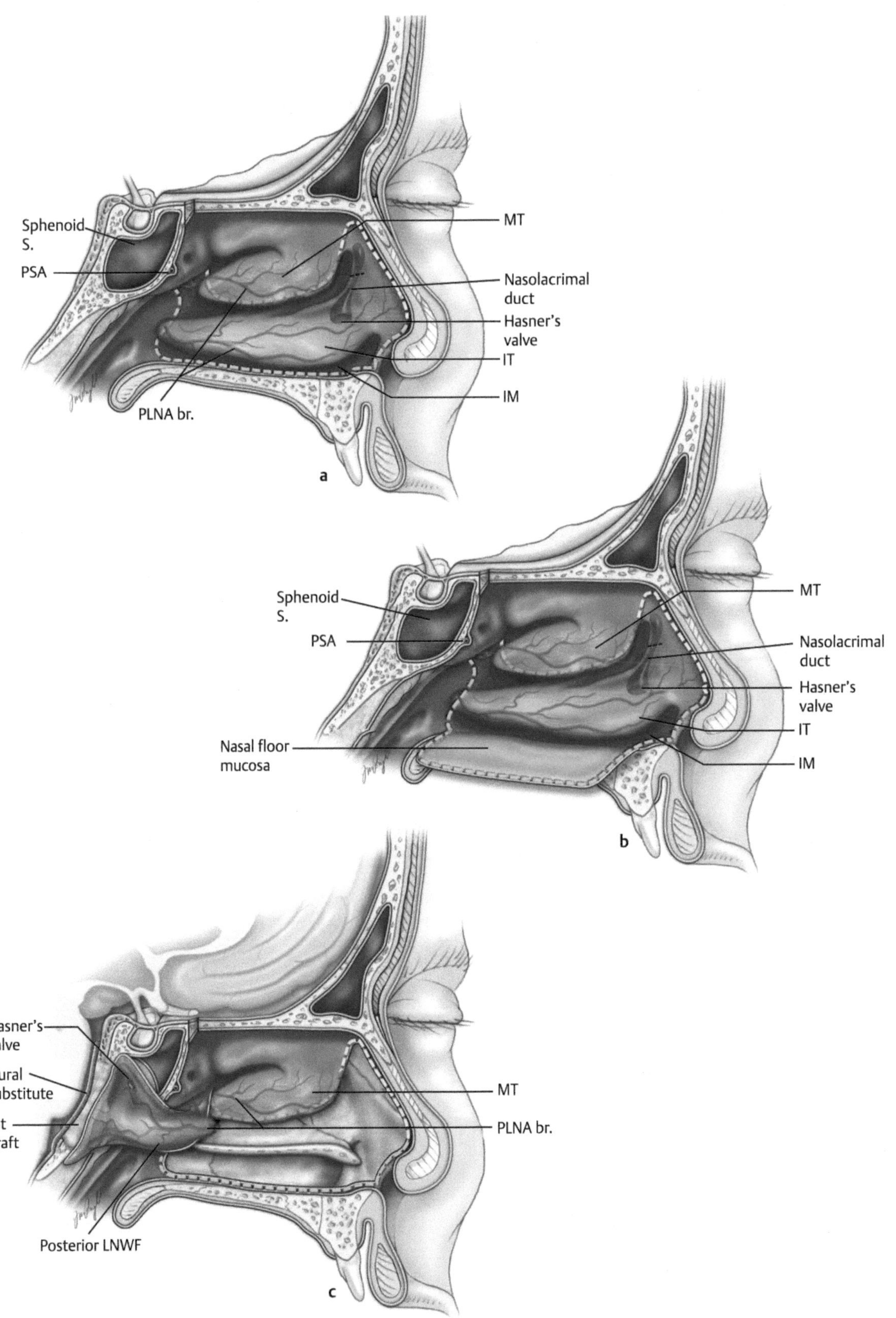

Fig. 10.2 Sagittal view of the left nasal cavity to illustrate the harvest of the posterior-based lateral nasal wall flap (posterior LNWF). **(a)** Incisions for the standard posterior LNWF. *Green dashed line*—inferior incision. *Blue dashed line*—anterior incision. *Yellow dashed line*—superior incision. Note the representation of the sharp incision (*black dashed line*) of the nasolacrimal duct. This step is important to elevate the flap from the lateral wall. **(b)** Extended posterior LNWF with inclusion of the nasal floor mucosa. The medial limit of the inferior incision (*green dashed line*) is made along the transition between the septum and the nasal floor. The flap can be extended further to include the mucosa of the septum if needed. **(c)** Flap inset for reconstruction of a clival defect. br., branch; IM, inferior meatus; IT, inferior turbinate; LNWF, lateral nasal wall flap; MT, middle turbinate; PLNA, posterior lateral nasal artery; PSA, posterior septal artery; S, sinus.

and is firmly adherent to the mucoperiosteum. The attachment of the concha to the lateral nasal wall is often thin and easily fractured.

- A Cottle elevator is used to dissect the mucoperiosteum in an anterior to posterior direction. Elevation of the flap is limited by the nasolacrimal duct anteriorly. The overlying bone is removed with a Kerrison rongeur to fully expose the duct (▶ Fig. 10.3). It is then sharply transected with microscissors. This necessarily leaves a small perforation in the flap that can be sutured but is typically not an issue since it is positioned over fascia or bone once the flap is transposed. The flap should be maximally mobilized to the pedicle posterior to the inferior concha.
- The flap may be rotated in a clockwise or counterclockwise direction depending on the reconstructive needs. For clival and sellar defects, the flap is usually rotated inferiorly and medially (clockwise on the left side; counterclockwise on the right side) (▶ Fig. 10.2).
- The mucosa investing the inferior concha retains its shape following dissection and does not conform well to the bone once it is transposed. It functions more as a vascular bridge for the mucosa of the lateral nasal wall or nasal floor/septum.
- Indocyanine green fluoroscopy is useful in assessing the vascularity of the flap at the time of reconstruction.[14] Postoperative MRI can also be used to assess the viability of the flap postoperatively (▶ Fig. 10.4).
- The reconstruction is supported with Gelfoam and Merocel tampons.

10.5.2 Extended Posterior LNWF

- With an extended flap, the flap incorporates the mucosa of the nasal floor.[4] An anterior incision runs across the nasal floor at the edge of the pyriform aperture. A medial incision is placed at the junction of the nasal floor and septum. Posteriorly, an incision runs transversely across the nasal floor at the posterior margin of the hard palate. It courses up the lateral nasal wall to the superior margin of the Eustachian tube, taking care to avoid injury to the vascular pedicle at the posterior attachment of the inferior turbinate (▶ Fig. 10.2b).
- When the flap is transposed, the nasal floor mucosa covers the superior aspect of the dural defect.
- ▶ Fig. 10.5 shows an anatomical dissection of the extended posterior LNWF for anterior cranial base reconstruction.

10.5.3 Extended Posterior LNWF with Nasal Septum

- The posterior LNWF may be further extended by including the mucosa of the nasal septum.[4] This is an option when the mucosa of the anterior septum is preserved but the posterior septal branches of the sphenopalatine artery are absent due to prior surgery or tumor involvement.
- Parallel vertical incisions are made on the nasal septum as extensions of the anterior and posterior nasal floor incisions. The superior incision is the same as an NSF, approximately 1 cm below the olfactory mucosa but including the superior septal mucosa anterior to the middle turbinate.

10.6 Postoperative Care

- Lumbar spinal drainage (approximately 10 mL/h) is used in high-risk patients for 3 days to decrease the risk of a postoperative CSF leak. Standard precautions include head of bed elevation and avoidance of strenuous activity and nose-blowing.
- There should be no passage of tubes through the nose (feeding tubes) unless it is performed with endoscopic visualization.
- Merocel tampons remain in the nasal cavity for up to 1 week. Antibiotic prophylaxis with a second-generation cephalosporin is maintained during that time.
- Frequent saline spray and lavage promote mucosalization of the exposed bone.
- Nasal endoscopy with removal of loose crusts is performed every few weeks until healing is complete (▶ Fig. 10.6).

10.7 Complications

- Due to the challenge of the reconstructions, the risk of a postoperative CSF leak is higher, especially for large clival defects that have already failed reconstruction with an NSF. In our experience, when the posterior LNWF was performed because an NSF was unavailable, the rate of postoperative CSF leak was 20% (2 out of 10 patients).[2] When the posterior LNWF was used in the setting of a postoperative CSF leak, the rate of postoperative CSF leak was 29% (4 out of 14 recurrent postoperative CSF leaks). Extended posterior LNWFs have been used in a minority of cases. Our initial experience included five cases (two with inclusion of the nasal septal mucosa) with only one postoperative CSF leak.[4]
- In our experience, most postoperative CSF leaks are solved with repositioning of the flap and augmentation with additional tissue (adipose tissue or fascia lata).
- An extracranial pericranial flap is an alternative reconstructive option when local flaps have failed.[15]
- Postoperative contrast-enhanced MRI, when available, showed posterior LNWF enhancement in 91.3% of cases (21 out of 23).[2] There were no instances of flap necrosis. Mobilization of the flap pedicle may increase the risk of flap necrosis.
- Postoperative epiphora may occur due to scarring of the nasolacrimal duct. This can be avoided by sharp transection of the duct without the use of electrocautery. We have not found it necessary to place lacrimal stents routinely.
- The exposed bone of the lateral nasal wall and nasal floor mucosalizes very well after a period of nasal crusting that may last several months. We have not observed long-term nasal morbidity such as empty nose syndrome related to this.

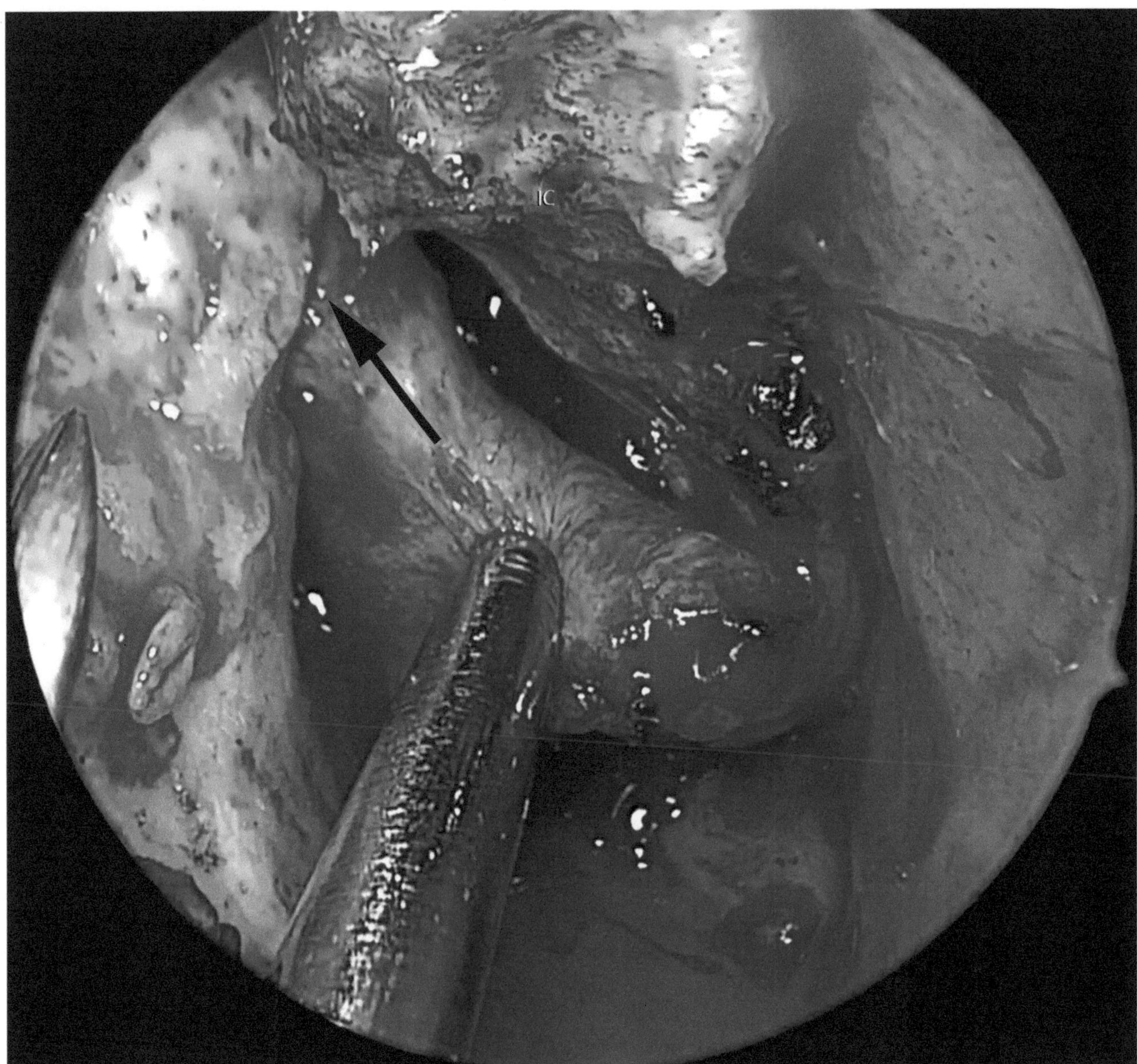

Fig. 10.3 Dissection of right posterior-based lateral nasal wall flap from the inferior concha (IC). The nasolacrimal duct (*arrow*) is exposed in the canal and transected sharply to prevent stenosis.

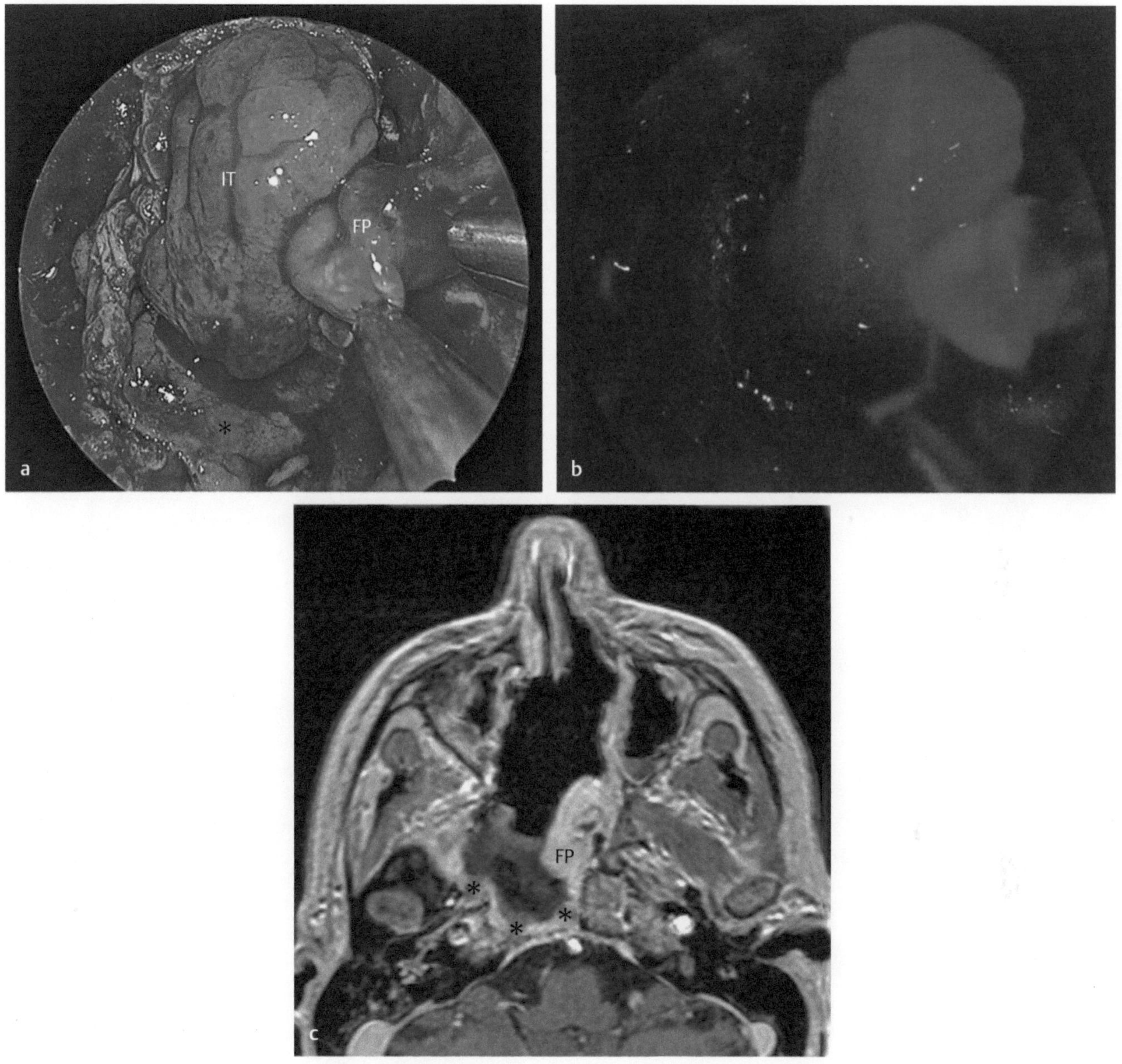

Fig. 10.4 (a, b) Intraoperative endoscopic view of a left posterior-based lateral nasal wall flap (posterior LNWF). (a) Flap covering a clival defect before indocyanine green (ICG) fluoroscopy and (b) during ICG fluoroscopy. Note excellent vascularity of the flap pedicle (FP) and inferior turbinate (IT). The distal portion of the flap (*asterisk*) has delayed uptake. (c) Postoperative magnetic resonance imaging (MRI) confirms viability of a left-sided posterior LNWF. FP, flap pedicle including inferior turbinate (IT); *asterisks*, distal flap mucosa. (a and b—Reproduced with permission from Lavigne et al[10].)

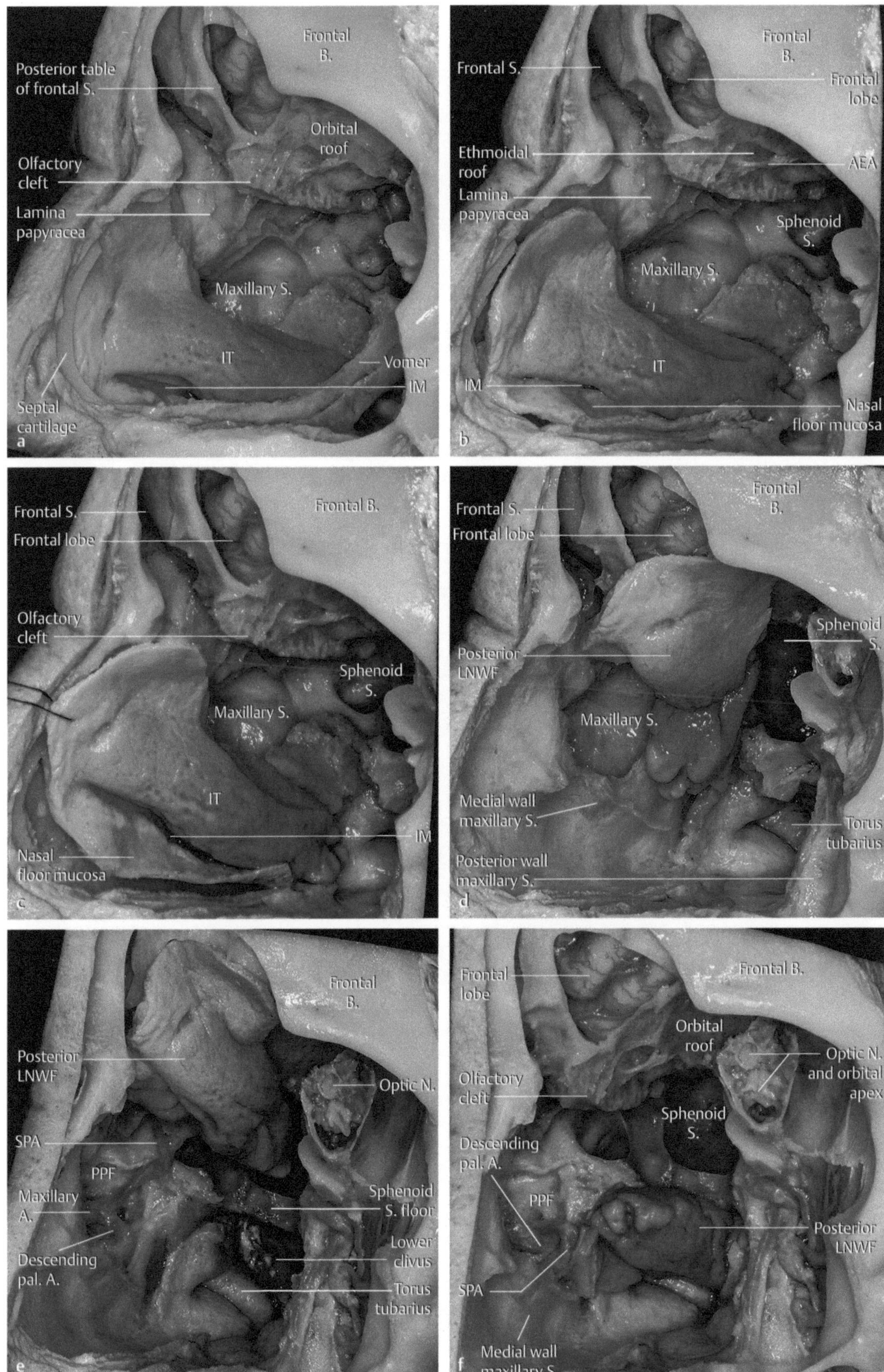

Fig. 10.5 Anatomical dissection after removal of the left hemiface, orbital contents, and exposure of the nasal cavity. **(a)** Right lateral nasal wall. **(b)** After the incisions for the extended posterior-based lateral nasal wall flap. Note the inclusion of the nasal floor mucosa to the flap. **(c)** Elevation of the flap in a subperiosteal plane. **(d)** Clockwise rotation of the flap toward the anterior cranial base. Observe the broad pedicle of the flap. **(e)** Similar to the nasoseptal flap, a pedicle release to free the maxillary artery can be performed to increase the reach of the flap. In this picture, the flap was mobilized anteriorly to cover a defect of the posterior table of the frontal sinus. **(f)** Counterclockwise rotation of the flap for clival reconstruction. A, artery; AEA, anterior ethmoidal artery; B, bone; IM, inferior meatus; IT, inferior turbinate; LNWF, lateral nasal wall flap; N, nerve; pal., palatine; PPF, pterygopalatine fossa; S, sinus; SPA, sphenopalatine artery.

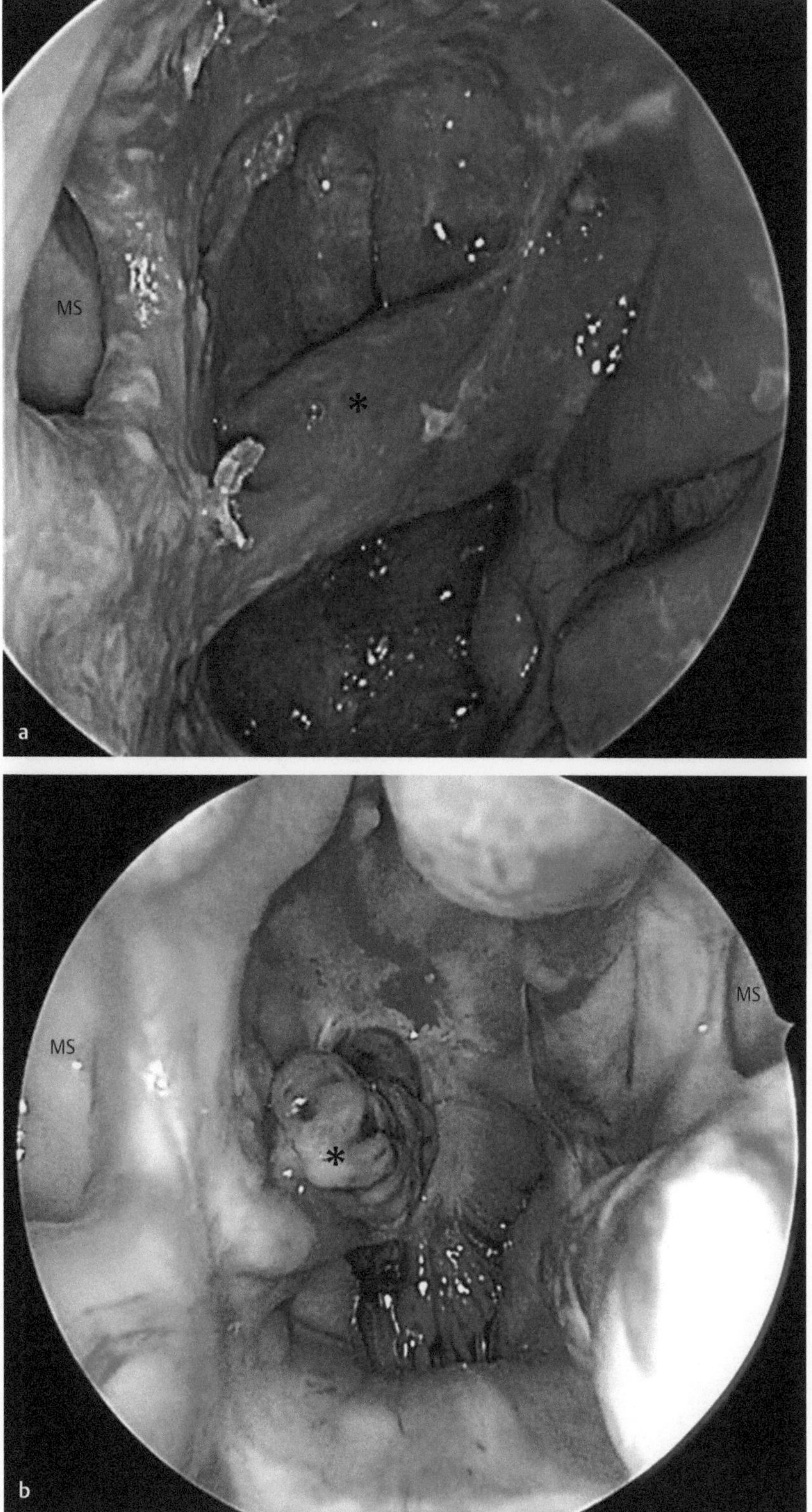

Fig. 10.6 Endoscopic view of a postoperative posterior-based lateral nasal wall flap (posterior LNWF) reconstruction of (a) suprasellar defect; (b) posterior fossa defect. *Asterisk*: posterior LNWF pedicle. MS, maxillary sinus. (Reproduced with permission from Lavigne et al.[10])

References

[1] Hadad G, Bassagasteguy L, Carrau RL, et al. A novel reconstructive technique after endoscopic expanded endonasal approaches: vascular pedicle nasoseptal flap. Laryngoscope. 2006; 116(10):1882–1886

[2] Harvey RJ, Parmar P, Sacks R, Zanation AM. Endoscopic skull base reconstruction of large dural defects: a systematic review of published evidence. Laryngoscope. 2012; 122(2):452–459

[3] Patel MR, Taylor RJ, Hackman TG, et al. Beyond the nasoseptal flap: outcomes and pearls with secondary flaps in endoscopic endonasal skull base reconstruction. Laryngoscope. 2014; 124(4):846–852

[4] Fortes FS, Carrau RL, Snyderman CH, et al. The posterior pedicle inferior turbinate flap: a new vascularized flap for skull base reconstruction. Laryngoscope. 2007; 117(8):1329–1332

[5] Harvey RJ, Sheahan PO, Schlosser RJ. Inferior turbinate pedicle flap for endoscopic skull base defect repair. Am J Rhinol Allergy. 2009; 23(5):522–526

[6] Rivera-Serrano CM, Bassagaisteguy LH, Hadad G, et al. Posterior pedicle lateral nasal wall flap: new reconstructive technique for large defects of the skull base. Am J Rhinol Allergy. 2011; 25(6):e212–e216

[7] Suh JD, Chiu AG. Sphenopalatine-derived pedicled flaps. Adv Otorhinolaryngol. 2013; 74:56–63

[8] MacArthur FJD, McGarry GW. The arterial supply of the nasal cavity. Eur Arch Otorhinolaryngol. 2017; 274(2):809–815

[9] Chabot JD, Patel CR, Hughes MA, et al. Nasoseptal flap necrosis: a rare complication of endoscopic endonasal surgery. J Neurosurg. 2018; 128(5): 1463–1472

[10] Lavigne P, Vega MB, Ahmed OH, Gardner PA, Snyderman CH, Wang EW. Lateral nasal wall flap for endoscopic reconstruction of the skull base: anatomical study and clinical series. Int Forum Allergy Rhinol. 2020; 10(5):673–678

[11] Snyderman CH. Inferior turbinate flap. In: Snyderman CH, Gardner PA, eds. Master techniques in otolaryngology-head and neck surgery: skull base surgery volume. Philadelphia, PA: Wolters Kluwer; 2015:429–426

[12] Choby GW, Pinheiro-Neto CD, de Almeida JR, et al. Extended inferior turbinate flap for endoscopic reconstruction of skull base defects. J Neurol Surg B Skull Base. 2014; 75(4):225–230

[13] Wu P, Li Z, Liu C, Ouyang J, Zhong S. The posterior pedicled inferior turbinate-nasoseptal flap: a potential combined flap for skull base reconstruction. Surg Radiol Anat. 2016; 38(2):187–194

[14] Gode S, Lieber S, Nakassa ACI, et al. Clinical experience with secondary endoscopic reconstruction of clival defects with extracranial pericranial flaps. J Neurol Surg B Skull Base. 2019; 80(3):276–282

[15] Geltzeiler M, Nakassa ACI, Turner M, et al. Evaluation of intranasal flap perfusion by intraoperative indocyanine green fluorescence angiography. Oper Neurosurg (Hagerstown). 2018; 15(6):672–676

11 Anterior-Based Lateral Nasal Wall Flaps

Carlos D. Pinheiro-Neto, Luciano C. P. C. Leonel, and Maria Peris-Celda

11.1 Anatomy

- The main blood supply to the lateral nasal wall posteriorly is provided by the posterior lateral nasal artery (PLNA), which is a branch of the sphenopalatine artery.[1]
- The PLNA bifurcates in inferior turbinate (IT) and middle turbinate arteries. The inferior turbinate branch is the main pedicle for the posterior-based lateral nasal wall flap (posterior LNWF).
- Anteriorly, the lateral nasal wall is supplied by the anterior lateral nasal artery (branch of the facial artery) and the lateral branch of the anterior ethmoidal artery.[2]
- The IT artery increases in diameter as it travels anteriorly, suggesting an important contribution from the anterior circulation to the vascularization of the IT.[3] The anterior-based lateral nasal wall flap (anterior LNWF) is based upon this anterior vascularization to the IT and lateral nasal wall.
- Transecting the IT in the coronal plane, three layers are noticeable: Medial (nasal) mucosal layer, lateral (meatal) mucosal layer, and a central osseous layer.[4]
- The bone of the IT is usually cancellous and accommodates most of the blood supply to the turbinate in its trabecular system.[5]
- The IT bone is thicker anteriorly and is absent along the inferior border and tail of the IT.[6]
- The nasolacrimal duct opening (Hasner valve) is a mucous fold within the anterior part of the inferior meatus, close to the attachment of the head of the IT.

11.2 Fundamentals

- The main anatomical structure present in this flap is the IT.
- Similar to the posterior LNWF, the anterior flap is tailored according to the size of the defect.
- The mucosa of the inferior meatus/nasal floor and also the septal mucosa, if available, can be included to increase the reconstructive area of the flap.
- The nasolacrimal duct should be exposed and sharply transected for the vast majority of anterior LNWF. In some cases of smaller skull base defects, a flap can be harvested from the medial surface of the IT or with incisions within the inferior meatus avoiding the region of the Hasner valve.
- The pedicle area of the flap is broad and corresponds to the mucosa that covers the ascending process of the maxilla, which is the area anterior to the middle turbinate.
- The mucosa of the region of the pedicle is elevated superiorly toward the nasal dorsum, between the ascending process of the maxilla and the septum to improve its rotation.
- In cases of cranialization of the frontal sinuses, the endonasal reconstruction is more complex as the posterior table of the frontal sinuses are completely removed and a large column of cerebrospinal fluid (CSF) forms anteriorly where frontal sinuses were located. To reinforce the reconstruction against this column of CSF pressure, the anterior LNWF may be an interesting option.

11.3 Indications

- The flap can be an option in cases of anterior cranial base defects, when the nasoseptal flap or the posterior LNWF are not available, especially when the defect is very anterior.[7]
- In cases of cranialization of the frontal sinus, this flap helps to seal the area corresponding to the frontal sinus recesses.
- In cases of obliteration of the frontal sinus, this flap can be used to seal the endonasal surface.

11.4 Limitations

- The complete removal of IT bone is technically challenging. It is preferable to leave small pieces of thin bone attached to the flap instead of risking mucosal lacerations with the complete bone removal.
- Severe bleeding during the elevation of the IT mucosa can occur.
- The transection of the nasolacrimal duct leaves an opening in the flap. This can be sutured or plugged with a fat/muscle graft. If possible, avoid opposing the opening toward the dural defect.
- Because of the broad pedicle and narrow area at the nasal dorsum, the rotation of the flap leaves a bulky tissue in the region of the pedicle.
- If the frontal sinus is not cranialized or obliterated, the flap may block the frontal sinus outflow.

11.5 Surgical Technique (*Video 11.1*)

11.5.1 Harvest

- Using a needle tip Bovie set at 10 W, an anterior incision is performed along the piriform aperture, anterior to the head of the IT.
- If the nasal floor mucosa is added to the flap, the anterior incision is progressed toward the septum. If available, the septal mucosa can also be added to the flap.
- A superior incision is performed along the anterior border of the uncinate process from superior to inferior. Then, the incision is progressed posteriorly along the posterior fontanelle toward the tail of the IT. If an uncinectomy and maxillary antrostomy were performed, most of the superior incision is completed with those procedures.
- The inferior incision can be performed at different levels depending upon the size of the flap desired:
  - Inferior border of the IT and inclusion of only the medial (nasal) surface of the turbinate. In this case, the IT is split in the sagittal plane and only its medial surface is elevated. A blunt dissector is used to elevate the medial surface of the IT from the underlying bone. Since the bone is absent in the inferior border and tail of the turbinate, endoscopic scissors are used to divide the IT in the sagittal plane in those areas. The IT bone and meatal surface are left attached to the lateral wall, keeping the inferior meatus, Hasner valve, and nasolacrimal duct intact (▸ Fig. 11.1).

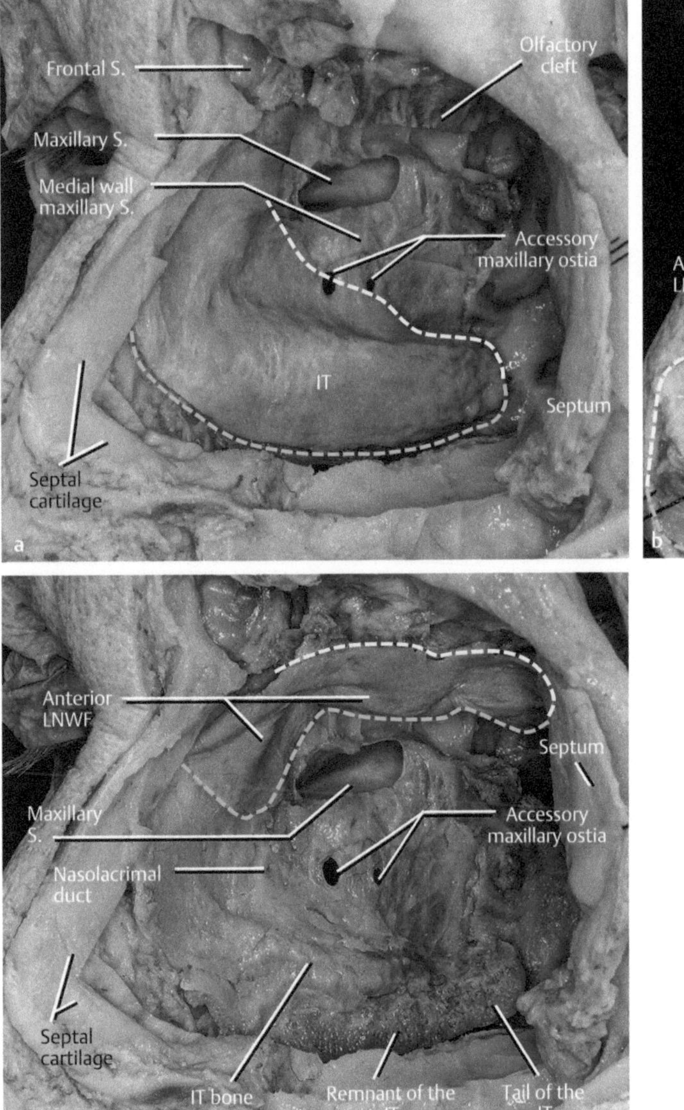

Fig. 11.1 Anatomical dissection after removal of the left hemiface, orbital contents, and exposure of the nasal cavity. **(a)** Right lateral nasal wall after maxillary antrostomy, complete ethmoidectomy, sphenoidotomy, and middle turbinectomy. Incisions to harvest an anterior-based lateral nasal wall flap (anterior LNWF) with inclusion of the medial (nasal) surface of the inferior turbinate (IT). *Blue dashed line*—anterior incision. *Yellow dashed line*—superior incision. *Green dashed line*—inferior incision along the inferior border of the IT. **(b)** Elevation of the flap with exposure of its subperiosteal surface. The IT bone, meatal (lateral) mucosa of the IT, and nasolacrimal duct are preserved. Note that there is no bone along the inferior border and tail of the IT. At those areas, the mucosal incision between the nasal surface and the lateral surface of the IT is performed sharply with endoscopic scissors. **(c)** Counterclockwise rotation of the right-sided flap to cover the anterior cranial base.
IT, inferior turbinate; LNWF, lateral nasal wall flap; S, sinus.

   - Inferior incision along the inferior meatus/nasal floor/ septum. In these cases, the IT is opened like a "book" to increase the reconstructive surface. It is important to elevate the mucosa from the turbinate before detaching it from the lateral wall to keep the turbinate stable during the mucosal elevation. Removal of the IT bone is laborious and is achieved with a combination of Cottle dissector, Kerrison rongeurs, and thru-cut forceps. Since there is no bone at the tail of the turbinate, this region should be incorporated to the flap as it is. The nasolacrimal duct should be sharply transected (▶ Fig. 11.2).
- In some cases, the inferior incision can also be designed to exclude the Hasner valve from the flap. However, the resultant shape and size of the flap are compromised.
- The superior and inferior incisions are united posteriorly along the tail of the IT.
- After the three incisions are completed, the mucosa is elevated from the lateral nasal wall starting from the anterior incision (piriform aperture) in a subperiosteal plane with elevation of the medial surface of the IT until identification of the superior incision.
- The IT bone is carefully removed with exposure of the mucoperiosteum of the meatal surface. At this region, the mucosal layer is very thin and careful dissection is required to avoid laceration.
- Anteriorly, the meatal mucosa of the IT is continuous with the nasolacrimal duct. Kerrison rongeurs are used to expose the nasolacrimal duct superiorly. Then, the transection of the nasolacrimal duct is performed below the lacrimal sac.
- The inferior meatus mucosa is elevated until the inferior incision of the flap is reached. The transition between the IT and the mucosa of the lateral wall of the inferior meatus is an area of high risk for laceration due to the sharp angle and thin mucosa between these two areas.
- Finally, the mucosa over the ascending process of the maxilla should be elevated toward the nasal dorsum in order to facilitate the rotation of the flap.

11.5.2 Reconstruction

- If the frontal sinus is not obliterated or cranialized, a Draf III frontal sinusotomy is recommended to allow drainage through the contralateral side.
- The usual rotation of the flap is clockwise for left-sided flap or counterclockwise for right-sided flap. In both cases, the posterior part of the flap is moved superiorly toward the anterior cranial base (▶ Fig. 11.1c and ▶ Fig. 11.2c).
- After the placement of the flap, pieces of oxidized cellulose are applied to its borders, followed by dural sealant and absorbable packing. Nonabsorbable packing is usually placed after the absorbable one, particularly for large and very anterior cranial base defects. Nasal splints are placed to prevent postoperative synechiae.
- ▶ Fig. 11.3 shows a surgical example of an anterior LNWF.

11.6 Postoperative Care

- Postoperative visits 1 week, 1 month, and 4 months after surgery for nasal debridement.
- During the first postoperative visit (1 week after surgery), the nasal splints are removed and the debridement is performed mostly to improve nasal breathing. The absorbable packing and crusting around the flap are not removed.
- Large-volume saline nasal irrigation is used during the first month to help with the removal of the absorbable packing and dural sealant.
- During the second postoperative visit (1 month after the surgery), the nasal debridement is performed next to the reconstruction area and the flap is visualized.
- During the following 3 months, large-volume saline irrigation is used as needed. The patient comes to the clinic for the third postoperative visit (4 months after the surgery) for final assessment of the healing. After that, the follow-up is scheduled accordingly to the baseline disease or if patient has any issue with nasal crusting or sinusitis.

11.7 Complications

- Transection of the nasolacrimal duct carries the risk of epiphora. The patient may need endoscopic dacryocystorhinostomy if symptomatic.
- Chronic nasal crusting and potential risk of atrophic rhinitis with the complete resection of the IT.
- Chronic frontal sinusitis due to blockage of the frontal sinus by the pedicle of the flap.
- Inadvertent opening of the inferior meatus lateral wall can lead to a fistula to the maxillary sinus and chronic maxillary sinusitis due to recirculation of mucus.[8]
- Injury to the greater palatine nerve during the flap elevation next to the tail of the IT can cause palatal and maxillary teeth numbness.
- Injury to the sphenopalatine artery can lead to severe bleeding.

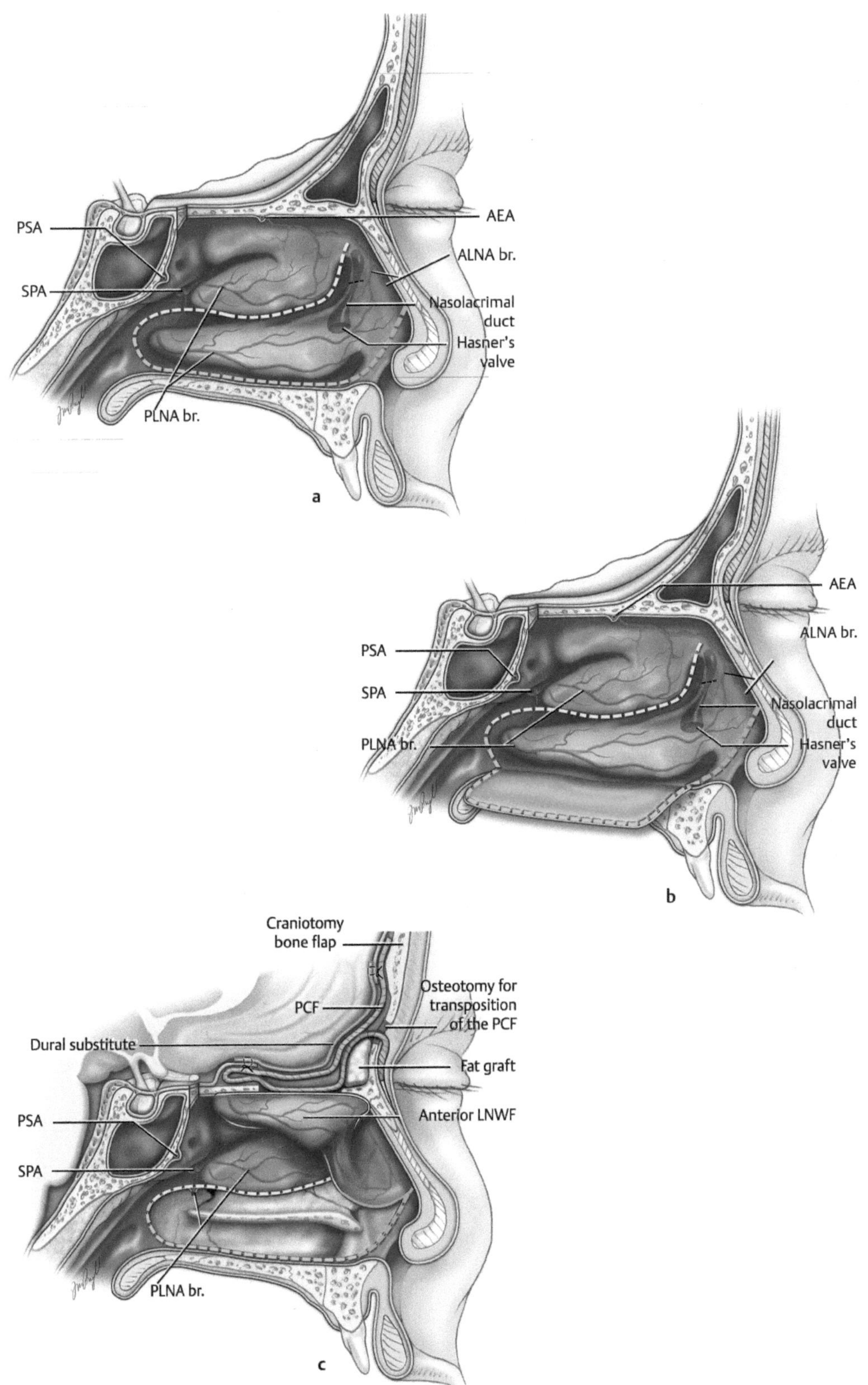

Fig. 11.2 Illustration of the left nasal cavity sagittal view. **(a)** Incisions to harvest an anterior-based lateral nasal wall flap (anterior LNWF). *Blue dashed line*—anterior incision. *Yellow dashed line*—superior incision. *Green dashed line*—inferior incision along the transition between the inferior meatus lateral wall and nasal floor. **(b)** Anterior LNWF with inclusion of mucosa of the nasal floor. *Green dashed line*—inferior incision along the transition between the septum and nasal floor. In both cases, the inferior turbinate (IT) is opened like a "book" to increase its reconstructive surface. It also requires transection of the nasolacrimal duct to fully elevate the mucoperiosteum of the lateral wall. **(c)** Flap inset to reinforce the anterior border of the cranial base reconstruction after a combined endoscopic endonasal approach and bifrontal craniotomy with cranialization of the frontal sinus. The cranialization of the frontal sinus increases the cerebrospinal fluid (CSF) pressure at the anterior border of the defect, particularly in combined approaches with removal of the frontal sinus floor. AEA, anterior ethmoidal artery; ALNA, anterior lateral nasal artery; br., branch; LNWF, lateral nasal wall flap; PCF, pericranial flap; PLNA, posterior lateral nasal artery; PSA, posterior septal artery; SPA, sphenopalatine artery.

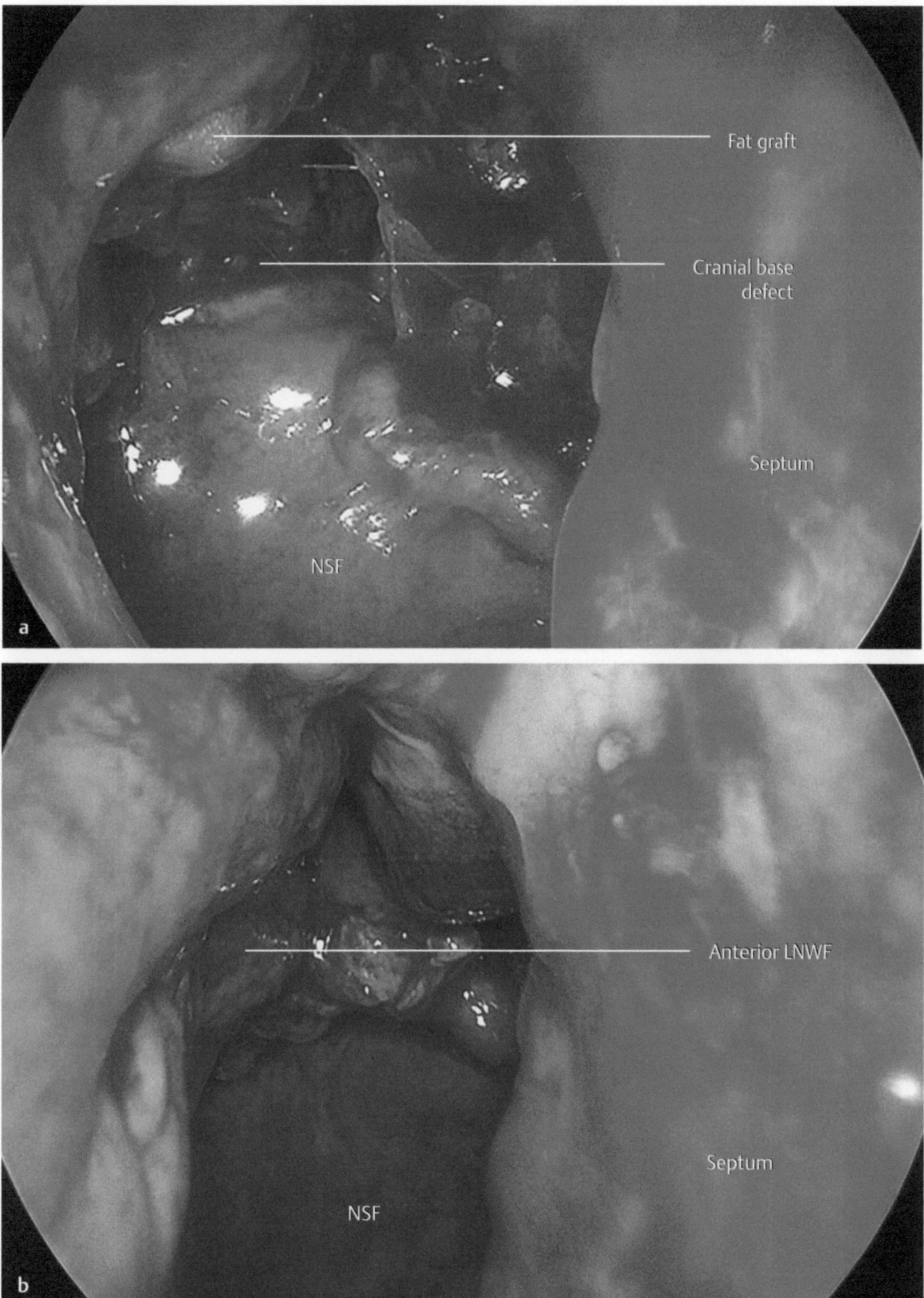

Fig. 11.3 Clinical case of a patient who had a combined endoscopic endonasal approach and bifrontal craniotomy for a large anterior cranial base meningioma. Cranialization of the frontal sinus was performed due to tumor involvement of the sinus. Initially, a nasoseptal flap (NSF) was used for the endonasal reconstruction and a pericranial flap for the intracranial reconstruction. The patient presented with a postoperative cerebrospinal fluid (CSF) leak 2 weeks after the surgery after blowing the nose. **(a, b)** Intraoperative pictures obtained with a 45-degree endoscope in the right nasal cavity during the CSF leak repair. **(a)** Note that the NSF contracted, exposing the fat graft that was originally placed intracranially filling the space where the frontal sinus floor was located. **(b)** This very anterior defect was reconstructed with an anterior-based lateral nasal wall flap. Only the nasal surface of the inferior turbinate was used in this case.
LNWF, lateral nasal wall flap; NSF, nasoseptal flap.

References

[1] Fortes FS, Carrau RL, Snyderman CH, et al. The posterior pedicle inferior turbinate flap: a new vascularized flap for skull base reconstruction. Laryngoscope. 2007; 117(8):1329–1332

[2] MacArthur FJ, McGarry GW. The arterial supply of the nasal cavity. Eur Arch Otorhinolaryngol. 2017; 274(2):809–815

[3] Murakami CS, Kriet JD, Ierokomos AP. Nasal reconstruction using the inferior turbinate mucosal flap. Arch Facial Plast Surg. 1999; 1(2):97–100

[4] Gindros G, Kantas I, Balatsouras DG, Kandiloros D, Manthos AK, Kaidoglou A. Mucosal changes in chronic hypertrophic rhinitis after surgical turbinate reduction. Eur Arch Otorhinolaryngol. 2009; 266(9):1409–1416

[5] Sahin-Yilmaz A, Naclerio RM. Anatomy and physiology of the upper airway. Proc Am Thorac Soc. 2011; 8(1):31–39

[6] El-Anwar MW, Hamed AA, Abdulmonaem G, Elnashar I, Elfiki IM. Computed tomography measurement of inferior turbinate in asymptomatic adult. Int Arch Otorhinolaryngol. 2017; 21(4):366–370

[7] Hadad G, Rivera-Serrano CM, Bassagaisteguy LH, et al. Anterior pedicle lateral nasal wall flap: a novel technique for the reconstruction of anterior skull base defects. Laryngoscope. 2011; 121(8):1606–1610

[8] Matthews BL, Burke AJ. Recirculation of mucus via accessory ostia causing chronic maxillary sinus disease. Otolaryngol Head Neck Surg. 1997; 117 (4):422–423

Section IV

Extranasal Flaps

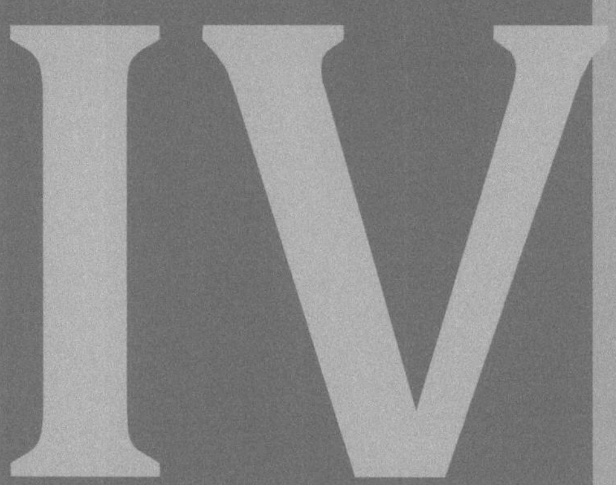

12 Pericranial Flap

Laura Salgado-Lopez, Maria Peris-Celda, and Carlos D. Pinheiro-Neto

12.1 Anatomy

- From superficial to deep, the layers of the scalp are: Skin, subcutaneous layer, aponeurotic layer (includes the temporoparietal fascia laterally, the galea superiorly with the frontalis muscle anteriorly, and the occipitalis muscle posteriorly), subaponeurotic layer (loose areolar tissue), and periosteal layer (contiguous with the temporal fascia)[1,2] (see Fig. 13.1 in Chapter 13).
- The "pericranium" is a surgical term defined as a combination of the subaponeurotic and periosteal scalp layers located between the superior temporal lines.[1,2]
- The anteriorly based frontal pericranial flap (PCF) is usually pedicled on the ipsilateral supraorbital and supratrochlear neurovascular bundles.[3]
- The supratrochlear and supraorbital nerves are two cutaneous branches of the ophthalmic division of the trigeminal nerve. The supraorbital nerve innervates the skin and conjunctiva of the upper eyelid and most scalp areas in the forehead, with some branches extending posteriorly to innervate the vertex and a small area of the parietal scalp. The supratrochlear nerve innervates the skin and conjunctiva of the upper eyelid and the skin of the lower forehead.[4]
- While the supraorbital nerve also divides into two to four superficial and deep branches near the orbital rim, usually following a parallel trajectory to the branches of the supraorbital artery, the supratrochlear nerve usually gives only one superficial branch after emerging onto the forehead that follows the supratrochlear artery.[4]
- The supraorbital and supratrochlear arteries are both terminal branches of the ophthalmic artery, which branches from the supraclinoid segment of the internal carotid artery as it emerges from the roof of the cavernous sinus.[3]
- The main trunk of the supraorbital and supratrochlear arteries course below the orbital roof and divide near or above the supraorbital rim into superficial and deep branches. The superficial branches run in the aponeurotic layer of the scalp, and the deep branches ascend in and supply the pericranium in an axial pattern.[1,3]
- Overall, the deep branches of the supraorbital artery comprise the major supply of a PCF and arise at the level of supraorbital rim (80%), but they can also arise within the aponeurotic layer and cross to the pericranium 5.5 to 15 mm (mean, 8.5 mm) above the supraorbital rim (20%).[3]
- The supraorbital artery and nerve leave the orbit passing around the free edge of the supraorbital rim or through the supraorbital notch or foramen, which is located approximately 22.2 mm from the midline.[3]
- The supratrochlear artery is smaller than the supraorbital artery, and it exits the orbit along with the supratrochlear nerve approximately 10.6 mm medial to the supraorbital notch through the frontal notch or foramen to enter the corrugator muscle at the level of the supraorbital rim.[4]
- The lateral pericranium also receives blood supply from the frontal branch of the superficial temporal artery, a terminal branch of the external carotid artery.[1,3]
- Both the supraorbital and supratrochlear arteries anastomose with each other and in some cases laterally along the superior temporal line with deep branches of the superficial temporal artery, forming anastomosis between the internal and external carotid arterial systems.[1]
- Both the deep veins from the pericranium and the superficial veins from the aponeurotic layer drain into the transverse portion of the supraorbital vein that courses between both layers near or above the supraorbital rim and joins the frontal vein at the medial angle of the orbit to form the angular vein.[3]
- The frontal branch of the facial nerve lies immediately underneath (or sometimes within) the temporoparietal fascia above the zygomatic arch and superficial to the superficial layer of the deep temporalis fascia.[1,2]

12.2 Fundamentals

- The PCF offers a reconstructive alternative to intranasal flaps, and it has been used extensively for anterior skull base and craniofacial reconstruction.[2,5,6]
- The PCF can be harvested by a traditional coronal incision or endoscopically and turned inward to separate the intracranial contents from the sinonasal cavity through a supranasion frontal osteotomy.[7,8]
- The advantage of harvesting the PCF endoscopically is less donor site morbidity, with a reduced scalp incision and minimal scalp edema and pain. However, the coronal incision may be more cosmetically appealing than a glabellar incision for some patients.[8]
- Preoperative computed tomography (CT) scan analysis may help to determine the size of the PCF required and facilitate incision planning, especially in minimally invasive endoscopic cases. Some of the initial length of the PCF is lost due to tissue contracture and surgical rotation of the flap; so, adding an additional 20 to 30 mm to the anticipated length is recommended.[8]
- The PCF can be harvested as a single flap pedicled on the ipsilateral supraorbital and supratrochlear bundles, or as two different flaps separated along the midsagittal plane, each of them based on its ipsilateral neurovascular bundles.[1,9,10]
- A broad PCF can also be harvested from one superficial temporal line to the other, pedicled bilaterally upon the supraorbital and supratrochlear arteries. This design is more commonly used in open craniotomy and combined approaches.
- When a unilateral PCF is selected, at least a 30 mm wide pedicle at the orbital rim is recommended, and the medial limit of the flap should not extend lateral to midline to avoid compromising the contralateral vessels for future salvage operations.[1,5,9]
- The PCF harvest can be extended posteriorly to the coronal incision using scalp retractors to achieve a length that will reach the middle and posterior skull base.[9]
- To preserve the arterial and venous supply of the PCF, care must be taken to not separate the aponeurotic layer from the pericranium closer than 10 mm of the orbital rim.[3]

- The PCF is easier to dissect than the temporoparietal fascia flap, it is closer to the anterior skull base and more suited for anterior skull base defects, and its transposition does not require transpterygoid dissection.[11]
- Because the PCF is a nonmucosal flap, it tends to form more crusting in the postoperative period compared to intranasal mucosal flaps. Nonmucosal flaps require a longer healing period for mucosalization of its endonasal surface, and the crusting is usually more adherent to the flap. In cases of complex reconstruction and combined approaches, the PCF can be inset intracranially and a nasoseptal flap can be used to resurface the endonasal surface of the PCF. This will improve the strength of the reconstruction, help with the mucosalization process, and decrease nasal crusting postoperatively.

12.3 Indications

- The PCF is a size-versatile flap ideal for anterior skull base defects that are too large for intranasal flaps or they are not available.[6,12]
- Skull base reconstruction from the frontal sinus to the upper one-third of the clivus after transcribiform, transsellar, and some transclival resections.[8]
- Large anterior skull base defects when intranasal pedicled flaps are not available because either they have been compromised, harvested in a previous surgery, and cannot be reused, or the tissue of the potential intranasal flaps is affected by neoplastic involvement.[8]
- Large skull base defects that require multiple flaps, such as defects that extend from the anterior skull base to the clivus.[1]
- When a combination of open and endoscopic approaches is needed, a PCF can be used inlay for the intracranial reconstruction and a nasoseptal flap used onlay to cover the endonasal surface of the PCF.[1]

12.4 Limitations

- Need for external incisions with the consequent morbidity and esthetical repercussion.
- Scalp numbness posterior to the incision.
- Previous radiation to the donor site.[9]
- Craniofacial trauma, particularly orbital rim fractures, or previous open cranial surgery may compromise the blood supply of the PCF (such as the subfrontal or supraorbital approaches). Preoperative Doppler assessment of the intended flap pedicle can be useful to address the patency of the vessels in these cases.[1,6]
- The posterior reach of the PCF is the sella/upper third of the clivus.[12] Middle or inferior clival or spinal defects overextend the limits of the PCF vasculature. For posterior fossa defects that require regional vascularized flaps, the temporoparietal fascia flap is a more suitable option.[11]

12.5 Surgical Technique

12.5.1 Pericranial Flap Harvest via Coronal Approach

- A scalp incision is performed from one preauricular region to the other, starting 1 to 2 cm posterior to the coronal suture and extending it first lateroinferiorly to the temporal line on both sides. Special care must be taken to avoid division of the underlying pericranium.
- Placing the scalp incision at that level maximizes the length of the PCF while providing a superior cosmetic outcome and avoids injury to the anterior branches of the superficial temporal artery. The pericranium incision can be placed posterior to the skin incision line, depending on the size of the defect to cover.
- The incision is then continued from the temporal line to the superficial layer of the deep temporal fascia into the preauricular region bilaterally.
- Hemostasis of the scalp can be achieved preferentially with Rainey clips to avoid excessive cauterization and injury to the hair follicles, although bipolar electrocautery may be necessary in some cases.
- Once the coronal incision has been made, the plane between the aponeurotic and the subaponeurotic layers is identified. Inclusion of the subaponeurotic layer (loose areolar tissue) in the PCF makes the flap more robust.
- The scalp is elevated separating the galea from the pericranium with scissors from posterior to anterior between the two superior temporal lines. Laterally at the preauricular region, the temporoparietal fascia is elevated from the superficial layer of the deep temporal fascia.
- The frontal branch of the facial nerve is preserved by performing an interfascial dissection. About 2 cm from the orbital rim, an incision parallel to the course of the frontal branch is performed in the superficial layer of the deep temporal fascia. This exposes the superficial temporal fat pad and the dissection is safely carried anteriorly in this plane between the two layers of the deep temporal fascia. The nerve courses superficially to the superficial layer of the deep temporal fascia.
- Anteriorly, the scalp should be separated from the underlying PCF toward the supraorbital rims only as far as needed to obtain adequate length of the flap and stopped at least 10 mm closer to the orbital rim. Separation of the PCF from the galea-frontalis muscle near the supraorbital rim should be done with caution to avoid damage to the supratrochlear and supraorbital neurovascular bundles, their anastomosis, as well as to the transverse supraorbital vein.
- The coronal flap is then reflected and secured anteriorly with scalp retraction hooks.
- If additional length of the PCF is needed, the scalp posterior to the coronal incision can be elevated in the subgaleal plane exposing further pericranium.
- The pericranium is then incised starting laterally along the ipsilateral temporal line, separating the periosteum from the margin of the deep temporal fascia. A second pericranial incision can be carried medially in a parallel manner, creating at least a flap with a 30 mm wide base. A third incision is made posteriorly to join the posterior edge of the previous two pericranial incisions (▶ Fig. 12.1a).
- The PCF is dissected and elevated with a blunt dissector from posterior to anterior, being careful not to perforate the flap. Special care must be taken to prevent damage of the supraorbital and supratrochlear pedicles as they exit the orbit through their respective foramen/notch or around the orbital rim. If there is a complete supraorbital foramen, the supraorbital neurovascular pedicle may be released performing an

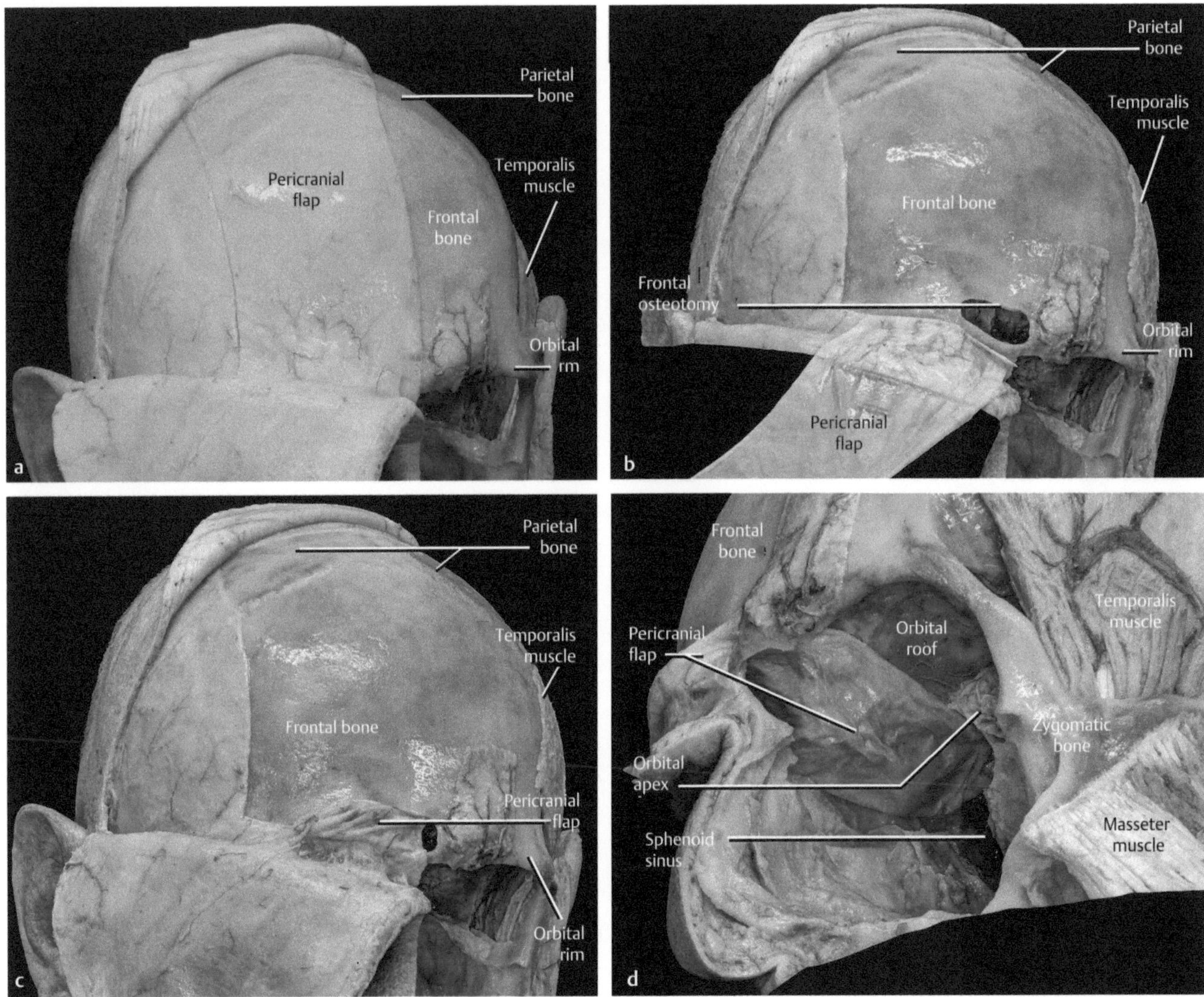

Fig. 12.1 Anatomical dissection after a coronal approach and removal of the left hemiface and orbital contents. **(a)** Right pericranial flap (PCF). The left pericranium was removed. **(b)** Supranasion frontal osteotomy for transposition of the PCF to the nasal cavity. **(c)** Frontal view of the flap transposition. **(d)** PCF inset onlay along the anterior cranial base. B, bone; M, muscle; PCF, pericranial flap; S, sinus.

inverted-V osteotomy with a 3 mm osteotome to avoid inadvertent traction injury to the pedicle (▶ Fig. 12.1b).

- The PCF is then reflected forward over the coronal scalp flap and covered with a wet gauze until it is needed (▶ Fig. 12.2a).
- An 8 × 20 mm frontal osteotomy is performed just above the nasion with a 3 mm high-speed drill, communicating the frontonasal area with the endonasal resection site (▶ Fig. 12.1b and ▶ Fig. 12.2a).
- An endoscopic Draf III frontal sinusotomy can be performed at this point if it was not done before to preserve the frontal sinus drainage and to prevent frontal sinus mucocele postoperatively (▶ Fig. 12.3a).
- The PCF is carefully transposed through the supranasion frontal osteotomy into the nasal cavity avoiding rotation of the neurovascular pedicle (▶ Fig. 12.1c). The superficial surface of the pericranium that was facing the scalp is placed against the defect, while the deeper surface which was in contact with the skull forms the endonasal surface of the flap.
- Synthetic dural substitute or fascia lata is used inlay to cover the defect (▶ Fig. 12.2b and ▶ Fig. 12.3b).
- Then, the PCF is applied covering the bone edges of the skull base defect and flattened to avoid dead space in an extradural extracranial onlay manner (▶ Fig. 12.1d, ▶ Fig. 12.2b, and ▶ Fig. 12.3b).
- Pieces of oxidized cellulose are placed on the edges of the PCF followed by dural sealant.
- Absorbable nasal packing is placed to support the PCF in place and fill the superior aspect of the nasal cavity. Then nonabsorbable expandable packing is used along the floor of the nasal cavity in each side.
- A suction drain is placed subcutaneously and the coronal incision is closed in a multilayered fashion after thorough hemostasis is achieved.

12.5.2 Pericranial Flap Harvest via Endoscopic Approach

- Preoperative CT scan analysis may guide incision planning to maximize optimal flap length.[8]
- The trajectory of the ipsilateral supraorbital and supratrochlear arteries at the orbital rim can be assessed by Doppler and marked with a marking pen.
- A unilateral 4 to 5 cm coronal incision is performed just behind the hairline between the midsagittal plane and superior temporal line.
- Dissection of the aponeurotic layer from the underlying pericranium can be done endoscopically from posterior to anterior to the level of the orbital rim using scalp retractors.
- The dissection is continued posteriorly to incision to maximize the length of the PCF.
- The pericranium is then incised in the same manner as the open procedure using a needle tip cautery with a bended tip under direct endoscopic visualization.
- The PCF is then elevated from the cranium from posterior to anterior.
- A 10 mm horizontal glabellar incision is made in a skin crease and dissected down with a needle tip cautery to expose the frontal bone. A subperiosteal dissection is then carried inferiorly toward the nasion and superiorly over the frontal bone until the PCF is reached.
- Once the frontal bone above the nasion is well exposed, a 8 × 20 mm osteotomy is performed with a 3 mm high-speed drill creating a bone window similar to the standard coronal approach. Skin edges must be protected from the heat created by the drill while the tip of the drill can be monitored endonasally with the endoscope.
- The PCF is then transposed through the glabellar incision under direct endoscopic visualization to prevent torsion of the vascular pedicle and passed through the supranasion frontal osteotomy into the endonasal surgical field.
- After inlay reconstruction is performed with fascia lata or synthetic dural substitute, the PCF is unfolded and applied onlay to cover the entire skull base defect (▶ Fig. 12.2b and ▶ Fig. 12.3b).
- The remaining steps are the same as for the reconstruction after a coronal PCF harvest. The glabellar incision is closed with a multilayer technique with an intradermal suture for the skin.

12.6 Postoperative Care

- Care must be taken when applying any dressing over the orbital rim to avoid compression of the vascular pedicle.
- The scalp subcutaneous suction drain is usually removed after 24 to 48 hours.
- Postoperative visits 1 week, 1 month, 3 months, and 6 months after the surgery for nasal debridement, which can be more often or longer, depending on the severity of the nasal crusting.
- Antibiotics are continued until the nasal packing is removed.
- Gently remove the nonabsorbable packing during the first postoperative visit. Also perform debridement of loose crusts to improve nasal breathing. There is no need to expose the flap during the first debridement.
- Since the PCF is a nonmucosal flap, it tends to form more adherent crusts over the flap during the mucosalization period.
- Staples or stitches are removed after 10 days.

12.7 Complications

- Besides the expected scalp numbness posterior to the coronal incision, numbness and paresthesia over the forehead can occur from injury to the supraorbital nerve.[6]
- Vascular failure and necrosis of the PCF.[10]
- Alopecia in the area of flap harvest, especially along the incision line due to injury of the hair follicles.[10]
- Postoperative radiation therapy can lead to necrosis or breakdown of the skin in the frontal/forehead area.[6]
- Injury to the frontal branch of the facial nerve during the scalp elevation.[6]
- Postoperative frontal sinus obstruction causing chronic sinusitis or mucocele. After the flap is well healed to the cranial base, the pedicle across the frontal sinus outflow can be transected to restore the frontal sinus drainage without compromising the reconstruction.[8]

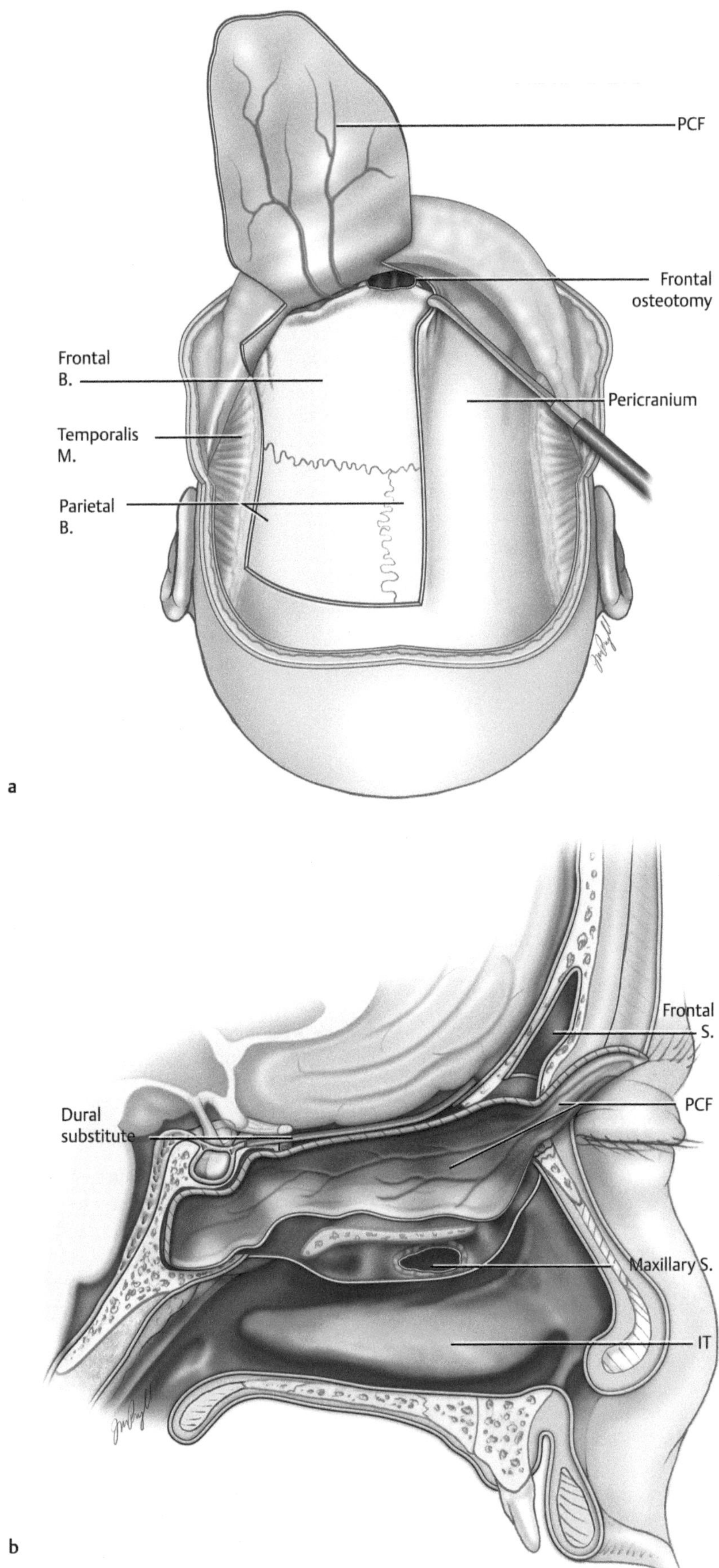

Fig. 12.2 **(a)** Illustration of a left pericranial flap harvest after a coronal approach. Note the supranasion frontal osteotomy for the flap transposition to the nasal cavity. **(b)** Sagittal view showing the flap inset onlay along the anterior cranial base. B, bone; IT, inferior turbinate; M, muscle; PCF, pericranial flap; S, sinus.

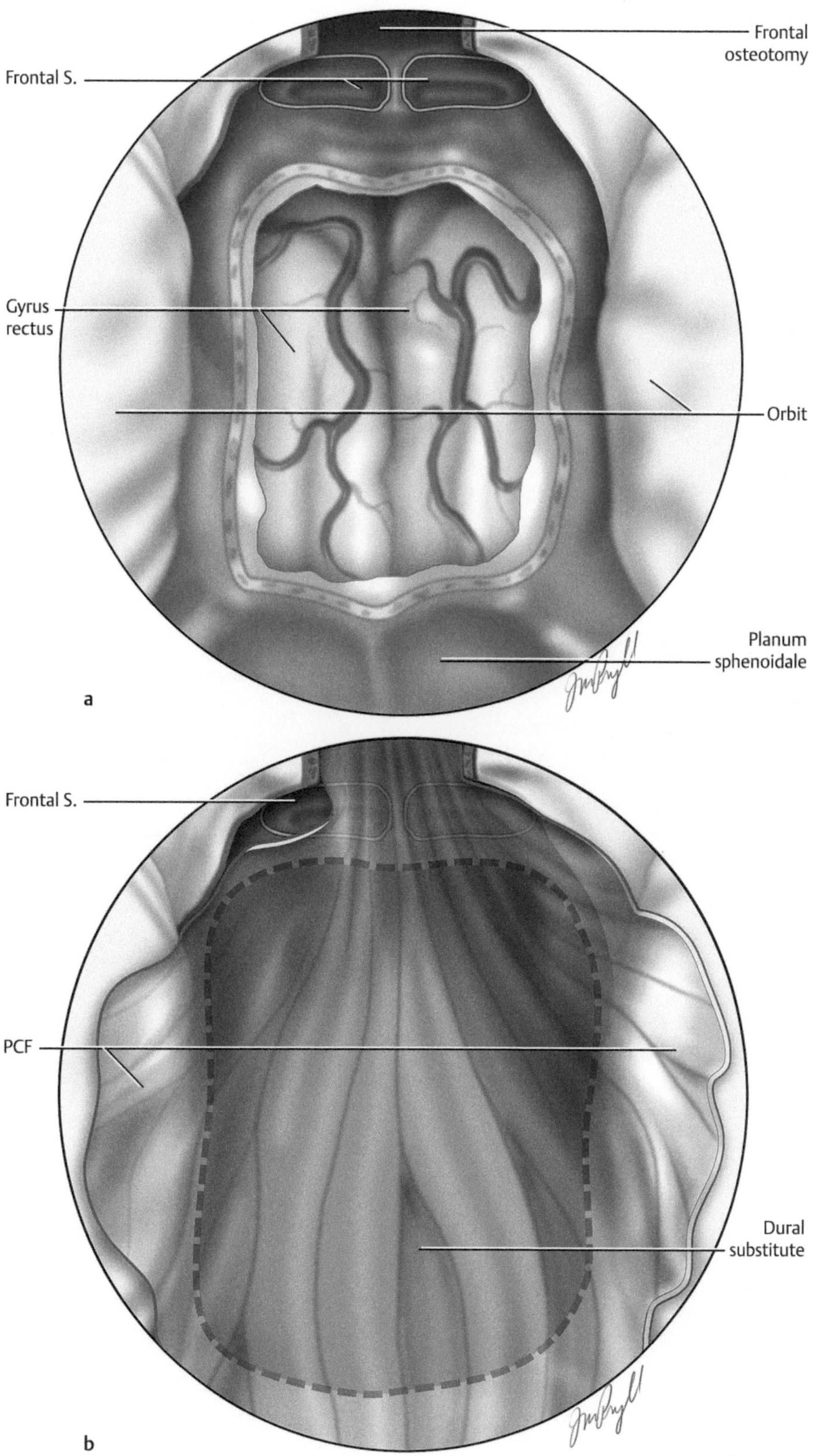

Fig. 12.3 (a) Illustration of the endoscopic endonasal view after an anterior cranial base resection. Observe the wide Draf III frontal sinusotomy and the mucosa of the frontal sinus preserved. **(b)** Inset of the pericranial flap (PCF). The flap is transposed through a supranasion frontal osteotomy. Note that the PCF is displaced to the left side at the level of the frontal sinuses in order to allow the drainage through the right side. The removal of the interfrontal septation during the Draf III frontal sinusotomy allows the drainage of left frontal sinus through the contralateral side. The PCF is illustrated partially transparent to highlight its relation with the frontal sinus and the anterior cranial base defect (*shaded dashed line*). The *purple* color inside the defect represents the dural substitute placed inlay. The PCF is placed onlay and covers the entire cranial base defect, part of the medial orbital walls and planum sphenoidale. S, sinus.

References

[1] Safavi-Abbasi S, Komune N, Archer JB, et al. Surgical anatomy and utility of pedicled vascularized tissue flaps for multilayered repair of skull base defects. J Neurosurg. 2016; 125(2):419–430

[2] Price JC, Loury M, Carson B, Johns ME. The pericranial flap for reconstruction of anterior skull base defects. Laryngoscope. 1988; 98(11):1159–1164

[3] Yoshioka N, Rhoton AL, Jr. Vascular anatomy of the anteriorly based pericranial flap. Neurosurgery. 2005; 57(1) Suppl:11–16, discussion 11–16

[4] Konofaos P, Soto-Miranda MA, Ver Halen J, Fleming JC. Supratrochlear and supraorbital nerves: an anatomical study and applications in the head and neck area. Ophthal Plast Reconstr Surg. 2013; 29(5):403–408

[5] Zanation AM, Snyderman CH, Carrau RL, Kassam AB, Gardner PA, Prevedello DM. Minimally invasive endoscopic pericranial flap: a new method for endonasal skull base reconstruction. Laryngoscope. 2009; 119(1):13–18

[6] Snyderman CH, Janecka IP, Sekhar LN, Sen CN, Eibling DE. Anterior cranial base reconstruction: role of galeal and pericranial flaps. Laryngoscope. 1990; 100(6):607–614

[7] Zanation AM, Thorp BD, Parmar P, Harvey RJ. Reconstructive options for endoscopic skull base surgery. Otolaryngol Clin North Am. 2011; 44 (5):1201–1222

[8] Patel MR, Shah RN, Snyderman CH, et al. Pericranial flap for endoscopic anterior skull-base reconstruction: clinical outcomes and radioanatomic analysis of preoperative planning. Neurosurgery. 2010; 66(3):506–512, discussion 512

[9] Smith JE, Ducic Y. The versatile extended pericranial flap for closure of skull base defects. Otolaryngol Head Neck Surg. 2004; 130(6):704–711

[10] Yano T, Tanaka K, Kishimoto S, Iida H, Okazaki M. Reliability of and indications for pericranial flaps in anterior skull base reconstruction. J Craniofac Surg. 2011; 22(2):482–485

[11] Fortes FS, Carrau RL, Snyderman CH, et al. Transpterygoid transposition of a temporoparietal fascia flap: a new method for skull base reconstruction after endoscopic expanded endonasal approaches. Laryngoscope. 2007; 117 (6):970–976

[12] Patel MR, Stadler ME, Snyderman CH, et al. How to choose? Endoscopic skull base reconstructive options and limitations. Skull Base. 2010; 20(6):397–404

13 Temporoparietal Fascia Flap

Carlos D. Pinheiro-Neto, Luciano C. P. C. Leonel, and Felipe S. G. Fortes

13.1 Anatomy

- Layers of the temporoparietal region from superficial to deep (▶ Fig. 13.1):
  - Skin.
  - Subcutaneous tissue: It contains numerous glands, capillaries, hair follicles, and fat.
  - Galea aponeurotica: In surgical terms, the temporoparietal fascia (TPF) is the inferior continuation of the galea aponeurotica below the level of the superior temporal line. The TPF represents the superior continuation of the superficial musculoaponeurotic system (SMAS) of the face. The TPF is also known as superficial temporal fascia.
  - Loose areolar connective tissue deep to the TPF (subgaleal plane).
  - Temporal fascia (also called deep temporal fascia in surgical terms) is divided into superficial and deep layers. Both layers of the temporal fascia cover the lateral surface of the temporalis muscle between the zygomatic arch and the superior temporal line. Above the superior temporal line, both layers of the temporal fascia fuse with the periosteum underneath the temporalis muscle and are contiguous with the pericranium. The superficial layer of the temporal fascia attaches to the lateral aspect of the zygomatic arch, while the deep layer is attached to its medial aspect. Both are continuous with the periosteum of the zygomatic arch. Above the arch, the two layers are separated by the superficial temporal fat pad.
  - Temporalis muscle.
  - Periosteum (below the superior temporal line) and pericranium (above the superior temporal line).
- The temporalis muscle originates at the temporal fossa and inserts in the coronoid process of the mandible.[1]
- The TPF is a strong fascial layer that is connected to the overlying fibrous septae of the subcutaneous tissue superficially, which makes the surgical separation of these two layers laborious due to the absence of a defined surgical plane (▶ Fig. 13.2a).
- The blood supply to the TPF comes from the superficial temporal artery (STA), which is one of the terminal branches of the external carotid artery (ECA).
- The STA courses through the retromandibular parotid gland, crosses the posterior root of the zygomatic process of the temporal bone, and becomes incorporated into the TPF at the level of the zygomatic arch.[1]
- The mean distance between the STA and the tragus is 16 mm. In most patients, the STA divides into an anterior (frontal) and a posterior (parietal) branches at the level of the zygomatic arch; however, the bifurcation point can be superior or inferior to the arch.[2]
- One or two veins follow the STA and are superficial to the artery.
- The frontal branch of the facial nerve courses immediately deep to the TPF as it crosses the lateral surface of the zygomatic arch running superficial to the superficial layer of the temporal fascia[1] (▶ Fig. 13.1).
- Part of the temporalis muscle (below the zygomatic arch) is located in the infratemporal fossa (ITF) and forms its lateral boundary. The ITF is an irregular-shaped space posterior to the maxilla and lateral to pterygoid plates. Between the ITF and temporal fossa, the temporalis muscle and the deep temporal fat pad are deep to the zygomatic arch.[3] The deep temporal fat pad is a superior extension of the buccal fat pad.
- The lateral and medial pterygoid muscles are located in the ITF medial to the temporalis muscle.

13.2 Fundamentals

- The temporoparietal fascia flap (TPFF) is one of the most reliable flaps for head and neck reconstruction because it is thin and pliable with a long pedicle and rich vascularity.
- When intranasal flaps are not available, the TPFF can be used for reconstruction of the ventral cranial base after endoscopic endonasal approaches.[4]
- Nonmucosal flaps such as the TPFF tend to form more crusting in the postoperative period since it requires a longer period for mucosalization of the endonasal surface of the flap.
- The TPFF used for endoscopic skull base reconstruction includes not only the TPF but also the galea superiorly in order to provide enough flap length for the transposition into the nasal cavity.
- A temporal–infratemporal soft tissue tunnel is dissected to transpose the flap into the nasal cavity.
- The transposition of the TPFF into the nasal cavity allows reconstruction of the ventral skull base without the need for maxillofacial osteotomies.
- The pedicle of the flap is located just anterior to the tragus, which is nearly at the same level of the clivus in the coronal plane. This makes the clival region ideal for reconstruction with this flap since the temporal–infratemporal tunnel brings the flap directly to the nasopharynx.
- The TPFF is a 2 to 4 mm thick fibrous network with a great arch of rotation. Over the parietal region, it extends in a fan-like manner from the preauricular area, comprising a surface as large as 17 × 14 cm.[5]
- Harvest and transposition of the TPFF to the nasal cavity is carried after the final defect size is determined.
- The TPFF should be harvested on the same side of the defect, unless contraindicated.
- Previous scalp incisions may alter availability and laterality of the harvest.

13.3 Indications

- When intranasal flaps are not available.
- Reconstruction of:
  - Clival defects.
  - Craniovertebral junction.
  - ITF.
  - Orbital defects.
- Reconstruction of anterior cranial base defects when the pericranial flap is not available.

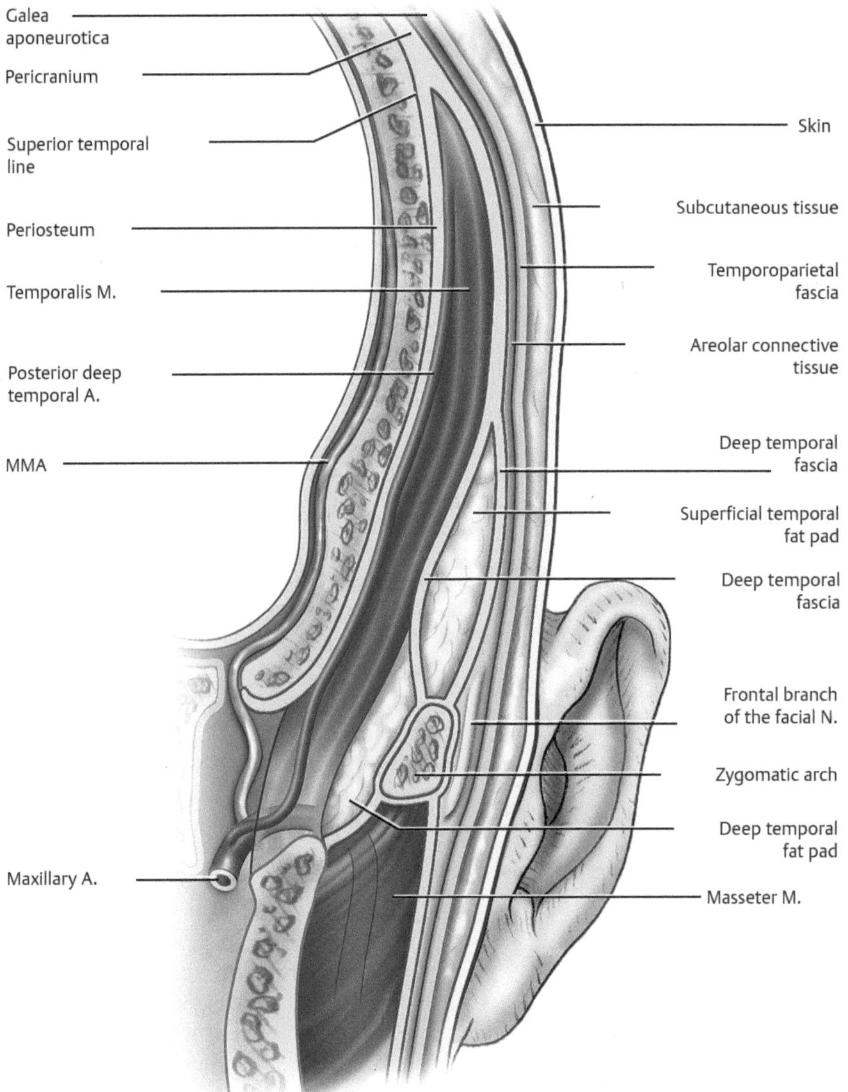

Fig. 13.1 Illustration of the left temporoparietal region (coronal view) to demonstrate the layers and key anatomical structures. *Temporoparietal fascia = also known as superficial temporal fascia.* A, artery; D, deep; M, muscle; MMA, middle meningeal artery; N, nerve; Sup, superficial.

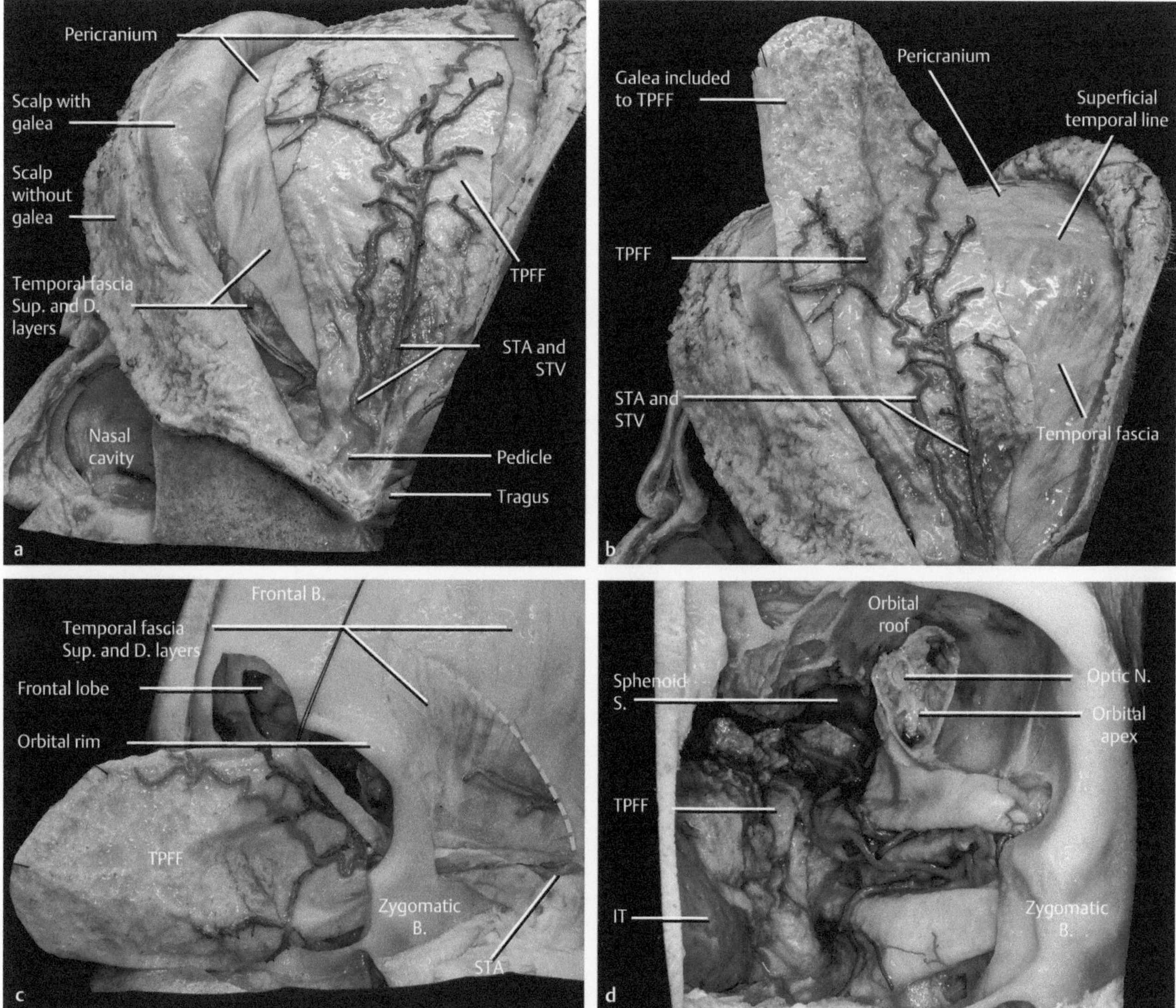

Fig. 13.2 Anatomical dissection after an extended hemicoronal incision. The left hemiface and orbital contents were removed to illustrate the transposition of the temporoparietal fascia flap (TPFF) to the nasal cavity. **(a)** Vascularization of the TPFF. The flap is composed of temporoparietal fascia (TPF) inferiorly and galea superiorly to the superior temporal line. Note the absence of galea/TPF in the scalp after the flap harvest. **(b)** Elevation of the flap from the underlying pericranium and superficial layer of the deep temporal fascia. **(c)** Transposition of the flap anterior to the temporalis muscle. Note the oblique incision (*green dashed line*) along the superficial layer of the deep temporal fascia to allow an interfascial dissection. This incision is performed at least 2 cm posterior to the orbital rim to avoid injury to the frontal branch of the facial nerve. The interfascial dissection through the superficial temporal fat pad (removed in the picture) also protects the facial neve, which courses superficially to the superficial layer of the deep temporal fascia. **(d)** TPFF inset to cover the clival region using the anterior corridor for the transposition of the flap. This corridor is anterior to the temporalis and pterygoid musculature, with no need of drilling of the pterygoid plates.
B, bone; D, deep; IT, inferior turbinate; N, nerve; STA, superficial temporal artery; STV, superficial temporal vein; Sup, superficial; TPFF, temporoparietal fascia flap.

13.4 Limitations

- It requires a hemicoronal incision and dissection through the ITF for the transposition of the flap into the nasal cavity.
- A well-defined dissection plane is absent between the TPF and the subcutaneous tissue.
- The closure of the scalp incision is harder after the TPF is separated from the subcutaneous tissue.

13.5 Surgical Technique

13.5.1 Endoscopic Infratemporal Fossa Approach

- The endoscopic ITF approach prepares the endonasal corridor for the TPFF transposition.

Posterior Corridor

- If not performed previously as a part of the approach/resection of the cranial base lesion, a complete anterior and posterior ethmoidectomy and a large maxillary antrostomy are performed.
- The nasal mucosa posterior to the maxillary antrostomy is elevated and the sphenopalatine artery (SPA) is identified at the sphenopalatine foramen.
- The orbital process of the palatine bone and the posterior wall of the maxillary sinus are removed with retrograde dissection of the SPA into the pterygopalatine fossa (PPF). Combination of high-speed drill and Kerrison rongeurs can be used for bone removal.
- The periosteal layer covering the PPF contents (medially) and ITF (laterally) is exposed.
- The neurovascular bundle formed by the descending palatine artery and greater palatine nerve is identified in its inferior vertical trajectory and is dissected from its canal. Partial posterior medial maxillectomy can be performed to free the descending palatine artery and greater palatine nerve all the way inferiorly toward the nasal floor. This step will help with the lateralization of the PPF contents and exposure of the pterygoid plates.
- The vertical plate of the palatine bone inferior to the SPA is also removed.
- The extensive bone removal allows the inferior and lateral displacement of the contents of the PPF and exposure of the pterygoid base and process.
- Transection of the vidian nerve allows further lateralization and wider exposure of the pterygoid base. Unless this step is required for the surgical approach, the vidian should be preserved during the transposition of the TPFF into the nasal cavity.
- The medial and lateral pterygoid plates are partially drilled with a high-speed drill to enlarge the space for the transposition of the TPFF.
- The entry point of the flap to cavity/nasopharynx is a window formed by the descending palatine artery and greater palatine nerve anteriorly; Eustachian tube posteriorly; the vidian nerve superiorly; and the soft palate inferiorly.
- In this corridor, the flap is transposed through the pterygoid musculature, which makes it ideal for reconstruction of the clivus and craniovertebral junction (▶ Fig. 13.3a).

Anterior Corridor

- A variation of this technique can be performed to avoid exposure and drilling of the pterygoid plates.
- The PPF and ITF periosteum are exposed in a similar manner as for the posterior corridor. However, for the anterior corridor, there is no need for drilling of the pterygoid plates and, consequently, no exposure and dissection of the descending palatine artery and greater palatine nerve are required.
- A sublabial transmaxillary approach is recommended to enlarge the opening of the posterior wall of the maxillary laterally.
- An incision is performed along the periosteum that encases the PPF and ITF. Care should be taken to avoid injury of the maxillary artery (MA). This incision marks the entry point of the TPFF into the sinonasal area.
- Through the anterior corridor, the TPFF will arise at the posterior aspect of maxillary sinus and anterior to the pterygoid musculature.
- The anterior corridor can be used for orbit, ITF, clival, and anterior cranial base reconstructions.[6]
- For clival and craniovertebral junction defects, the flap lays anterior to the descending palatine artery and greater palatine nerve before turning posteriorly toward the clivus.
- The advantages of the anterior corridor compared to the posterior one are no need of removal of the pterygoid plates and less risk of neurovascular injury within the PPF. The anterior corridor is a much easier and faster dissection.
- The disadvantage of the anterior corridor for clival and craniovertebral junction defects is that the TPFF needs to be longer. The posterior corridor provides a more direct route from the pedicle to the clivus compared to the anterior corridor (▶ Fig. 13.3b).

13.5.2 Temporoparietal Fascia Flap Harvest and Transposition

- The TPFF is harvested from the ipsilateral side of the ITF approach.
- A hemicoronal incision is carried down to the level of the hair follicles. Care must be taken to avoid injuring the pedicle at the inferior aspect of the incision.
- An extended hemicoronal incision can be performed, which progresses the incision to the contralateral superior temporal line. This allows the harvest of a longer flap.
- The skin and subcutaneous tissue are gradually elevated, leaving the TPF attached to the deep layers of the scalp. This is a laborious dissection since there is no well-defined plane between the TPF and the subcutaneous tissue. The dissection has to stop anteriorly approximately 2 cm behind the orbital rim to avoid injury to the frontal branch of the facial nerve.
- After enough exposure of the TPF and galea, the flap incisions are made superiorly, anteriorly, and posteriorly.
- Superiorly, the flap is carefully elevated with or without the pericranium (part of the flap above the superior temporal line).
- The elevation of the TPFF is continued inferiorly toward the zygomatic arch with great exposure of the superficial layer of the temporal fascia.

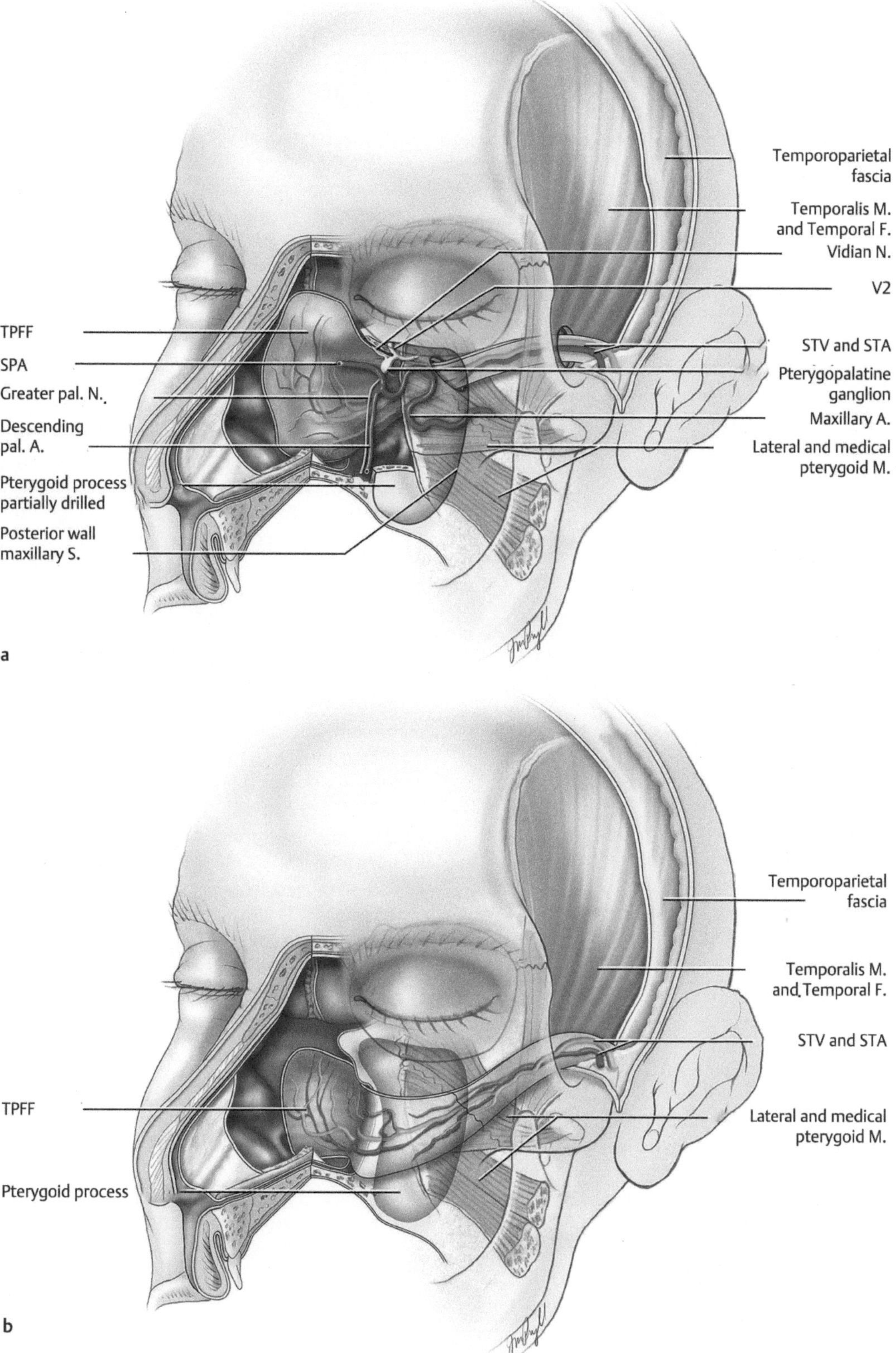

Fig. 13.3 Illustration showing the transposition of a left temporoparietal fascia flap (TPFF) to reconstruct the clival region. **(a)** Posterior transposition. A tunnel is created through the temporal fossa to the nasopharynx passing through the temporalis and pterygoid musculature using percutaneous tracheotomy dilators. The entry point window into the nasopharynx is created with partial removal of the pterygoid plates and is located in between the descending palatine artery/greater palatine nerve and the Eustachian tube. **(b)** Anterior transposition. Note the flap passing from the temporal fossa to the maxillary sinus anterior to the temporalis muscle. The TPFF is placed in front of the pterygoid musculature and pterygoid plates before turning posteriorly toward the clivus. In such cases, there is no need for dissection of the descending palatine artery/greater palatine nerve or pterygoid plates drill out. A, artery; F, fascia; M, muscle; N, nerve; pal., palatine; SPA, sphenopalatine artery; STA, superficial temporal artery; STV, superficial temporal vein; TPFF, temporoparietal fascia flap.

- The superficial layer of the temporal fascia is incised about 2 cm posterior to the orbital rim and parallel to the course of the frontal branch of the facial nerve. This incision exposes the superficial temporal fat pad and allows interfascial dissection to further elevate the scalp anteriorly. The frontal branch of the facial nerve is superficial to this plane of dissection.
- The anterior elevation of the scalp in this region allows wide exposure of the deep layer of the temporal fascia (► Fig. 13.2).

Posterior Corridor

- At the level of the zygomatic arch, the deep layer of the temporal fascia is incised, exposing the deep temporal fat pad and giving access to the ITF and pterygoid musculature.
- A guidewire is passed into the nose through the temporalis/pterygoid musculature. The guidewire enters the nose through the window previously created with the drilling of the pterygoid process (lateral and medial pterygoid plates).
- The pterygoid musculature is subsequently blunt dissected using percutaneous tracheotomy dilators of increasing sizes through the guidewire to create a wide soft tissue tunnel and avoid compression of the flap.
- Then the superior border of the flap is tied to the guidewire, which is gently pulled out from the nose bringing the TPFF to the nasal cavity. The mobilization of the flap through the tunnel is assisted with external manipulation. It is important to avoid torsion of the flap in its longer axis because this may compromise its blood supply.
- The external incisions are closed after insertion of a suction drain.

Anterior Corridor

- For the transposition through an anterior corridor, instead of incising the deep layer of the temporal fascia at the level of the zygomatic arch, the anterior edge of the temporalis muscle is elevated posteriorly from the lateral orbital rim to expose the lateral orbital wall.
- The temporalis muscle is retracted posteriorly and the dissection is carried inferiorly toward the inferior orbital fissure until identification of the wide opening at the posterior wall of the maxillary sinus, which was performed during the endoscopic ITF approach.
- Part of the anterior border of the temporalis muscle can be removed to enlarge the transposition tunnel and decrease the risk of flap compression.
- The flap can be easily transposed to the maxillary sinus and will lie anterior to the pterygoid musculature and descending palatine artery/greater palatine nerve.

13.5.3 Reconstruction

- All mucosa around the edges of the defect should be removed.
- Placement of an inlay dural substitute or fascia lata.
- For clival defects, fat graft is placed to fill the space of the clivectomy after the inlay reconstruction.
- The TPFF is placed over the defect.
- Dural sealant is used after the flap is in position, followed by absorbable packing and possible nonabsorbable packing for large defects.
- The hemicoronal incision is sutured with 2-0 Vicryl for the subcutaneous tissue. Because of the absence of the TPF/galea, it is recommended the inclusion of dermis in this suture. Suturing only the subcutaneous fat without the TPF/galea underneath or the dermis superficially is nearly impossible to approximate the incision. Then staples are applied. Other option is using only Prolene stitches that include the epidermis, dermis, and subcutaneous fat.

13.6 Postoperative Care

- Postoperative visits 1 week, 1 month, 3 months, and 6 months after surgery for nasal debridement, which can be more often or longer, depending on the severity of the nasal crusting.
- Loose crusts should be removed in the first postoperative visit to improve nasal breathing. There is no need to expose the flap during the first debridement.
- Since the TPFF is a nonmucosal flap, it tends to form more adherent crusts compared to intranasal mucosal flaps.
- The suction drain is usually removed after 24 to 48 hours.
- Staples or Prolene stitches are removed after 10 days.

13.7 Complications

- Injury to the hair follicles during the separation of the TPF from the subcutaneous tissue can lead to alopecia in the affected area.
- Injury of the frontal branch of the facial nerve during the scalp elevation.
- Palatal numbness from injury of the greater palatine nerve.
- Injury to the vidian nerve causing xerophthalmia.
- Facial numbness from injury of the maxillary division of the trigeminal (V2) nerve.
- Eustachian tube dysfunction from trauma to the tube during the flap transposition or the flap covering the nasopharyngeal ostium of the tube.
- MA injury during the flap transposition.

References

[1] Casoli V, Dauphin N, Taki C, et al. Anatomy and blood supply of the subgaleal fascia flap. Clin Anat. 2004; 17(5):392–399

[2] Pinar YA, Govsa F. Anatomy of the superficial temporal artery and its branches: its importance for surgery. Surg Radiol Anat. 2006; 28(3):248–253

[3] Cavallo LM, Messina A, Gardner P, et al. Extended endoscopic endonasal approach to the pterygopalatine fossa: anatomical study and clinical considerations. Neurosurg Focus. 2005; 19(1):E5

[4] Fortes FS, Carrau RL, Snyderman CH, et al. Transpterygoid transposition of a temporoparietal fascia flap: a new method for skull base reconstruction after endoscopic expanded endonasal approaches. Laryngoscope. 2007; 117(6):970–976

[5] David SK, Cheney ML. An anatomic study of the temporoparietal fascial flap. Arch Otolaryngol Head Neck Surg. 1995; 121(10):1153–1156

[6] Lee DD, Kenning T, Pinheiro-Neto CD. Use of composite osteotemporoparietal fascia flap for midface reconstruction after en bloc resection of squamous cell carcinoma involving the zygomaticomaxillary complex. Plast Reconstr Surg Glob Open. 2016; 4(8):e835

14 Composite Extranasal Flaps: Osteopericranial and Osteotemporoparietal Fascia Flaps

Carlos D. Pinheiro-Neto and Maria Peris-Celda

14.1 Anatomy

- See Chapters 12 and 13 to review the anatomy of the pericranial flap (PCF) and temporoparietal fascia flap (TPFF), respectively.
- The blood supply of each composite flap is the same as their correspondent standard soft tissue flap.
- The skull is a frequent donor site of bone graft in reconstructive surgery. The parietal and frontal bones are the most commonly used.
- The frontal and parietal bones have an external cortical, a diploe (spongy cancellous bone), and an internal cortical.
- The frontal bone is the thicker skull bone.[1]
- The coronal suture is located between the frontal and parietal bones.
- The thicker area of the parietal bone is located 2 cm anterior to the lambdoid suture.[1]
- The sagittal suture unites the two parietal bones and is used as a landmark for the superior sagittal sinus.

14.2 Fundamentals

- Advantages of the calvarial bone graft are easy access during craniofacial reconstruction due to the proximity to the surgical field, large grafts can be obtained, and relatively painless donor site.
- The osteopericranial and osteotemporoparietal fascia flaps are composite flaps where a piece of calvarium bone is kept attached to the respective flap.
- A split osteotomy within the cancellous bone is performed to separate the external cortical from the internal cortical of the calvarium maintaining the vascularized flap attached and the periosteum intact.[2]
- This technique provides additional support, especially for osseous defects of the head and neck.[3]
- The relatively thin bony consistency of this flap aids in the restoration of a viable skeletal framework in poor recipient sites.[3]
- Successful head and neck reconstructions have been done using free grafts from the iliac crest, fibula, radius, rib, and scapula. Although these are acceptable options, vascularized flaps are reported to be more reliable, have lower rates of infection, and allow earlier bone integration.[4]
- Free flaps require revascularization, necessitating expertise in microvascular techniques and prolonged operative times.
- Composite calvarium flaps do not require microvascular anastomosis. Their proximity to the defects allows their use as local flaps that remain vascularized from perforators within the pericranium and temporoparietal fascia (TPF).[5]
- The osseous component of the osteopericranial flap (OPF) is harvested from the frontal bone just anterior to the coronal suture in the parasagittal region to avoid injury to the superior sagittal sinus. If a longer pedicle is needed, the bone component of the OPF can be harvested from the parietal bone.
- The osseous component of the osteotemporoparietal fascia flap (OTPFF) is harvested from the parietal or frontal bone between the superior temporal line and the midsagittal plane.
- The osseous component of the OTPFF can be harvested from the contralateral side to avoid the sagittal sinus in the midline and leave a long pedicle for the transposition into the nasal cavity. For the majority of zygomatic or orbital reconstruction, the osseous component of the flap can be harvested ipsilaterally.
- The osseous component of the OTPFF is actually attached to the pericranium, that remains connected to the galea and TPF. See Fig. 13.1 in Chapter 13 to review the anatomy of the layers of this region.

14.3 Indications

- Composite calvarium flaps are mainly indicated for orbitomaxillary, palatal, mandibular, and zygomatic defects.[6]
- Potentially, these flaps can be used for anterior cranial base reconstruction (OPF) or clival defects (OTPFF).

14.4 Limitations

- Rigid reconstruction should be carefully used next to neurovascular structures such as carotid arteries and optic nerves.
- It requires a larger tunnel for transposition into the nasal cavity compared to the standard PCF or TPFF.
- The sagittal sinus and temporalis muscle limit the amount of bone that can be added to the OTPFF. If a larger bone component is required, part of the temporalis muscle can be left attached connecting the TPF to the bone harvested.

14.5 Surgical Technique

14.5.1 Harvest

- The harvest techniques of the OPF and OTPFF are similar to the techniques used for the standard PCF and TPFF, respectively.
- The shape and size of the bone piece desired is drawn on the flap and the elevation of the pericranium or galea/TPF is performed centripetally until it reaches the marked area in the center.
- At this point, a high-speed drill is used to perform a U-shaped osteotomy, leaving the open part of the "U" toward the pedicle (proximal part) (▶ Fig. 14.1a and ▶ Fig. 14.2a).
- The pericranium or galea/TPF is carefully folded and protected with a malleable retractor during the drilling.
- Once the diploe is exposed along the U-shaped osteotomy, a curved osteotome and curved drill are used to separate the outer cortical from the inner.
- Finally, the proximal outer cortical (open part of the U-shaped osteotomy) is separated with an osteotome. The osseous

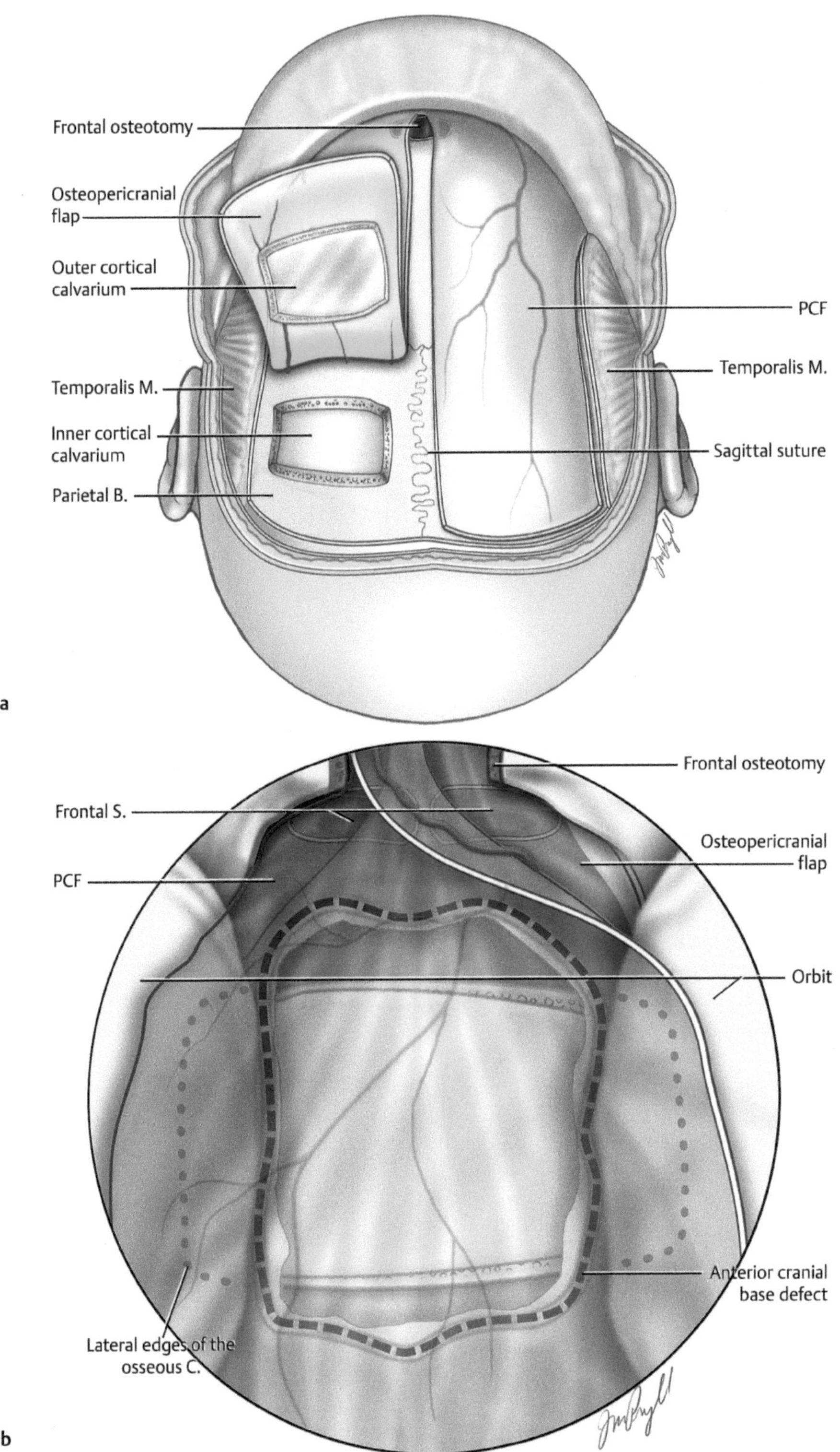

Fig. 14.1 (a) Illustration showing a bicoronal approach to harvest of a composite osteopericranial flap (*green*) on the left side and a standard pericranial flap on the right (*pink*). The "U"-shaped osteotomy is performed with a high-speed drill along the sides and distal border of the osseous part of the flap. The separation of the outer cortical from the inner cortical of the calvarium is performed using association of curved osteotome and curved drill. Finally, the proximal outer cortical is separated with an osteotome. **(b)** Flaps inset through a supranasion frontal osteotomy to cover an anterior cranial base defect. First the composite flap is transposed and placed inlay. The lateral edges of the osseous component are placed above the orbital roofs (*dotted line*). Note that the bone component is larger than the defect on its laterolateral dimension and shorter on its anterior–posterior dimension. Since the bone does not completely cover the defect, two gaps are present: anterior and posterior. The pericranial component of the flap is placed inlay covering those gaps. Because the extra pericranium of the composite flap is used to cover the spaces along the skull base defect, the pericranium cannot be used to wrap the bone and a second pericranial flap (*pink*) is required and placed onlay covering the entire defect. *Dashed line*—anterior cranial base defect. *Dotted line*—lateral edges of the osseous component of the flap placed on top of the orbital roof bilaterally. B, bone; C, component; M, muscle; PCF, pericranial flap; S, sinus.

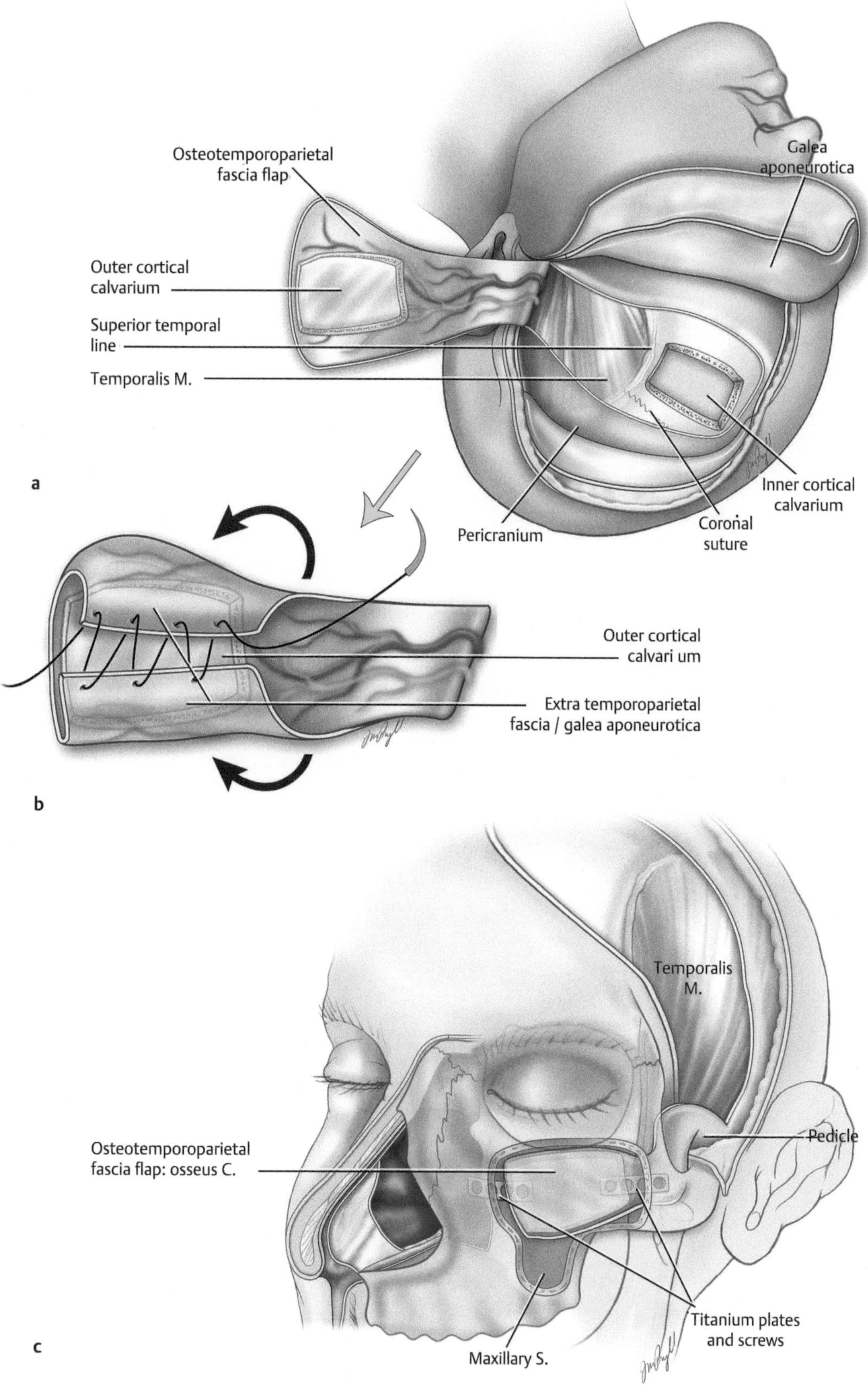

Fig. 14.2 **(a)** Illustration showing the harvest of a composite osteotemporoparietal fascia flap. Note that the osseous component of the flap is harvested between the superior temporal line and the sagittal suture. It is important to avoid the calvarial split close to the sagittal suture due to risk of injury to the superior sagittal sinus. The "U"-shaped osteotomy is initially performed to expose the diploe, which creates the space to separate the outer cortical from the inner cortical. **(b)** For orbital, palatal, or maxillary defects, the extra fascia can be folded and sutured to envelope the osseous component of the flap. This decreases the risk of exposed bone or need for a second flap, especially when the flap is used toward the sinonasal or oral cavity. **(c)** Flap inset to reconstruct a zygomaticomaxillary complex defect. Note that titanium plates and screws are used to secure the osseous component of the flap. C, component; M, muscle; S, sinus.

component is kept attached to the pericranium or galea/TPF, which is elevated as usual toward the pedicle.

14.5.2 Reconstruction

- The composite flap is used to restore osseous defects.
- The transposition of the OPF to the nasal cavity requires a larger supranasion frontal osteotomy.
- For anterior cranial base reconstruction, ideally the bone should be placed on top of the orbits. The anterior–posterior dimension of the bone should be smaller than the anterior–posterior dimension of the defect.
- The pericranial surface of the flap stays superior and facing the brain/inlay reconstruction. A contralateral PCF should be harvested and placed onlay to cover the osseous component of the OPF (▶ Fig. 14.1b).
- Rotation of the flap to oppose the osseous surface toward the defect is not recommended due to the consequent pedicle torsion and risk of flap necrosis.
- A technique that can be used to cover the osseous component of the flap and avoid the use of a second flap is harvesting extra pericranium or TPF to wrap the bone part with this extra tissue. The edges are sutured and the osseous component stays completely enveloped with pericranium or TPF for the reconstruction (▶ Fig. 14.2b).
- This is performed before the transposition to the nasal cavity and helps to prevent the exposure of the osseous component of the flap during the healing process.[6]
- The wrapping technique is ideal for reconstruction of defects of the facial skeleton/orbit but should be avoided to seal intradural defects since the flap would lack extra tissue to appropriately fill the gaps between the bone and the defect.
- If possible, titanium plates and screws can be used to secure the bone component of the flap in craniomaxillofacial reconstructions (▶ Fig. 14.2c).
- ▶ Fig. 14.3 illustrates a surgical example of an OPF used for nasal reconstruction.
- ▶ Fig. 14.4 shows a case of patient who had an OTPFF for zygomaticomaxillary complex reconstruction. Titanium meshes can be used to reconstruct the calvarium donor site.

14.6 Postoperative Care

- Scalp subcutaneous suction drain is kept for 24 to 48 hours.
- Removal of scalp staples in 10 days.
- Postoperative visits 1 week, 1 month, 3 months, and 6 months after surgery for nasal debridement.

14.7 Complications

- See complications of the PCF (Chapter 12) and TPFF (Chapter 13).
- Violation of the inner cortical of the calvarium during the bone harvest with consequent dural laceration, cerebrospinal fluid (CSF) leak, and possible brain injury.
- Injury to the sagittal sinus if the bone is harvested too close to the midline can lead to catastrophic complications including death due to venous congestion of the brain.
- Possibility of osteoradionecrosis of the osseous component in patients who undergo postoperative radiation.

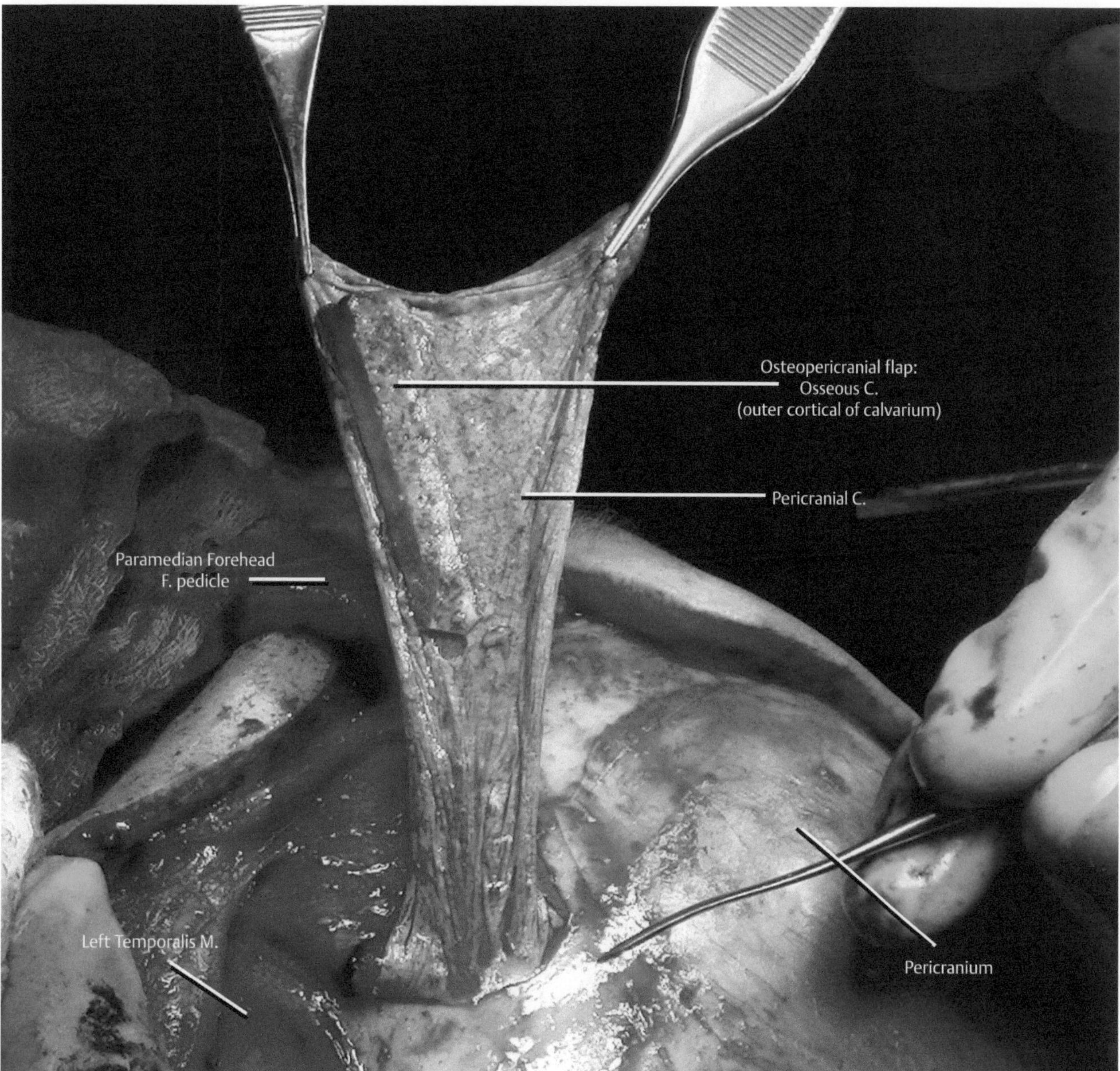

Fig. 14.3 Surgical illustration of a composite osteopericranial flap used for nasal reconstruction after partial rhinectomy. A right-sided paramedian forehead flap was used for the skin coverage. The medial-superior edge of the paramedian forehead flap incision was extended to the contralateral side in the coronal plane and a left-sided composite flap was harvested and used to reconstruct the framework of the nose (osseous component) and the endonasal lining (pericranial component). C, component; F, flap; M, muscle.

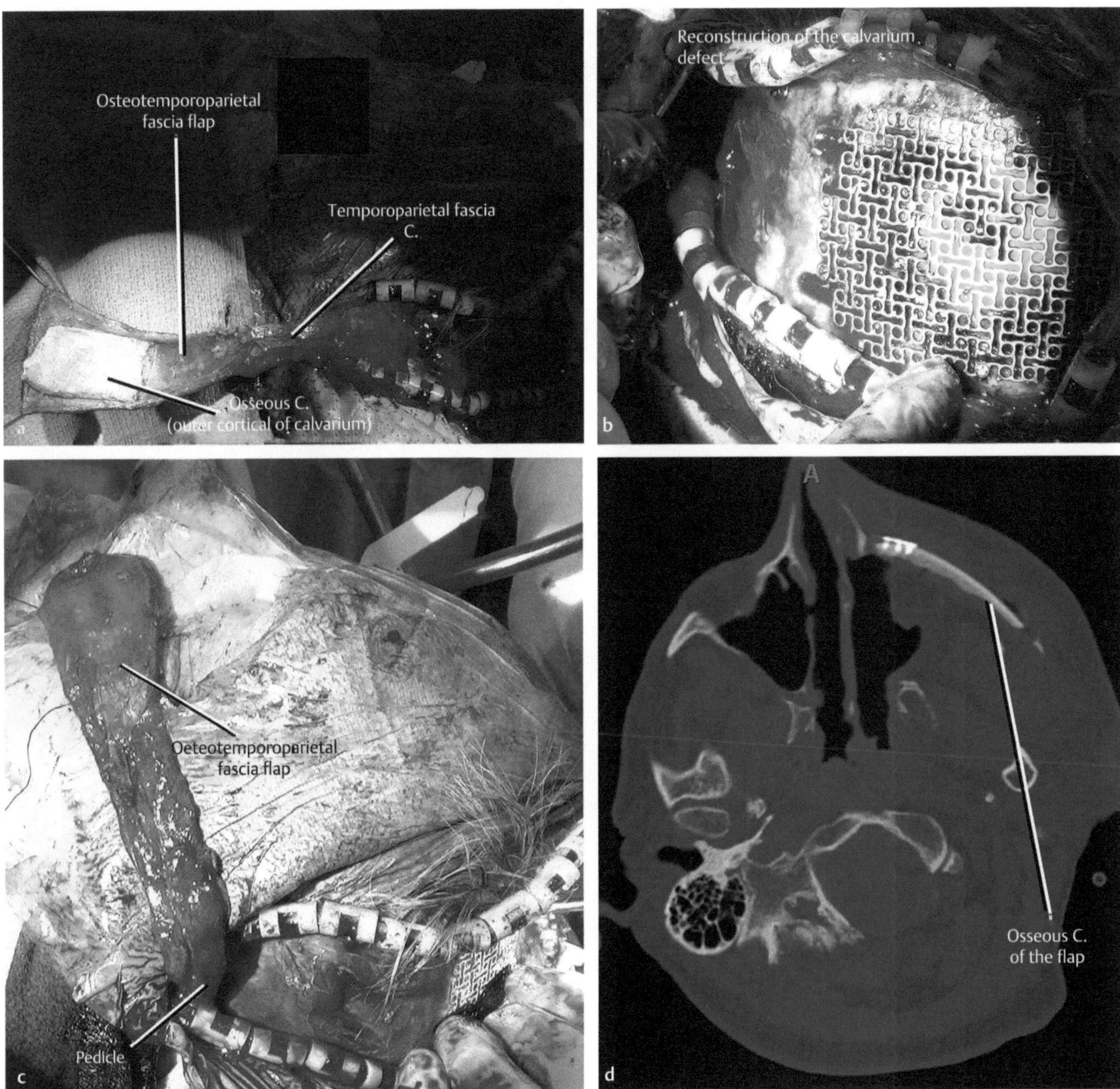

Fig. 14.4 Surgical case of a left-sided osteotemporoparietal fascia flap used for reconstruction after resection of a carcinoma involving the zygoma and maxilla. **(a)** Harvest of the flap. **(b)** Reconstruction of the calvarium donor site with titanium mesh. **(c)** Before the flap transposition to show the rotation of the flap toward the maxilla. Note that the extra fascia was sutured to wrap the osseous component. **(d)** Postoperative computed tomography (CT) scan 4 months after surgery axial view showing the osseous part of the flap integrated. Observe the titanium plate used to secure the bone.
C, component.

References

[1] Moreira-Gonzalez A, Papay FE, Zins JE. Calvarial thickness and its relation to cranial bone harvest. Plast Reconstr Surg. 2006; 117(6):1964–1971

[2] Engle RD, Butrymowicz A, Peris-Celda M, Kenning TJ, Pinheiro-Neto CD. Split-calvarial osteopericranial flap for reconstruction following endoscopic anterior resection of cranial base. Laryngoscope. 2015; 125(4):826–830

[3] Parhiscar A, Har-El G, Turk JB, Abramson DL. Temporoparietal osteofascial flap for head and neck reconstruction. J Oral Maxillofac Surg. 2002; 60 (6):619–622

[4] Davison SP, Mesbahi AN, Clemens MW, Picken CA. Vascularized calvarial bone flaps and midface reconstruction. Plast Reconstr Surg. 2008; 122(1):10e–18e

[5] Davison SP, Boehmler JH, Ganz JC, Davidson B. Vascularized rib for facial reconstruction. Plast Reconstr Surg. 2004; 114(1):15–20

[6] Lee DD, Kenning T, Pinheiro-Neto CD. Use of composite osteotemporoparietal fascia flap for midface reconstruction after en bloc resection of squamous cell carcinoma involving the zygomaticomaxillary complex. Plast Reconstr Surg Glob Open. 2016; 4(8):e835

15 Temporalis Muscle Flap

Roberto M. Soriano and C. Arturo Solares

15.1 Anatomy

- The temporalis muscle (TM) originates from the superior temporal line, passes medial to the zygomatic arch, and inserts onto the coronoid process of the mandible.
- The TM lies in the temporal fossa, which is delimited anteriorly by the frontozygomatic rim, which forms part of the lateral orbital wall.
- Anteriorly, the TM attaches to the lateral orbital rim and anterior temporal crest. Medially, the TM overlies the cranial periosteum.
- Going from a superficial to a deep plane, the TM can be found below the skin, subcutaneous tissue, subgaleal (loose areolar connective tissue) layer, temporoparietal fascia (TPF), and temporal fascia (TF), respectively (see the anatomy section in Chapter 13).
- Important: The temporal branch of the facial nerve (CN VII) passes through the parotid gland below the zygomatic arch and lies deep to the TPF after passing over the zygomatic arch.
- The TF (or deep TF) directly overlies the TM. It is contiguous with the pericranium superiorly, and splits into a deep and superficial layer, at approximately the level of the superior orbital rim, which attach to the medial and lateral aspects of the zygomatic arch, respectively.
- The superficial temporal fat pad (STFP) is contained in between the deep and superficial layers of the deep TF.
- The TM has dual blood supply provided by the deep temporal (anterior and posterior) and the middle temporal arteries.
- The deep temporal arteries (DTAs) are branches of the maxillary artery and supply the anterior two-thirds of the TM. They lie deep to the TM, in between the periosteum and the TM.[1]
- The middle temporal artery is a branch of the superficial temporal artery (STA) arising below the zygomatic arch and perforates the TF. It provides the vascular supply to the posterior third of the TM and anastomoses to the DTAs within the TM.
- The TM has a length of 12 to 16 cm if completely harvested with a 0.5 to 1 cm thickness and its pedicle tolerates up to 135 degrees of rotation.[2,3,4,5]

15.2 Fundamentals

- Gillies was the first to use a true temporalis muscle flap (TMF) in 1917 as a transposition flap for midfacial deformities following traumatic loss of the zygomatic bone.[3,6]
- Since its first use, the TMF has been used in the reconstruction of oral, palatal, and maxillary defects, facial reanimation surgery, midfacial augmentation, and obliteration of orbital defects.[1,2,3,4,7]
- More relevantly, it has been extensively used to reconstruct a variety of skull base defects and has proven to be a reliable reconstructive alternative.[1,3,4,5,7,8,9]
- The TMF is a nonbulky, versatile, and well-perfused flap that can be accustomed to fit a variety of defect sizes and results in minimal to no functional morbidity and mild aesthetic deformity of the donor site.[3,4]
- Additionally, the TM usually lies near skull base defects and can be harvested as part of the exposure in open approaches.[1,3]
- The TMF can be harvested as a complete flap for large defects and can also be split based on the anterior or posterior circulation to accommodate smaller defects.[3,5]

15.3 Indications

- A complete TMF can be used for defects up to 20 square cm,[3,5] while a single split TMF can reliably cover defects up to 12 square cm.[5]
- The TMF provides moderately thick muscular tissue and can be used for a variety of skull base defects in the anterior, middle, and posterior fossa as well as cribriform plate, ethmoid sinus, sphenoid sinus, and orbit.[3]
- It is a well-vascularized pedicled flap that is adequate for reliable closure of large skull base defects, contains a reliable blood supply, provides a strong barrier for future radiation, and separates intracranial contents from the upper aerodigestive tract.[5,10]
- It can be used in cases were a moderately thick, flexible, and adaptable flap is required.
- Primary reconstruction of the orbit following orbital exenteration can be performed with a TMF. It provides an acceptable aesthetic outcome[11] (▶ Fig. 15.1a).
- Although its use in endoscopic surgery is limited, like the TPF flap, it is indicated in patients undergoing endoscopic surgery where nasoseptal flaps are not available due to previous surgeries, tumoral invasion, previous radiation, or where resection of septum, pterygopalatine fossa, or sphenoid sinuses is required for an oncologically sound resection[9,12] (▶ Fig. 15.1b).
- If the need for a TMF arises, ideally, a preoperative evaluation should be performed to assess[1,4]:
  - Temporal artery circulation (Doppler/palpation).
  - TM function (clench teeth) with noticeable bulging in the temporal fossa.
  - History of previous surgeries, trauma, or radiation of the temporozygomatic region and adjacent areas.
- An abnormal examination or a positive surgical traumatic history, as mentioned above, constitutes a contraindication for the use of a TMF.

15.4 Limitations

- External incision is required for harvest.
- Possible zygomatic arch osteotomy.
- Small size relatively to free microvascular free flaps.
- Temporal hollowing following harvest of complete TMF.
- Primarily used in open skull base approaches.

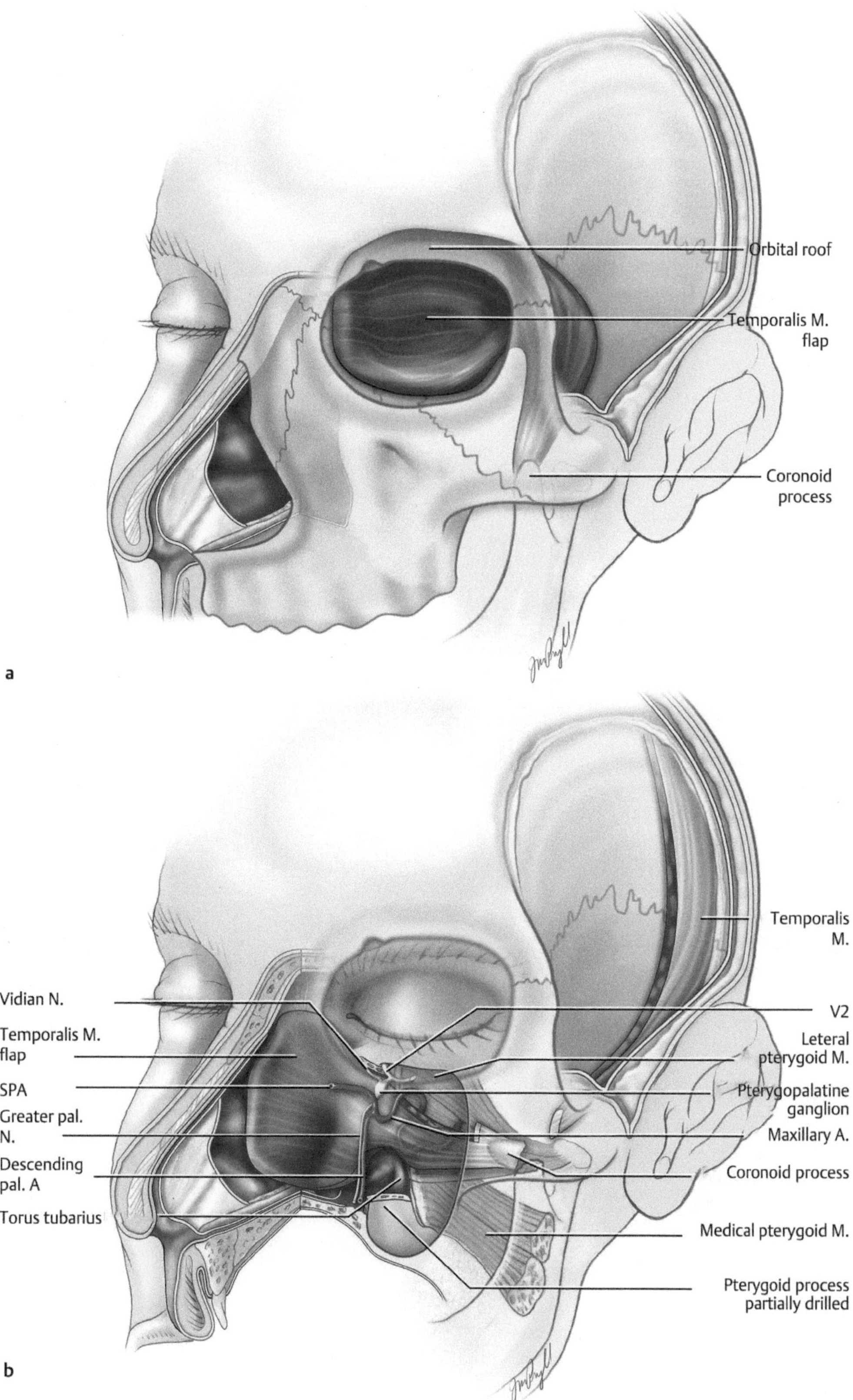

Fig. 15.1 (a) Illustration showing the inset of a left temporalis muscle flap (TMF) for orbital reconstruction through a lateral orbitotomy. Note that the entire muscle was harvested to fill the orbital cavity. This transposition can also be used for anterior cranial base defects after orbital exenteration with removal of the orbital roof. **(b)** Inset of the TMF through the infratemporal fossa for reconstruction of the clivus. Note that a partial muscle flap was harvested for this reconstruction. The osteotomy of the coronoid process and its medial mobilization improve the reach of the flap. Drilling of the pterygoid plates is needed to create a window for the flap transposition to the clivus between the greater palatine nerve/descending palatine artery and Eustachian tube. This route allows a more direct course of the flap to the clival region. A, artery; M, muscle; N, nerve; pal., palatine; SPA, sphenopalatine artery.

15.5 Surgical Technique

15.5.1 Widening of Pterygoid Passage

- If not already performed, various steps must be performed prior to harvest of the TMF.
- A complete ethmoidectomy (anterior and posterior) and maxillary antrostomy must be performed, followed by removal of the posterior maxillary wall to expose the pterygopalatine fossa contents.
- Sphenopalatine artery ligation, dissection of the palatine neurovascular bundle from its canal, separation of the vidian nerve, and removal of the lateral maxillary wall are performed to allow for inferolateral displacement of pterygopalatine fossa contents in order to expose the pterygoid plates (▶ Fig. 15.2a).
- The anterior portion of the pterygoid plates is then exposed and drilled to allow for greater space when transposing the flap (▶ Fig. 15.2b).

15.5.2 Temporalis Muscle Flap Harvest

- A hemicoronal incision is created from approximately 2 cm posterior to the hairline to the preauricular region no more than 8 mm anterior to the tragus to prevent injury of the facial nerve (CN VII).
- As an alternative, using the same preauricular incision as for the hemicoronal incision, a smaller incision can be made with the superior limb over the superior temporal line (▶ Fig. 15.3a).
- Care must be taken in the preauricular area to prevent injury of the STA.
- Superiorly, a plane of dissection is established in the subgaleal layer in between the galea and the pericranium (the galea is contiguous with the TPF inferiorly and the pericranium is contiguous to the deep TF) (▶ Fig. 15.3b).
- Dissection is carried anteriorly to the supraorbital ridge to raise the superior portion of the skin flap.
- Dissection is continued inferiorly until the STFP underlying the superficial layer of the deep TF is identified and incised along its superior border (▶ Fig. 15.3c). The zygomatic arch can be reached with inferior dissection along this plane to protect CN VII (▶ Fig. 15.3d).
- Attention is then turned to the preauricular region. The incision is taken down through the posterior portion of the STFP to the zygomatic root, where we can establish a subperiosteal plane along the zygomatic arch.
- Subperiosteal dissection is continued anteriorly along the zygoma. This helps us dissect the STFP and superficial layer of the deep TF off the zygoma in order to protect CN VII traveling along the TPF. Subperiosteal dissection is also performed on the medial zygomatic arch.
- Once the zygoma has been exposed, we make an incision through the deep TF along the temporal crest anteriorly, and it is carried posteriorly along the superior temporal line to delineate the TM.
- Blunt subperiosteal dissection is then performed in order to separate the TM and underlying periosteum from the skull. During this step, care must be taken to not damage the DTAs and preserve the flap pedicle.
- Once the flap has been harvested, it can be transposed and rotated to fill the necessary defect.
- The coronoid process can be removed or mobilized medially after osteotomy to increase the arc of rotation.
- The zygomatic arch can also be removed for easier elevation of the TMF, extra length, reduced trauma to flap, and facilitate coronoidectomy.[9]
- If a split TMF is desired, the procedure can be carried in the same manner. Once the flap is raised, it can be split coronally into a posterior portion. The anterior portion can be used for the reconstruction and the posterior portion is used to fill the remaining anterior TM defect.[4,5,8]
- Following flap harvest, a drain is placed in the donor site and closure is performed in a multilayer fashion.

15.5.3 Flap Transposition and Inset

Endoscopic Endonasal Reconstruction (*Video 15.1*)

- The TMF can be transposed endonasally following extended endonasal resections via transpterygoid or a transmaxillary approach.[9,12]
- It is mobilized medial to the zygomatic arch and transposed anterior to the previously drilled anterior surface of the pterygoid plates.
- The flap is then mobilized into the nasal cavity as would be done with a TPF flap (▶ Fig. 15.4a, b).
- Following, placement of preferred inlay graft, it is inset over the defect as an onlay flap.
- Dead spaces between the flap and the skull base are then eliminated to prevent flap migration and postoperative cerebrospinal fluid leak (▶ Fig. 15.4c, d).
- Surgicel, tissue glue, and Gelfoam can be placed over the flap with placement of bilateral nasal packing for flap bolstering.

Orbital Reconstruction

- The TMF can be used for orbital reconstruction following orbital exenteration as well as defects involving the orbital walls.[4,5]
- Following orbital exenteration and TMF harvest, a lateral orbitotomy is performed by drilling and removing the lateral orbital wall (▶ Fig. 15.5a–c).
- This creates a communication between the temporal fossa and orbital cavity that will allow for transposition of the TMF.
- The TMF is then transposed medially, through the lateral orbitotomy to fill the orbital defect (▶ Fig. 15.5d, e).
- This can also be used for anterior cranial base defects created following resection of the orbital roof.
- If the eyelid is preserved, it can be sutured to the flap. Otherwise, a full-thickness skin graft can be harvested to suture over the muscle.[11]

15.6 Postoperative Care

- Surgical drains should be placed posterior to the incision for adequate drainage.[4]
- Drain is removed on postoperative day 2 when no temporal fossa implant is used.[4]

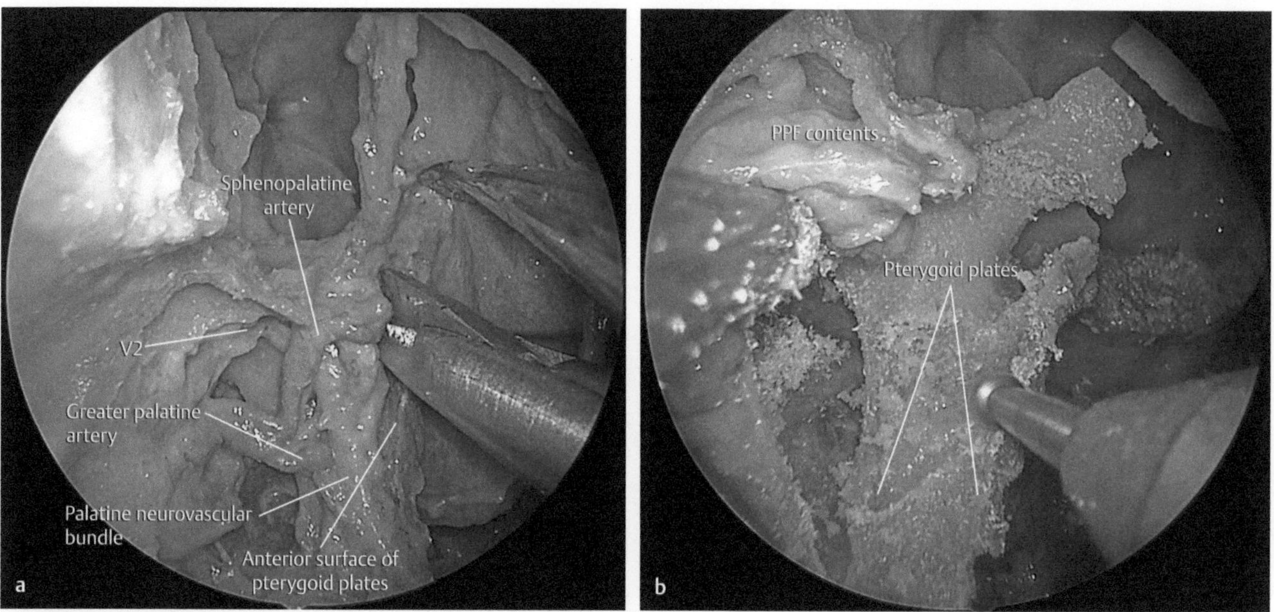

Fig. 15.2 Endoscopic endonasal anatomical dissection demonstrating exposure of the right pterygopalatine fossa (PPF) contents following removal of the posterior maxillary wall **(a)** and lateralization of PPF contents with drilling of the anterior surface of the pterygoid plates **(b)**.

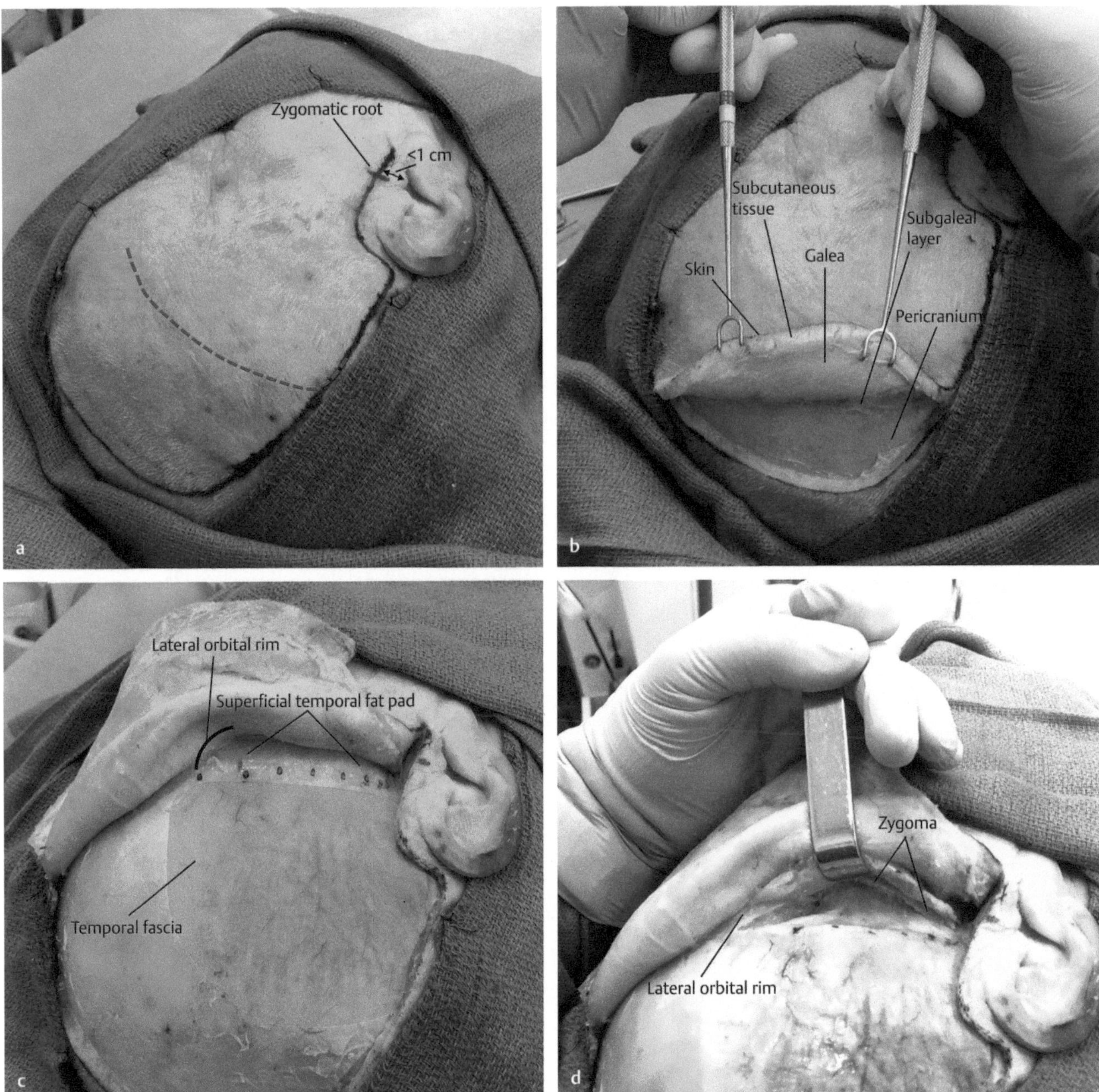

Fig. 15.3 **(a)** Anatomical dissection demonstrating a right hemicoronal (*blue continuous line*) and superior temporal incision (*blue dashed line*) that can be used for harvest. **(b)** Planes of dissection that must be identified prior to proceeding inferiorly and anteriorly with scalp elevation. **(c)** Exposure of superficial temporal fat pad (STFP) following raising of scalp flap. **(d)** Exposure of zygoma following incision of superficial temporal fascia and dissection through the STFP.

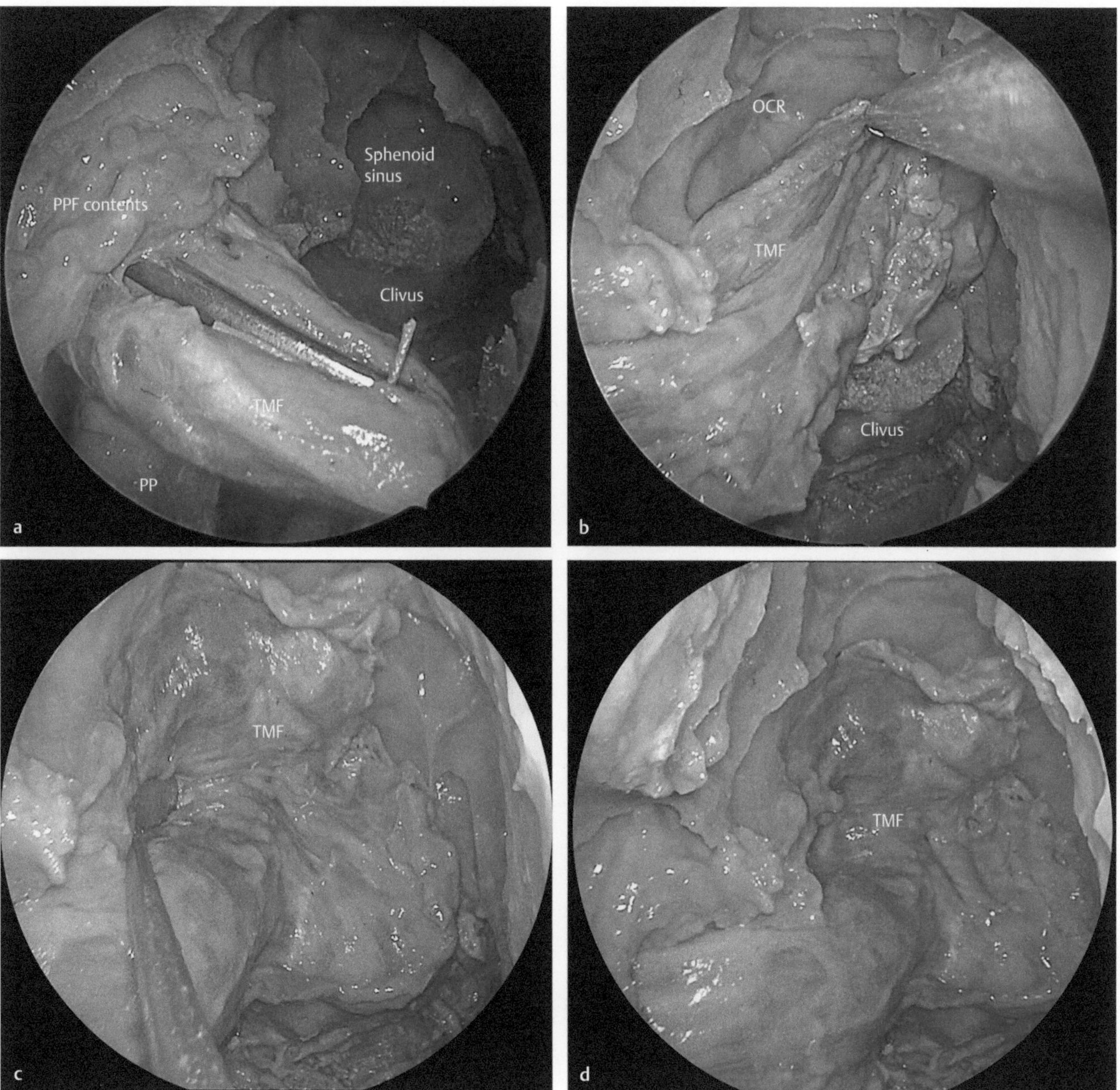

Fig. 15.4 (a) Anatomical dissection to show the endoscopic endonasal transposition of a right temporalis muscle flap (TMF). Note the flap passing posterior to the pterygopalatine fossa contents, which includes at that level the greater palatine nerve and descending palatine artery. **(b)** Inset of the flap over the defect. **(c)** Elimination of dead spaces between flap and skull base. **(d)** Final view after the inset of the flap covering the sella and clival region.
OCR, opticocarotid recess; PP, pterygoid plates, PPF, pterygopalatine fossa; TMF, temporalis muscle flap.

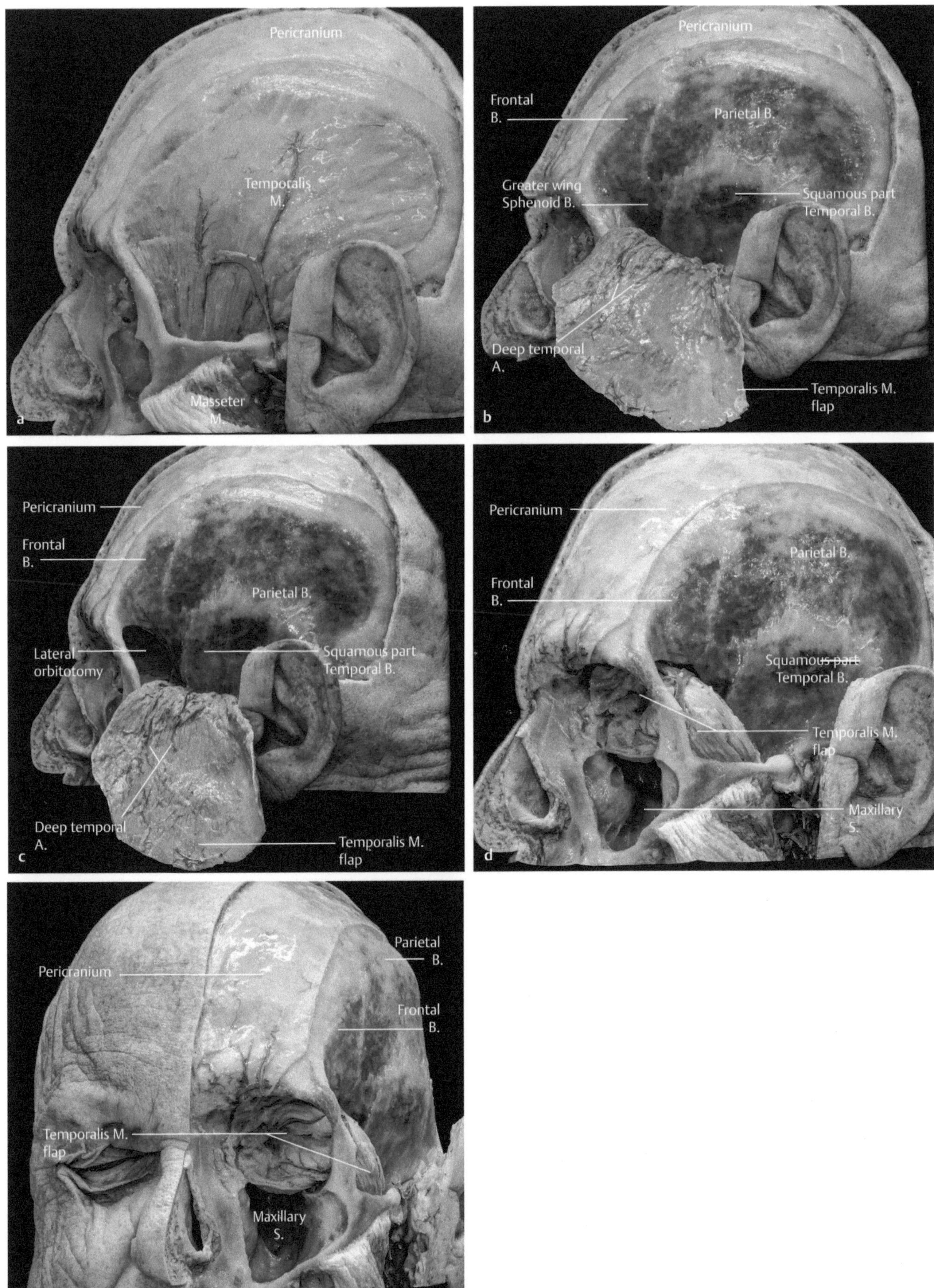

Fig. 15.5 **(a)** Anatomical dissection after removal of the left facial skin, scalp, anterior wall of the maxillary sinus, and orbital contents. **(b)** Harvest and inferior reflection of the temporalis muscle flap. **(c)** Lateral orbitotomy. **(d)** Transposition of the flap to reconstruct the orbital defect. **(e)** Frontal view of the flap inset. A, artery; B, bone; M, muscle; S, sinus.

- Consider delayed removal of drains when temporal fossa implant is placed.[4]
- Staples and/or sutures are removed on postoperative day 10.
- There is no need to place graft when in the oral or nasal cavity.[2]
- After endonasal skull base reconstruction, postoperative nasal debridement is required until complete mucosalization of the flap is achieved.

15.7 Complications

- *Flap necrosis*[1,4,8]:
  - Very infrequent (less than 2% failure rate).
  - Partial necrosis and dehiscence rate of less than 15%.
  - Caused by trauma to the vascular pedicle during flap harvest or severe tension created while transposing the flap.
  - Can be prevented by careful subperiosteal dissection and identification of DTAs and creating an anterior split TMF or removing zygomatic arch to decrease tension necessary to transpose it.
- *Facial nerve injury*:
  - Frontal branches (transient 10%,[1] resolves at 4–5 months[1,4]; permanent damage 3%).
  - Caused by excessive retraction during surgery and/or inexperience with surgical anatomy.[1]
  - Prevented by performing adequate dissection of the temporal fat pad and exposure of zygoma as described earlier.
  - The hemicoronal incision can also be extended anteriorly for less retraction on the scalp.[1,2,4]
  - Treatment for postoperative CN VII weakness includes: Massage, oral corticosteroids for 1 week, and artificial teardrops.
  - Surgical intervention (e.g., gold-weight implant) necessary if persistent > 6 months.[1]
- *Seroma/Hematoma*:
  - Preventable with adequate placement and removal of drains.
  - Higher incidence of seroma when temporal fossa reconstruction is performed (implants, cement); therefore, delayed removal of drains should be considered.[3,4]
- *Restricted mouth opening*:
  - 10% of cases.[1]
  - Initially due to postoperative edema.
  - Recommend physiotherapy for restoration of mouth opening (jaw stretching exercises).
  - Most patients resolve in 6 to 9 weeks with physiotherapy.
- *Temporal hollowing*[1,3,4,7]:
  - Most common aesthetic donor site morbidity.[4]
  - Most significant with complete rotation of TMF.
  - Prevented by:
    - Mobilizing the posterior portion of the muscle anteriorly in split TMF.
    - Preservation of STFP.
    - Temporal fossa implants.
    - Fat graft.

References

[1] Lam D, Carlson ER. The temporalis muscle flap and temporoparietal fascial flap. Oral Maxillofac Surg Clin North Am. 2014; 26(3):359–369

[2] Smith JE, Ducic Y, Adelson R. The utility of the temporalis muscle flap for oropharyngeal, base of tongue, and nasopharyngeal reconstruction. Otolaryngol Head Neck Surg. 2005; 132(3):373–380

[3] Smith JE, Ducic Y, Adelson RT. Temporalis muscle flap for reconstruction of skull base defects. Head Neck. 2010; 32(2):199–203

[4] Eldaly A, Magdy EA, Nour YA, Gaafar AH. Temporalis myofascial flap for primary cranial base reconstruction after tumor resection. Skull Base. 2008; 18 (4):253–263

[5] Lesavoy MA, Lee GK, Fan K, Dickinson B. Split, temporalis muscle flap for repair of recalcitrant cerebrospinal fluid leaks of the anterior cranial fossa. J Craniofac Surg. 2012; 23(2):539–542

[6] Speculand B. The origin of the temporalis muscle flap. Br J Oral Maxillofac Surg. 1992; 30(6):390–392

[7] Cordeiro PG, Wolfe SA. The temporalis muscle flap revisited on its centennial: advantages, newer uses, and disadvantages. Plast Reconstr Surg. 1996; 98 (6):980–987

[8] Hanasono MM, Utley DS, Goode RL. The temporalis muscle flap for reconstruction after head and neck oncologic surgery. Laryngoscope. 2001; 111 (10):1719–1725

[9] Thomas R, Girishan S, Chacko AG. Endoscopic transmaxillary transposition of temporalis flap for recurrent cerebrospinal fluid leak closure. J Neurol Surg B Skull Base. 2016; 77(6):445–448

[10] Kim YO, Park BY. Reverse temporalis muscle flap: treatment of large anterior cranial base defect with direct intracranial-nasopharyngeal communication. Plast Reconstr Surg. 1995; 96(3):576–584

[11] Uyar Y, Kumral TL, Yıldırım G, et al. Reconstruction of the orbit with a temporalis muscle flap after orbital exenteration. Clin Exp Otorhinolaryngol. 2015; 8(1):52–56

[12] Fortes FS, Carrau RL, Snyderman CH, et al. Transpterygoid transposition of a temporoparietal fascia flap: a new method for skull base reconstruction after endoscopic expanded endonasal approaches. Laryngoscope. 2007; 117 (6):970–976

16 Other Extranasal Flaps: Facial Artery Buccinator Flap and Palatal Flap

Garret W. Choby

16.1 Anatomy

- The pedicled facial artery buccinator (FAB) flap is based upon the facial artery:
  - The facial artery crosses the inferior border of the mandible and ascends toward the nasolabial fold, just lateral to the corner of the mouth.[1,2,3]
  - Its distal aspect is located along the anterior aspect of the buccinator, approximately 1 to 1.5 cm from the oral commissure[4,5]:
    - The artery runs along the superficial surface of the buccinator muscle.[1]
    - Variations of this vascular anatomy can occur and have been documented.[4,5]
  - The common facial artery typically branches into the inferior and superior labial artery, then terminates near the nasal ala, branching into the lateral nasal artery and angular artery.
  - This flap is sometimes alternatively referred to in the literature as the facial artery myomucosal (FAMM) flap.[1,6,7]
  - The buccinator muscle is located along the lateral wall of the oral cavity and serves to pull the angle of the mouth laterally and flatten the cheek area during chewing:
    - The muscle arises from the alveolar process of the maxilla and inserts near the oral commissure, often interdigitating with fibers of the orbicular oris muscle.[2,3]
    - It is innervated by the facial nerve.
- The palatal flap is based on the greater palatine artery (GPA) as it passes through the greater palatine foramen (GPF) from the pterygopalatine fossa (PPF) into the mucosa of the palate[8]:
  - The GPA is a branch of the descending palatine artery, which arises from the maxillary artery, as it enters into the PPF.
  - After entering into the GPF, its name changes to the GPA and it primarily supplies the mucosa of the hard palate.[9]
  - At its most distal portion, it anastomoses with branches of the sphenopalatine artery via the incisive canal to supply a portion of the nasal septum.[10]

16.2 Fundamentals

- FAB flap:
  - The FAB flap has been used for intraoral reconstruction; however, it is largely an experimental flap for skull base reconstruction and may be utilized in salvage scenarios.
  - This flap can be raised as a muscular flap or a myomucosal flap, depending on the situation and clinical need.
  - Depending on the location of the defect, this can either be an inferiorly based flap (allowing for anterograde arterial flow) or superiorly based flap (allowing for retrograde arterial flow).[1,3,6]
  - When retrograde arterial flow is incorporated, this occurs via the angular artery, or in some cases, via the lateral nasal artery.[3]
  - For skull base reconstruction, a superiorly based flap is generally preferred due to the proximity of the arterial pedicle to the skull base.
- Palatal flap:
  - The palatal flap is more commonly utilized for repair of cleft palate defects or other defects in the oral cavity.
  - The primary risk of the palatal flap is development of an oral-antral fistula, potentially with severe long-term functional consequences:
    - For this reason, as well as the technical challenges of raising the flap, make this a last-line option for skull base reconstruction.[11]

16.3 Indications

- FAB flap:
  - The indications for this flap are largely defects in the anterior cranial base, when the more commonly utilized options are not available, such as the nasoseptal flap or pericranial flap.
  - Cadaveric studies suggest that this flap can reach as far posterior as the planum sphenoidale,[3] although transposition to this region is a far reach.
- Palatal flap:
  - The indications for this flap are usually in salvage situations for defects arising near the clivus or sella.
  - Given its inferoposterior pedicle, it has a limited reach for defects of the anterior cranial fossa. Pedicle dissection within the PPF may be required to improve the reach.

16.4 Limitations

- FAB flap:
  - Limited reach due to the pedicle location in the gingivobuccal sulcus and translocation via the maxillary sinus.
  - Necessity of extensive intraoral dissection.
- Palatal flap:
  - Limited reach anteriorly toward the anterior cranial fossa.
  - Necessity of intraoral dissection.
  - Risk of postoperative oral-antral fistula.

16.5 Surgical Technique

- FAB flap (superiorly based flap with retrograde arterial flow):
  - The parotid duct should be identified intraorally and care should be taken to not disrupt this when planning incisions. The parotid duct is the marker for the most superior extent of the flap.
  - The size of the flap can be tailored to the defect size and location:
    - The most anterior border is typically 1 cm from the oral commissure.

- The posterior border is typically at the level of the second molar.
- The flap is elevated in the plane of the traditional FAMM flap, just superficial to the facial artery, along the buccal fat pad.
- This flap can be harvested to include mucosa and buccinator muscle (myomucosal flap), or buccinator alone (muscular flap).
- The facial artery is located and clipped adjacent to the inferior incision.
- The flap is introduced into the nasal cavity via the maxillary sinus, usually with a combination of a generous Caldwell-Luc osteotomy and endoscopic medial maxillectomy (▸ Fig. 16.1).

- Palatal flap:
  - The palatal flap can incorporate mucosa from the entire hard palate or the ipsilateral half of the hard palate, depending on the size and location of the defect:
    - Palatal mucosal incisions are carried out with the desired size of the flap with a needle point cautery, ensuring to leave at least 5 mm of mucosa between the incision and dentition.
    - The posterior limit of the flap is the hard–soft palate junction.
    - The flap is raised in a submucoperiosteal plane with careful preservation of the ipsilateral neurovascular bundle.
    - After the flap is elevated, a high-speed diamond drill is used transorally to enlarge the GPF, with care to ensure that the neurovascular bundle is not injured.
  - Attention is then turned transnasally, as a wide medial maxillectomy is created and the bone over the posterior maxillary sinus wall is removed:
    - PPF exploration is then undertaken to identify the junction of the sphenopalatine and greater palatine vasculature within the PPF.
    - The posterior half of the inferior turbinate, along with the nasal floor mucosa are then elevated toward the junction of the nasal floor and septum.
    - The bony osteotomy is expanded enough to allow transposition of the flap and neurovascular bundle into the nasal cavity (▸ Fig. 16.2).
    - The nasal floor and inferior turbinate mucosa are then carefully repositioned over the bony defect of the hard palate/nasal floor.[9]
    - This mucosa is secured with fibrin glue sealant.
  - The hard palate mucosal defect can be covered with an acellular dermal graft or skin graft, and secured in place with an Aquaplast splint (Qfix, Inc., Avondale, PA) that is then secured via screws to the hard palate for approximately 2 weeks postoperatively.[10]

16.6 Postoperative Care

- FAB flap:
  - Postoperative care for the intranasal portion of this procedure mimics that of other pedicled rotational flaps for skull base reconstruction:
    - Postoperative debridement is routinely carried out two to three times during the initial postoperative period.
    - Patients are instructed to use intranasal saline sprays or high-volume rinses, depending on the clinical scenario.
  - For the oral cavity portion of the procedure, patients are maintained on a soft diet for the first 2 weeks following surgery:
    - After the initial healing phase, some patients may develop trismus.
    - The utilization of a TheraBite device (Atos Medical, Inc., New Berlin, WI) may help to prevent this sequelae.
- Palatal flap:
  - Postoperative care for the intranasal portion of the procedure mimics that of the above.
  - For the oral cavity portion of the procedure, the patient is maintained on a liquid or soft diet for approximately 2 weeks postoperatively:
    - The Aquaplast splint (Qfix, Inc., Avondale, PA) is removed at 2 weeks postoperatively.

16.7 Complications

- FAB flap:
  - Incisional dehiscence can occur at the donor site, leading to risk of infection.
  - The parotid duct may be injured during dissection.
  - Postoperative epistaxis from branches of the sphenopalatine artery.
  - Numbness in the V2 distribution, most commonly from injury during the Caldwell-Luc portion of the procedure.
- Palatal flap:
  - The most deleterious complication of the palatal flap is development of an oroantral/oronasal fistula:
    - This risk may be mitigated by careful reconstruction of the nasal floor portion of the defect with nasal floor and inferior turbinate mucosa.
    - However, mucosal breakdown can occur, perhaps more commonly in patients who have undergone previous radiation.[10]
  - Flap necrosis, particularly in large flaps with incorporation of contralateral mucoperiosteum.
  - Long-term exposed bone of the hard palate if remucosalization is not complete.
  - Damage to dentition if incisions are carried to far anteriorly or laterally, near the dental roots.

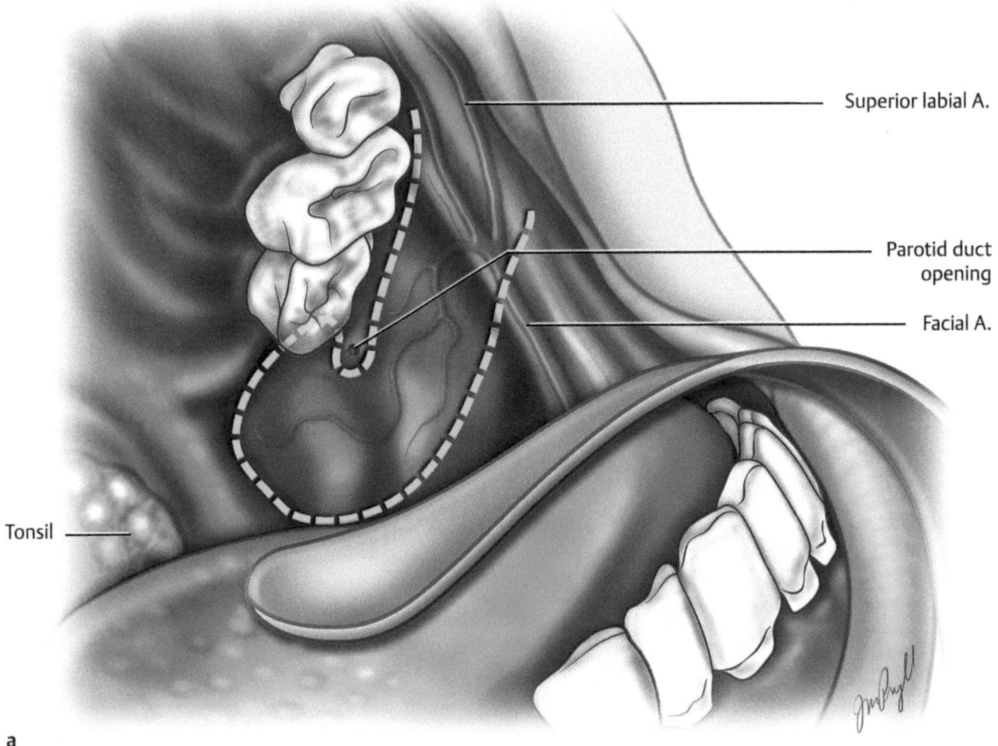

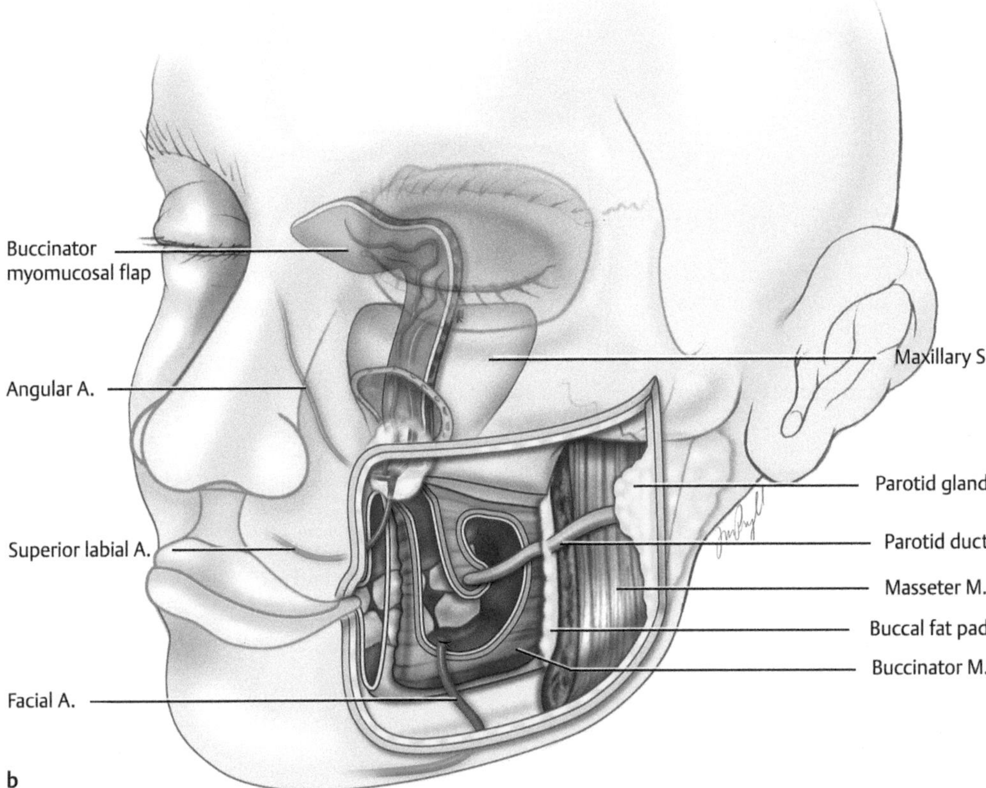

Fig. 16.1 (a) Illustration of the left buccal mucosa showing the incisions for the reverse-flow facial artery buccinator myomucosal flap (*green dashed line*). Note the relation of the incisions and the opening of the parotid duct. **(b)** Inset of the flap to cover an anterior skull base defect. Observe that the facial artery was transected inferiorly and the vascularization of the flap is based on the reverse flow from the superior labial and angular arteries. The anterior wall of the maxilla was opened for the transposition of the flap. A, artery; M, muscle; S, sinus.

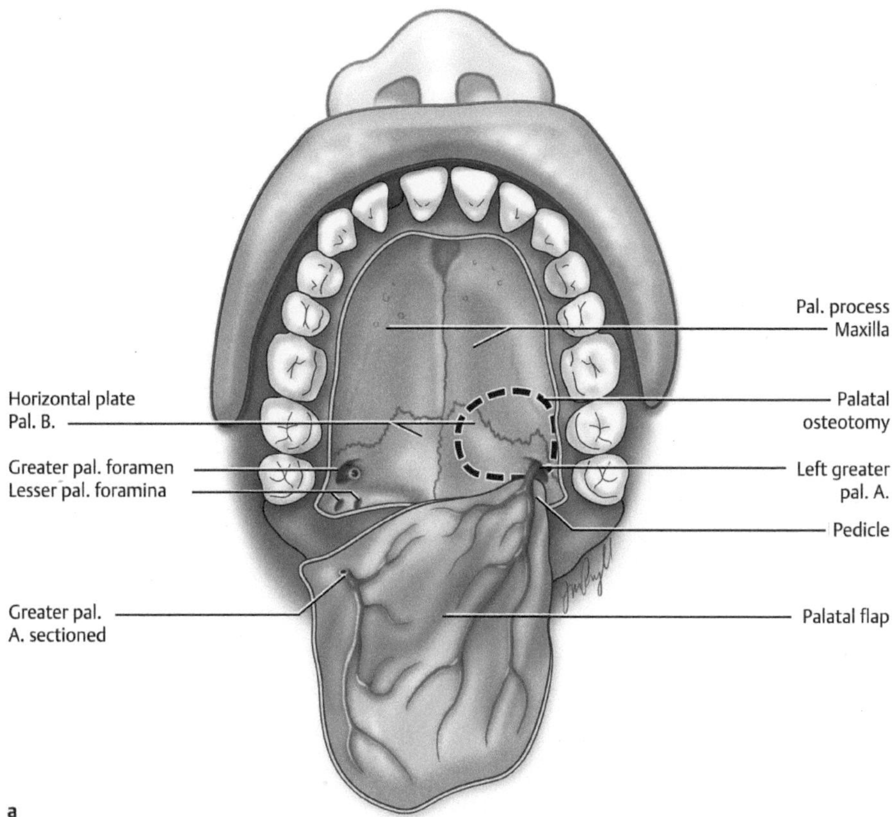

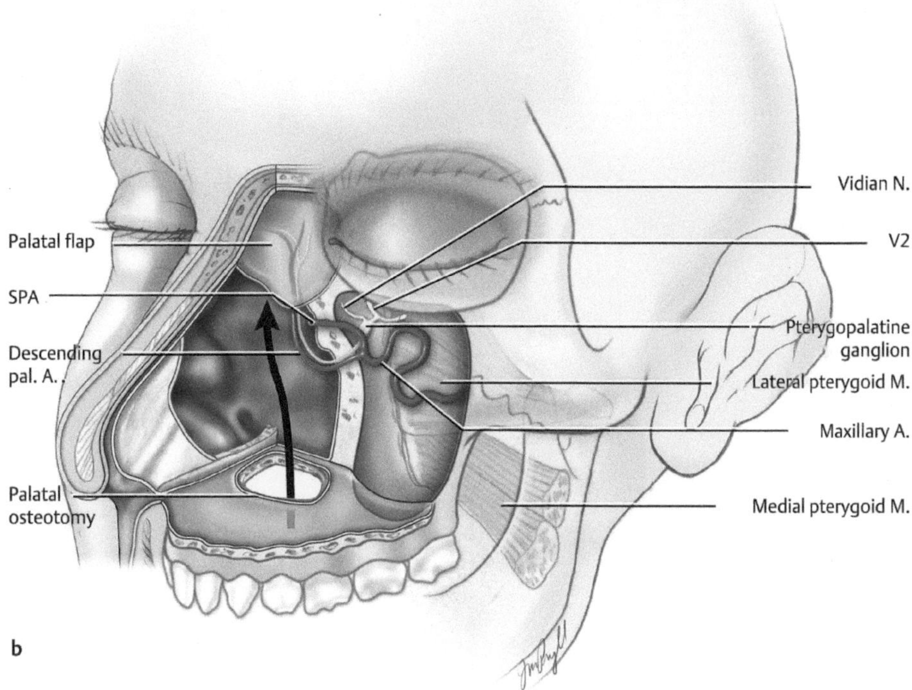

Fig. 16.2 **(a)** Illustration showing the harvest of the palatal flap. Note that the flap involves most of the mucoperiosteum of the hard palate and is pedicled on the left side requiring transection of the greater and lesser palatine neurovascular bundles on the contralateral side. *Black dashed line*—palatal osteotomy for the flap transposition to the nasal cavity. **(b)** Inset of the palatal flap to reconstruct an anterior cranial base defect. In this case, dissection within the pterygopalatine fossa (PPF) releases the vascular pedicle and allows superior mobilization of the flap toward the anterior cranial base. *Arrow*—movement of the flap toward the skull base. The descending palatine artery (DPA) is a branch of the maxillary artery. The DPA is named greater palatine artery after passing through the greater palatine foramen to supply the palate mucoperiosteum. A, artery; B, bone; M, muscle; N, nerve; SPA, sphenopalatine artery.

References

[1] Farzal Z, Lemos-Rodriguez AM, Rawal RB, et al. The reverse-flow facial artery buccinator flap for skull base reconstruction: key anatomical and technical considerations. J Neurol Surg B Skull Base. 2015; 76(6):432–439

[2] Franco D, Rocha D, Arnaut M, Jr, Freitas R, Alonso N. Versatility of the buccinator myomucosal flap in atypical palate reconstructions. J Craniomaxillofac Surg. 2014; 42(7):1310–1314

[3] Rivera-Serrano CM, Oliver C, Prevedello D, et al. Pedicled facial buccinator (FAB) flap: a new flap for reconstruction of skull base defects. Laryngoscope. 2010; 120 Suppl 4:S234

[4] Dupoirieux L, Plane L, Gard C, Penneau M. Anatomical basis and results of the facial artery musculomucosal flap for oral reconstruction. Br J Oral Maxillofac Surg. 1999; 37(1):25–28

[5] Zhao Z, Li S, Yan Y, et al. New buccinator myomucosal island flap: anatomic study and clinical application. Plast Reconstr Surg. 1999; 104(1):55–64

[6] Xie L, Lavigne F, Rahal A, Moubayed SP, Ayad T. Facial artery musculomucosal flap for reconstruction of skull base defects: a cadaveric study. Laryngoscope. 2013; 123(8):1854–1861

[7] Xie L, Lavigne P, Lavigne F, Ayad T. Modified facial artery musculomucosal flap for reconstruction of posterior skull base defects. J Neurol Surg Rep. 2016; 77(2):e98–e101

[8] Moore BA, Magdy E, Netterville JL, Burkey BB. Palatal reconstruction with the palatal island flap. Laryngoscope. 2003; 113(6):946–951

[9] Oliver CL, Hackman TG, Carrau RL, et al. Palatal flap modifications allow pedicled reconstruction of the skull base. Laryngoscope. 2008; 118(12):2102–2106

[10] Hackman T, Chicoine MR, Uppaluri R. Novel application of the palatal island flap for endoscopic skull base reconstruction. Laryngoscope. 2009; 119 (8):1463–1466

[11] Patel MR, Taylor RJ, Hackman TG, et al. Beyond the nasoseptal flap: outcomes and pearls with secondary flaps in endoscopic endonasal skull base reconstruction. Laryngoscope. 2014; 124(4):846–852

Section V

Free Grafts

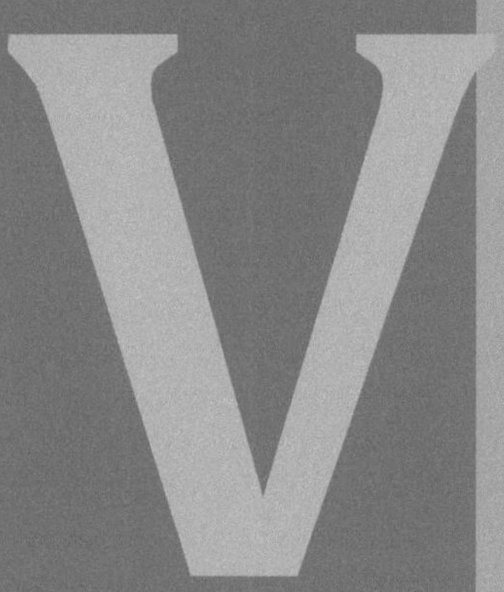

17 Mucosal Grafts

Ramón Moreno-Luna, Maria Peris-Celda, and Carlos D. Pinheiro-Neto

17.1 Fundamentals

- The most common areas to harvest intranasal mucosal grafts are nasal floor, middle turbinate (MT), nasal septum, inferior turbinate, and lateral nasal wall (anterior to the MT) (▶ Fig. 17.1).
- Free mucosal grafts (FMGs) usually involve a smaller area of harvest compared to the flap in the same anatomical region.
- Our work-horse graft is FMG from the nasal floor.
- In general, FMGs from the nasal cavity have been frequently used to reconstruct skull base defects with good outcomes.[1,2]
- The sinus mucosa is thinner and usually not commonly used as a graft.
- The selection of the site to harvest the graft is based on surgeon's experience, availability, and impact on postoperative quality of life.
- Our first choice is the nasal floor because of the easy harvest, homogenous mucosal thickness, and no increased postoperative nasal morbidity associated with the denuded bone at the nasal floor (measured with sinonasal outcome test-22). Maybe the lack of significant airflow along the nasal floor contributes to less crusting when compared to the denuded septum after nasoseptal flap harvest.[3]
- The MT FMG usually requires the resection of the turbinate with compromise of nasal airflow and heat transport.[4]
- Anterior nasal septum FMG is associated with more crust formation during the healing process of the exposed septal cartilage.
- Most of the intranasal mucosal grafts are mucoperiosteal grafts (nasal floor, inferior and MTs, anterior lateral nasal wall).
- For the graft inset, the subperiosteal/subperichondrial surface is oriented toward the defect and the mucosal surface toward the nasal cavity.
- The graft size is tailored according to the size of the defect and can be augmented with inclusion of an adjacent area.
- Mucosal grafts tend to contract during the healing process. Its reuse in reoperations is possible, but it can be challenging due to the memory that the mucosa assumes along the defect and risk of laceration of the graft during its elevation.
- At 3-month postoperative magnetic resonance imaging (MRI), mucosal grafts used for sellar reconstruction show enhancement with contrast. The grafts also maintain stable thickness over the years as observed in follow-up MRIs.[5]
- The harvest of FMG may preclude the use of a pedicled flap from the correspondent area in the future.

17.2 Indications

- In general, dural defects < 1.5 cm with low-flow intraoperative CSF leak. In some cases of larger defects, FMG can still be used successfully, such as for reconstruction of sellar defects after resection of large pituitary tumors.
- Meningoencephaloceles of the lateral recess of the sphenoid sinus.
- Defects involving the cribriform plate and its lateral lamella.
- Posterior table of frontal sinus defects.
- Sellar defects after resection of pituitary tumors, including defects > 1.5 cm.[6]
- FMG can also be used to resurface the septum donor site after nasoseptal flap harvest or the skull base bone after radical polypectomy.[7]

17.3 Limitations

- Longer time for healing (nonvascularized reconstruction).
- Sinonasal pathologies such as nasal polyposis, hypertrophy/atrophy of turbinates, deviated septum, septal perforation, and chronic inflammatory diseases may impact the dimensions, thickness, and/or quality of the mucosal graft.
- Anatomical variations such as paradoxical MT and bone hyperostosis may increase the risk of lacerations during the harvest.
- Hypertrophy of the inferior turbinate may restrict the space within the inferior meatus for the harvest of a nasal floor FMG. Inferior turbinoplasty can be performed to improve the inferior meatus space.
- History of inferior maxillary antrostomy compromises the lateral extension of the nasal floor FMG.

17.4 Surgical Technique

17.4.1 Nasal Floor Free Mucosal Graft (*Videos 17.1 and 17.2*)

- Mucosal vasoconstriction is achieved with topical oxymetazoline or epinephrine. Submucosal infiltration of 0.5% xylocaine with 1:200,000 epinephrine is not necessary but may facilitate the graft harvest.
- The nasal floor FMG can be elevated exclusively from the nasal floor (▶ Fig. 17.1a) or include the mucosa of the inferior meatus lateral wall (▶ Fig. 17.1b) and/or nasal septum (extended nasal floor mucosal graft).
- A vertical incision can be performed at the head of the inferior turbinate with an endoscopic sinus scissors to allow upward movement of the turbinate and better access to the inferior meatus.
- Four incisions are performed to harvest the graft.
- The incisions are done with a needle tip Bovie set at 10 W.
- The posterior incision is performed in the coronal place from septum to the tail of the inferior turbinate along the transition between the soft palate and hard palate. This transition can be identified by palpation with the tip of the Bovie bent at 45 degrees.
- The lateral incision is performed along the attachment of the inferior turbinate to the lateral wall of the inferior meatus. Anteriorly, it is very important to avoid injury of the Hasner valve. At the posterior aspect of the incision, there is a potential risk of injury to the descending palatine artery or even the greater palatine nerve traveling through the greater palatine canal.

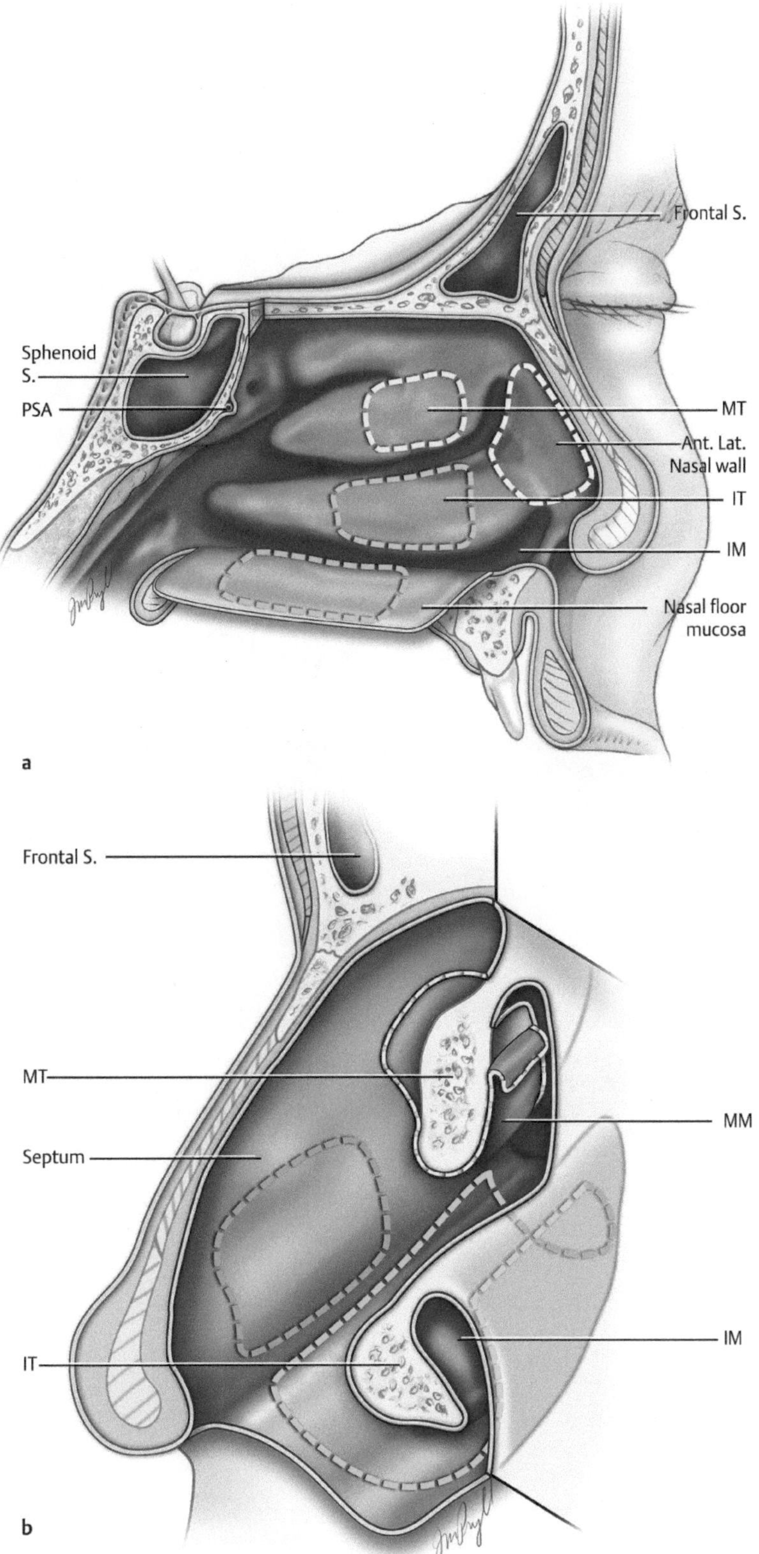

Fig. 17.1 (a) Illustration of the left nasal cavity sagittal view to show the areas of harvest of free mucosal grafts (FMGs). *Yellow dashed line*—middle turbinate (MT) graft. In this case, the turbinate is left attached to the skull base and the mucosa of its nasal surface is harvested. Careful dissection should be taken to avoid fracture of the turbinate and possible cerebrospinal fluid (CSF) leak. *White dashed line*—graft from the anterior lateral nasal wall. *Green dashed line*—inferior turbinate mucosal graft. *Blue dashed line*—graft from the nasal floor. **(b)** Cross-section view of the left nasal cavity. *Yellow dashed line*—MT graft with inclusion of the nasal and meatal surfaces. For this harvest, the turbinate is removed from the nasal cavity and the mucosal elevation is performed on the back table. *Green dashed line*—nasal floor FMG with inclusion of the mucosa of the lateral wall of the inferior meatus. *Blue dashed line*—graft from the nasal septum. This is the only mucoperichondrial graft represented while all the previous ones are mucoperiosteal grafts. A mucoperiosteal graft from the nasal septum can be elevated from the posterior part of the septum (not illustrated).
Ant, anterior; Lat, lateral; IM, inferior meatus; IT, inferior turbinate; MM, middle meatus; MT, middle turbinate; PSA, posterior septal artery; S, sinus.

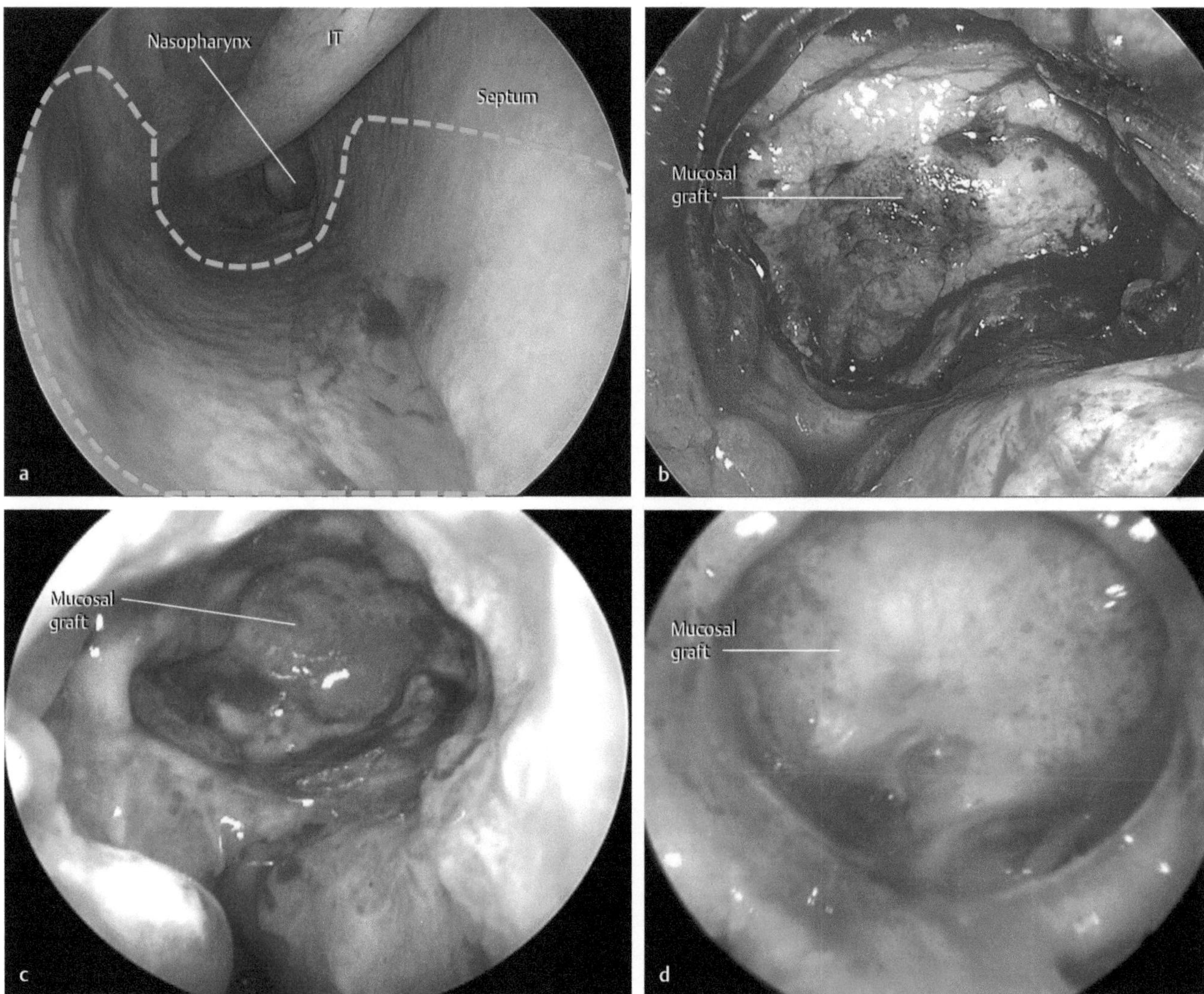

Fig. 17.2 (a, b) Intraoperative pictures obtained with a 0 degree endoscope of the right nasal cavity. **(a)** *Blue dashed line*—incisions to harvest an extended nasal floor mucosal graft with inclusion of the lateral wall of the inferior meatus mucosa and also part of the septal mucosa. A vertical incision at the head of the inferior turbinate was performed to allow great mobilization of the turbinate superiorly and wide access to the inferior meatus. **(b)** Inset of the graft to cover a sellar defect after pituitary tumor resection. **(c, d)** Postoperative pictures obtained with 0-degree endoscope through the right nasal cavity during follow-up visits in clinic. **(c)** One-month postoperative visit after nasal debridement showing the graft well healed to the skull base. **(d)** Four-month postoperative picture. IT, inferior turbinate. (Reproduced with permission from Peris-Celda et al.[6])

- The medial incision varies according to the desired size of the graft. This incision can be performed along the transition between the septum and the nasal floor. If a larger graft is needed, the medial incision is made along the septal mucosa.
- For sellar reconstruction, the medial incision is performed along the septal mucosa about 5 to 8 mm superior to the nasal floor. This should provide sufficient coverage for most sellar reconstructions and enough extra mucosa to contact the bone edges of the defect.
- The anterior incision is made in the coronal plane immediately posterior to incisive foramen region from the head of the inferior turbinate toward the septum. If a larger graft is needed, the anterior incision can be performed at the mucocutaneous junction of the nasal vestibule, along the piriform aperture. The incisive artery is identified 1 cm posterior to the nasal spine and transected with the needle tip Bovie.
- After all four incisions are completed, the nasal floor FMG is elevated in a subperiosteal plane with a Cottle dissector, leaving the underlying bone denuded.
- The harvest is performed from anterior to posterior in a centripetal fashion, starting along the incision lines (anterior, medial, and lateral) and elevating the mucosa toward the center and posteriorly until the posterior incision is reached.
- Endoscopic microscissors may be used to sharply divide some areas of mucosa not completely incised by the Bovie. It is important to confirm that the mucosa is completely separated before pulling out the graft to prevent mucosal lacerations.
- The graft is removed from the nasal cavity and its mucosal surface is marked with a marking pen to facilitate its identification during the graft inset. The graft should be kept in saline solution until the time for the reconstruction.
- Before placement of the graft, the mucosa around the skull base defect should be completely removed to allow appropriate contact of the subperiosteal surface of the graft to the bone.
- Fascia lata or synthetic collagen dural graft is placed inlay and the FMG is placed onlay (▸ Fig. 17.2).
- The average surface area of the graft with inclusion of part of the septal mucosa is 8 square cm. This allows adequate reconstruction of unilateral anterior cranial base defects, covering the ethmoidal roof from the anterior ethmoidal artery to the planum sphenoidale.[8] In the coronal plane, the graft covers from the superior septum/cribriform plate, ethmoidal roof, and part of the lamina papyracea.
- Oxidized cellulose pieces are placed at the borders of the graft for stabilization, followed by dural sealant and absorbable packing.
- Silastic septal splints are placed bilaterally and secured anteriorly with a 2–0 Prolene. The splints help to prevent synechiae.

17.4.2 Middle Turbinate Free Mucosal Graft

- The harvest of the MT FMG can be done from its medial (nasal) surface, maintaining the turbinate attached. The mucosa is elevated in a subperiosteal plane from the vertical portion of the MT. Care should be taken to avoid fracture of the MT at the skull base and risk of CSF leak (▸ Fig. 17.1a).
- If a larger graft is needed, the entire mucosa can be harvested (▸ Fig. 17.1b). The MT is removed and the mucosal harvest is completed at the surgical back table. A Cottle dissector is used to carefully remove the bone of the vertical portion of the MT. The meatal and the nasal surfaces of the mucosa of the turbinate are open like a "book."
- The MT FMG inset follows the same concepts previously described.

17.4.3 Nasal Septum Free Mucosal Graft

- It can be harvested anteriorly (mucoperichondrium) or posteriorly (mucoperiosteum) (▸ Fig. 17.1b).
- Mucoperiosteal graft harvest is preferable due to less crust formation postoperatively.
- For the anterior harvest, 1 cm of mucosa bellow the nasal dorsum should be preserved to avoid scarring and risk of saddle nose.
- To minimize nasal crusting, the exposed cartilage or bone may be removed, and the subperichondrial or subperiosteal surface of the contralateral mucosa is left exposed.

17.4.4 Inferior Turbinate Free Mucosal Graft

- The nasal (medial) surface of the inferior turbinate can be harvested and used as an FMG (▸ Fig. 17.1a).[9]
- The mucosa is elevated off the inferior turbinate bone.
- The inferior border and tail of the inferior turbinate are boneless. The separation of the nasal and metal surface is usually performed sharply with endoscopic sinus scissors.
- Due to the high vascularization of the inferior turbinate, the harvest can be bloody and the identification of the surgical plane is difficult.
- Total inferior turbinectomy is not recommended for graft harvest due to its negative impact on nasal physiology, risk of paradoxical nasal obstruction, and nasal crusting.

17.4.5 Lateral Nasal Wall Free Mucosal Graft (Anterior)

- The FMG is elevated from the ascending process of the maxilla just anterior to the MT (▸ Fig. 17.1a).
- Avoid harvest mucosa anterior to the ascending process of the maxilla to prevent injury to the upper lateral cartilage and risk of collapse of the internal nasal valve and/or saddle nose.

17.5 Postoperative Care

- Postoperative visits 1 week, 1 month, and 4 months after surgery for nasal debridement.
- Large-volume saline nasal irrigation is used until the nasal mucosa is completely healed.
- The nasal floor donor site is usually near-totally mucosalized or covered with granulation tissue at 1 month postoperative visit.[2,10]

17.6 Complications

- Usually, intranasal FMGs have lower morbidity compared to vascularized flaps.[6]

17.6.1 Nasal Floor Free Mucosal Graft

- Anterior dissection within the inferior meatus carries risk of injury of the Hasner valve and consequent epiphora. It is a very low risk if careful dissection within the inferior meatus is performed. After more than 400 nasal floor FMGs harvested for sellar reconstruction, we haven't had any case of epiphora or dacryocystitis postoperatively.
- Dissection around the incisive foramen can damage sensory fibers to the upper incisors causing numbness. Usually the numbness is transitory, but it may last for few months or even be permanent.
- Synechiae between the inferior turbinate and septum may occur. Use of plastic splints is recommended during the first postoperative week to avoid complication.

17.6.2 Middle Turbinate Free Mucosal Graft

- CSF leak during the middle turbinectomy or inadvertent fracture of the MT.[11]
- Anosmia or hyposmia due to injury of olfactory filaments near the cribriform plate.

17.6.3 Nasal Septum Free Mucosal Graft

- Septal perforation.
- Synechiae.
- Saddle nose.

17.6.4 Inferior Turbinate Free Mucosal Graft

- Atrophic rhinitis.
- Paradoxical nasal obstruction.
- Nasal crusting.
- Synechiae.

17.6.5 Lateral Nasal Wall Free Mucosal Graft (Anterior)

- Trauma to upper lateral cartilages if dissection is too anterior.
- Synechiae.

References

[1] Schlosser RJ, Bolger WE. Nasal cerebrospinal fluid leaks: critical review and surgical considerations. Laryngoscope. 2004; 114(2):255–265

[2] Dadgostar A, Okpaleke C, Al-Asousi F, Javer A. The application of a free nasal floor mucoperiosteal graft in endoscopic sinus surgery. Am J Rhinol Allergy. 2017; 31(3):196–199

[3] Scagnelli RJ, Patel V, Peris-Celda M, Kenning TJ, Pinheiro-Neto CD. Implementation of free mucosal graft technique for sellar reconstruction after pituitary surgery: outcomes of 158 consecutive patients. World Neurosurg. 2019; 122: e506–e511

[4] Patel V, Viswanathan R, Ruffner R, Peris-Celda M, Pinheiro-Neto CD. Comparing nasal physiology after superior ethmoidal and traditional endoscopic anterior cranial base approaches. Rhinology. 2020; 58(6):629–631

[5] Kim CS, Patel U, Pastena G, et al. The magnetic resonance imaging appearance of endoscopic endonasal skull base defect reconstruction using free mucosal graft. World Neurosurg. 2019; 126:e165–e172

[6] Peris-Celda M, Chaskes M, Lee DD, Kenning TJ, Pinheiro-Neto CD. Optimizing sellar reconstruction after pituitary surgery with free mucosal graft: results from the first 50 consecutive patients. World Neurosurg. 2017; 101:180–185

[7] Moreno-Luna R, Gonzalez-Garcia J, Maza-Solano JM, et al. Free nasal floor mucosal grafting after endoscopic total ethmoidectomy for severe nasal polyposis: a pilot study. Rhinology. 2019; 57(3):219–224

[8] González-García J, Moreno-Luna R, Palacios-García J, et al. Radioanatomical study of the extended free nasal floor mucosal graft and its clinical applications. Laryngoscope Investig Otolaryngol. 2020; 5(6):1011–1018

[9] Cassano M, Felippu A. Endoscopic treatment of cerebrospinal fluid leaks with the use of lower turbinate grafts: a retrospective review of 125 cases. Rhinology. 2009; 47(4):362–368

[10] Suh JD, Ramakrishnan VR, DeConde AS. Nasal floor free mucosal graft for skull base reconstruction and cerebrospinal fluid leak repair. Ann Otol Rhinol Laryngol. 2012; 121(2):91–95

[11] Chakravarthi S, Gonen L, Monroy-Sosa A, Khalili S, Kassam A. Endoscopic endonasal reconstructive methods to the anterior skull base. Semin Plast Surg. 2017; 31(4):203–213

18 Nonmucosal Grafts: Fat, Muscle, Fascia Lata, and Septal Cartilage

Laura Salgado-Lopez, Maria Peris-Celda, and Carlos D. Pinheiro-Neto

18.1 Anatomy

- Abdominal subcutaneous fat:
  - The subcutaneous fat layer is located immediately below the skin.
  - The superficial and deep fasciae are encountered below the subcutaneous fat. The superficial fascia overlies the entire anterior abdominal wall and the deep fascia surrounds the rectus abdomini muscles.
  - The deep inferior epigastric artery provides the main blood supply to the lower abdominal wall. It branches off the external iliac artery and follows a variable trajectory along the internal surface of the rectus abdomini muscle. Its musculocutaneous perforator branches pierce both fasciae to reach the skin and are more abundant in the area located 4 cm lateral to the umbilicus.[1]
- Muscle:
  - Muscle graft can be harvested from the temporalis muscle, rectus abdomini, or vastus lateralis. The latter two grafts can be harvested in combination with the fat graft and also in combination with fascia lata in the case of vastus lateralis or temporal fascia in the case of the temporalis muscle. Usually, muscle grafts are used to plug small dural openings or to fill limited dead space.
- Fascia lata:
  - The fascia lata constitutes the deep fascia of the thigh and arises superiorly from the tensor fascia lata and gluteus medius and maximus muscles to insert distally on the lateral condyle of the tibia.[2]
  - The fascia is thickened laterally to form the iliotibial band, which is harvested for use as graft.
  - The vastus lateralis head of the quadriceps femoris lies underneath the fascia lata.
  - The lateral femoral cutaneous nerve pierces the fascia lata beneath the inguinal ligament and runs laterally and distally within the deep subcutaneous tissue of the anterolateral region of the thigh to give terminal cutaneous branches.[3]
- Septal cartilage:
  - The nasal septum is formed by the septal (quadrangular) cartilage, perpendicular plate of the ethmoid, vomer, and maxillary crest.
  - The septal cartilage is covered by a mucoperichondrium. The subperichondrial plane is an avascular plane.
  - The septal cartilage is composed by hyaline cartilage, which has more collagen than elastin compared to elastic cartilage but fewer collagen fibers compared to fibrocartilage.[4]

18.2 Fundamentals

- Optimal cranial base reconstruction is achieved with multilayer technique.
- The flaps and grafts described in the previous chapters are mostly used to cover the endonasal lining of the defect (onlay reconstruction).
- The autologous nonmucosal grafts are usually used for inlay repairing, filling of dead space, or improving rigidness of the reconstruction.
- The dural repair is also largely performed with synthetic dural substitutes to avoid donor site morbidity. However, in more complex reconstructions, autologous grafts are superior and recommended instead of synthetic materials.
- Different tissues with specific characteristics can be used as free grafts in cranial base reconstruction with distinct purposes.
- Mucosal grafts may be used to cover small nonmucosal grafts. The mucosal graft should be large enough to cover not only the nonmucosal graft surface but also to establish adequate contact to the surrounding vascularized recipient site for appropriate healing.
- In some cases of large defects and complex reconstruction, areas of exposed nonmucosal grafts to the nasal cavity may be inevitable. All effort should be directed to maximize the coverage with vascularized flap, leaving minimal area of nonmucosal graft exposure.
- Do not use nonmucosal grafts over mucosal surfaces. It is imperative to remove all the mucosa around the defect. The graft will not heal over mucosa.

18.3 Indications

- Fat/muscle grafts:
  - Extradural filling of the clivus after clivectomy. Fat graft is the most commonly used.
  - Intracranial filling of the frontal sinus after its cranialization. Small defects can be filled with either fat or muscle, large defects are usually filled with fat graft.
  - Intracranial filling of dead space after resection of large anterior cranial base tumors. In such cases, the tumor leaves an empty space intracranially which complicates the inset of the inlay and onlay reconstruction. Fat graft can be used to partially fill the space, particularly along the anterior border of the defect. Care should be taken to avoid overpacking with fat and consequent mass effect.
  - Plug of small dural tears.
  - Patch internal carotid wall tear after injury (muscle graft only).
- Fascia lata graft:
  - Suprasellar defects (inlay–onlay button graft).
  - Clival defects (inlay–onlay button graft).
  - Anterior cranial base defects (usually inlay single layer).
- Septal cartilage graft:
  - Meningoencephalocele/spontaneous cerebrospinal fluid (CSF) leak. The buttress of cartilage improves the protection of the intracranial space and increases the strength of the reconstruction against the CSF pressure, which is particularly important in patients with high intracranial pressure.
  - Orbital defects. Medial or inferior orbital wall defects to contain orbital fat. Orbital roof to minimize brain pulsation over the eye globe.

18.4 Limitations

- History of prior radiation therapy increases the risk of graft failure. Vascularized flaps are recommended.[5]
- It is common for cartilage and fat grafts to suffer reabsorption. Fat grafts often reduce in volume by over 50%.[6]
- Additional incision and donor site morbidity.
- Prolonged healing process compared to vascularized flaps.

18.5 Surgical Technique

- Abdominal fat graft/abdominal muscle graft:
  - A 2 cm transverse paraumbilical incision.
  - Routinely done on the left side to prevent confusion with possible future appendectomy or other abdominal surgery on the right side.
  - Care is taken to limit the dissection superficially to the abdominal superficial fascia.
  - One-piece fat graft is preferred to assure a watertight seal.
  - A small incision can be made at the abdominal superficial fascia and a piece of fascia or abdominis rectus muscle can be harvested if needed for the reconstruction.
  - No synthetic material should be interposed between the graft and the skull base bone.[7]
  - The fat graft can be placed in the intracranial compartment to close dead spaces as part of a multilayered reconstruction.
  - Small pieces can be used as plug to seal small dural tears or holes in a flap.
  - A dermal fat graft can also be harvested to increase stability of the adipose tissue and facilitate its inset. Dermal fat grafts are particularly interesting for filling volume.
  - Pieces of oxidized cellulose can be used to wrap the fat graft to facilitate its manipulation and inset.
- Temporalis muscle:
  - A 3 cm scalp incision is made behind the hairline, starting superiorly at the superior temporal line in a coronal plane.
  - The temporoparietal fascia and deep temporal fascia are then incised in the same manner and a temporalis muscle graft is harvested.
  - The temporalis muscle graft is usually used as a plug to seal small dural tears as part of a multilayered reconstruction.[8]
  - It can also be used intracranially to fill dead space.
  - Alternatively, the temporalis muscle patch can be positioned directly over an injured internal carotid artery (ICA) to stop an intraoperative bleeding. After placing the temporalis muscle, gentle pressure has to be applied with overlying cotton patties for 10 minutes.[9]
- Fascia lata graft (Video 18.1):
  - A 4 to 8 cm skin incision is made in the lateral thigh above the iliotibial band, starting 10 cm superior to the lateral femoral epicondyle. The incision length depends on the desired length of the graft.
  - The subcutaneous tissue and the fat are dissected to expose the underlying fascia lata fibers running parallel to the axis of the leg. Further exposure of the anterior surface of the fascia can be achieved by superior and inferior blunt dissections.
  - A rectangular piece of fascia is then incised and removed. The size of the fascia graft can be tailored depending on the size of the skull base defect.
  - An additional small piece of the underlying vastus lateralis muscle can be harvested if needed for the skull base reconstruction.
  - Fat can also be harvested from the subcutaneous layer if needed.
  - The fascial defect is usually left unreconstructed especially if a large graft was harvested. If the fascial defect is small, the edges can be loosely approximated to prevent muscle herniation, leaving a generous hiatus between the fascia lata edges to avoid compartmental syndrome.
  - The fascia lata graft can be positioned alone in an inlay manner as part of a multilayered reconstruction.
  - Alternatively, two grafts of fascia lata can be sutured together with a hemitransfixation stitch in the center to create an inlay–onlay button graft.[10] The onlay fascia is slightly larger than the inlay graft. One of the layers is marked with a marking pen to help identification of the layers during the inset (▶ Fig. 18.1).
  - The fascia lata inlay–onlay button graft can be used for primary dural repair in conjunction with the nasoseptal flap for high-flow intraoperative CSF leaks, such as suprasellar defects. The onlay graft covers completely the defect but should not be larger than the nasoseptal flap. The flap should cover the onlay fascia and bone around the fascia for appropriate healing to the skull base[10,11] (▶ Fig. 18.2).
  - The fascia lata graft can also be used to create a "gasket seal" around a bone buttress (i.e., a piece of vomer). The fascia lata graft is fashioned to be larger than the bone defect and centered over the defect. Then a piece of bone roughly the size of the cranial base defect is centered over the fascia lata. The bone buttress is then wedged in place and the redundant fascia lata is wrapped around the bone, creating a watertight seal.[12]
- Septal cartilage:
  - The mucosa is incised at the caudal border of the septum and elevated in a subperichondrial plane toward the vomer.
  - Leaving a 1 cm strut at the nasal dorsum, a cartilaginous incision parallel to the nasal dorsum is performed from superior to inferior. At 1 cm from the caudal border of the septum, this incision is turned posteriorly toward the nasal spine. This technique will preserve a 1 cm L-shaped strut to support the nose.[13]
  - The contralateral mucosa is elevated from the cartilage in a subperichondrial plane, and the cartilage graft is disarticulated from the perpendicular plate of the ethmoid, vomer, and maxillary crest inferiorly.
  - The cartilage is removed from the nose and the septal incision sutured with absorbable stitches.
  - The cartilage is carved to assume the ideal size to cover the defect: Usually larger on the laterolateral dimension and shorter on the anterior-posterior dimension of the defect.
  - Next, the cartilage graft is positioned. One side of the cartilage is pushed intracranially and placed above the lateral edge of the defect to be supported by the bone. Then, the medial side of the cartilage graft is pushed intracranially and gently moved medially until it is supported along the medial bone edge of the defect.
  - Once the cartilage graft is well placed, a mucosal reconstruction is performed with onlay free mucosal graft or nasoseptal flap depending on the size of the defect and intensity of the CSF flow.

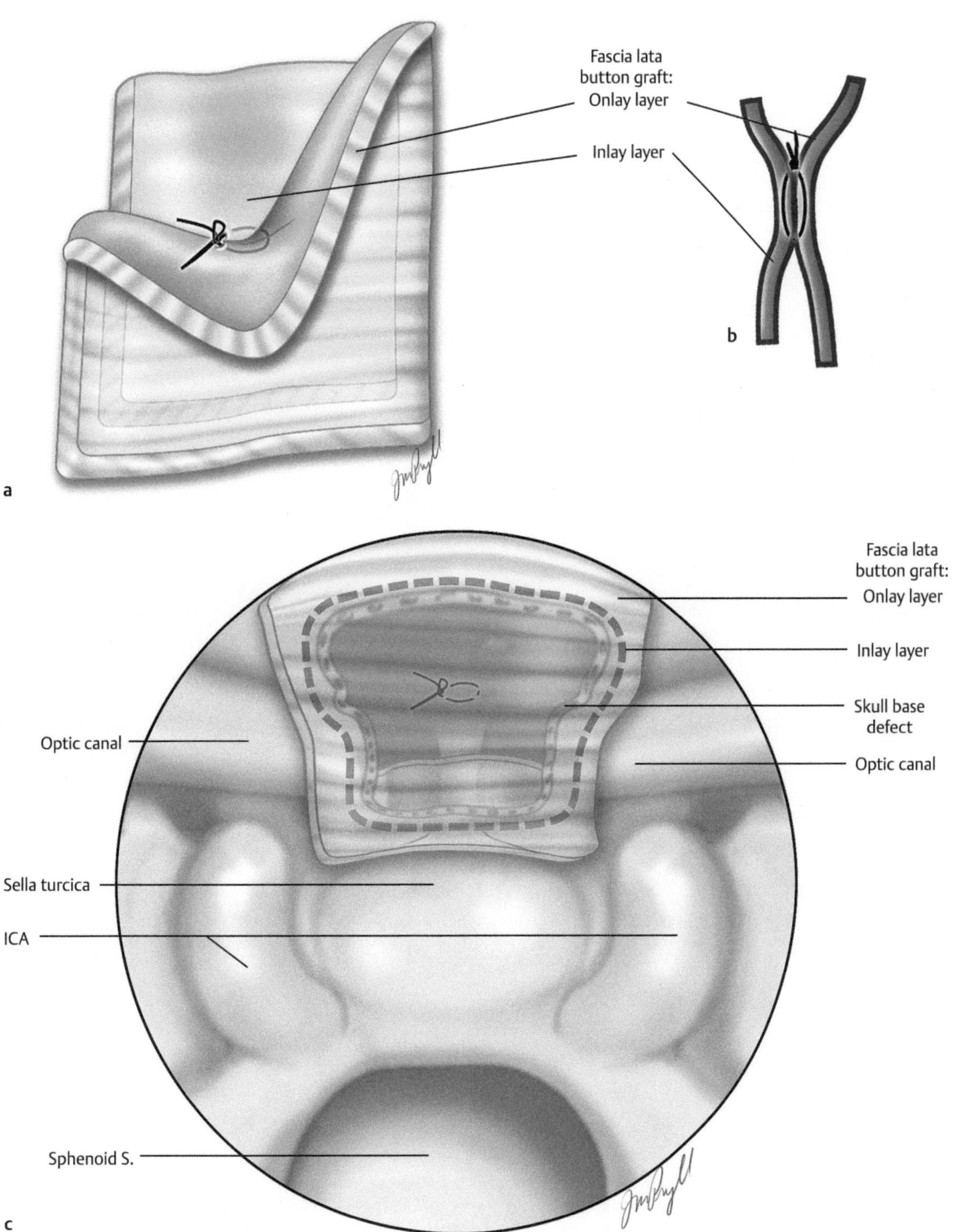

Fig. 18.1 **(a)** Fascia lata button graft: Inlay and onlay layers. A hemitransfixation suture is placed in the center between the two layers. **(b)** Sagittal view showing that the stitch does not fully transect any of the layers of the fascia. This technique avoids violation or laceration of the fascia decreasing the risk of postoperative cerebrospinal fluid (CSF) leak through the region of the suture. **(c)** Illustration of an endoscopic view of the sphenoid sinus after a transplanum and transtuberculum approach to the suprasellar space. *Black dashed line* represents the margins of the inlay layer of the fascia lata button graft. Note that the inlay layer is smaller than the onlay graft but still larger than the dural defect which helps securing the onlay graft in place. After the inset of the button graft, a vascularized flap (not shown) is used to cover the defect. ICA, internal carotid artery; S, sinus.

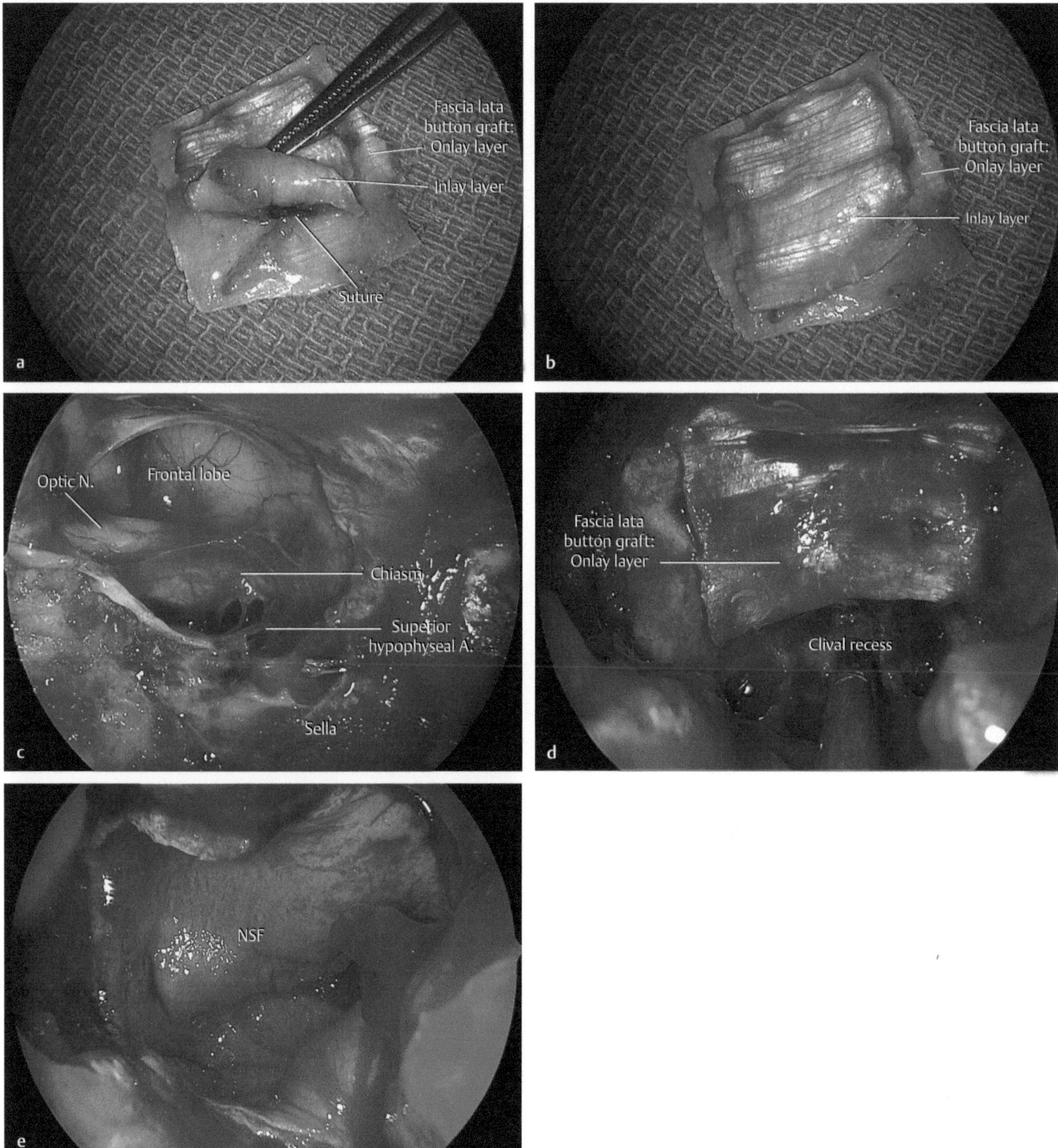

Fig. 18.2 Surgical example of application of the fascia lata inlay–onlay button graft to reconstruct a suprasellar defect after resection of a craniopharyngioma. **(a, b)** Preparation of the fascia lata button graft at the back table. The inlay graft was marked with a marking pen to help identifying the layers during the graft inset. Note that the onlay layer is slightly larger than the inlay graft. **(c)** Endoscopic view of a suprasellar defect obtained with a 0 degree endoscope. **(d)** View of the onlay layer after inset of the fascia lata button graft. **(e)** Inset of the nasoseptal flap. Observe that the flap is larger than the onlay graft which allows effective bone contact of the flap around the edges of the fascia. N, nerve; NSF, nasoseptal flap.

18.6 Postoperative Care

- Postoperative visits 1 week, 1 month, and 4 months after surgery for nasal debridement.
- Skin stitches/staples on the harvest site are removed at the 1-week postoperative visit.
- Saline nasal irrigation is used until the nasal mucosa is completely healed.

18.7 Complications

- Hypertrophic, keloid scar.
- Hematoma, seroma, wound infection.
- Abdominal fat graft:
  - Ileus (rare).
  - Inadvertent peritoneal perforation (rare).
  - Lipoid meningitis (rare).
- Muscle graft:
  - Temporalis muscle graft: Injury to the frontal branch of the facial nerve, trismus, alopecia around the incision line.
  - Rectus abdominis muscle graft: Ventral hernia (rare).
- Fascia lata:
  - Muscle herniation.
  - Hypoesthesia, pain, meralgia paresthetica (lateral femoral cutaneous nerve injury/compression).
  - Compartmental syndrome (rare), usually when the fascia lata edges are tightly sutured.
  - Seroma, large fluid area with no redness or fever, usually not painful to touch, usually resolves in weeks to months after the operation with conservative treatment. Differentiate from cellulitis or abscess in which the area is red, tender, inflammation markers are elevated, and usually courses with fever, in this case will need surgical drainage (if it is an abscess) and antibiotic treatment.
- Septal cartilage:
  - Septal perforation.
  - Saddle nose.

References

[1] El-Mrakby HH, Milner RH. The vascular anatomy of the lower anterior abdominal wall: a microdissection study on the deep inferior epigastric vessels and the perforator branches. Plast Reconstr Surg. 2002; 109(2):539–543, discussion 544–547

[2] Fiorindi A, Gioffrè G, Boaro A, et al. Banked Fascia lata in sellar dura reconstruction after endoscopic transsphenoidal skull base surgery. J Neurol Surg B Skull Base. 2015; 76(4):303–309

[3] Hanna A. The lateral femoral cutaneous nerve canal. J Neurosurg. 2017; 126 (3):972–978

[4] Krishnan Y, Grodzinsky AJ. Cartilage diseases. Matrix Biol. 2018; 71–72:51–69

[5] Dixon BJ, Vescan AD. Skull base reconstruction. In: Kountakis SE, ed. Encyclopedia of otolaryngology, head and neck surgery. Berlin, Heidelberg: Springer; 2013:2501–2507

[6] Bleier BS. Comprehensive techniques in CSF leak repair and skull base reconstruction. S. Karger AG; 2012

[7] Snyderman CH, Kassam AB, Carrau R, Mintz A. Endoscopic reconstruction of cranial base defects following endonasal skull base surgery. Skull Base. 2007; 17(1):73–78

[8] Spaziante R, de Divitiis E, Cappabianca P. Reconstruction of the pituitary fossa in transsphenoidal surgery: an experience of 140 cases. Neurosurgery. 1985; 17(3):453–458

[9] Duek I, Sviri GE, Amit M, Gil Z. Endoscopic endonasal repair of internal carotid artery injury during endoscopic endonasal surgery. J Neurol Surg Rep. 2017; 78(4):e125–e128

[10] Luginbuhl AJ, Campbell PG, Evans J, Rosen M. Endoscopic repair of high-flow cranial base defects using a bilayer button. Laryngoscope. 2010; 120(5):876–880

[11] Khatiwala R, Shastri K, Peris-Celda M, Kenning T, Pinheiro-Neto C. Endoscopic endonasal reconstruction of high-flow cerebrospinal fluid leak with fascia lata "button" graft and nasoseptal flap: surgical technique and case series. J Neurol Surg B Skull Base. 2020; 81(6):645–650

[12] Leng LZ, Brown S, Anand VK, Schwartz TH. "Gasket-seal" watertight closure in minimal-access endoscopic cranial base surgery. Neurosurgery. 2008; 62 (5) Suppl 2:ONSE342–ONSE 343, discussion E343

[13] Kim DW, Gurney T. Management of naso-septal L-strut deformities. Facial Plast Surg. 2006; 22(1):9–27

Section VI

Free Flaps

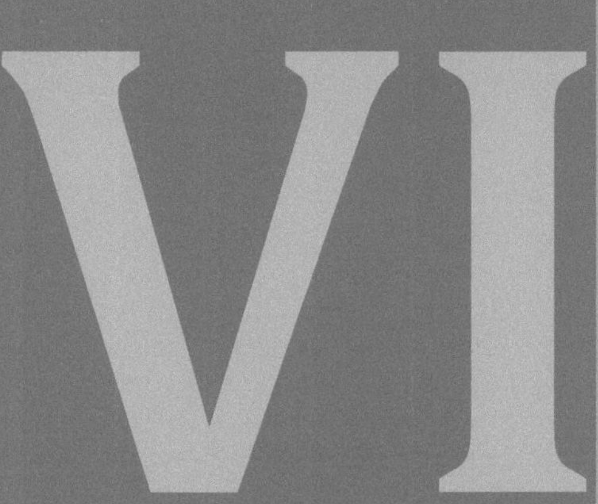

19 Endoscopic Cranial Base Free Flap Reconstruction

Akina Tamaki, Abdulaziz Alrasheed, Daniel Prevedello, Enver Ozer, Ricardo L. Carrau, and Stephen Y. Kang

19.1 Anatomy

- Endoscopic free flap reconstruction can be used to reconstruct a wide range of defects spanning from the anterior cranial fossa to the clivus and nasopharynx. The anatomy of the defect will largely be dictated by the pathology.
- There are various types of free tissue donor sites used in endoscopic cranial base reconstruction, the most frequent being anterolateral thigh, radial forearm, and rectus abdominus free flaps.
- The authors prefer using the anterolateral thigh as the primary donor site for microvascular reconstruction of endoscopic skull base defects.

19.2 Fundamentals

- Increasingly complex and advanced skull base tumors are being removed endoscopically, which has created a need for novel advanced reconstructive options.
- The majority of cranial base defects can be successfully reconstructed using free grafts, local flaps, and regional flaps.[1,2,3]
- However, when less invasive methods are not available or fail to successfully reconstruct a defect, it may become necessary to move up the reconstructive ladder to free microvascular flap reconstruction. The use of free flaps in the reconstruction of cranial base defects has been well described in the literature.[4,5]
- A variety of free flaps have been used in skull base reconstruction. These include, but are not limited to, anterolateral thigh, radial forearm, latissimus dorsi, serratus, and rectus abdominus free flaps.[5,6,7,8,9]
- Each donor site has advantages and disadvantages that can dictate use.
- Rectus abdominus myocutaneous flaps have a long vascular pedicle and reliable skin paddle. However, there is significant donor site morbidity, including ventral hernias, and adipose tissue can be excessive in patients with high BMI.[10]
- Radial forearm free flaps are thin, pliable, and have a long vascular pedicle, making it an excellent option for endoscopic repair.[11,12]
- Anterolateral thigh flaps, and its variations including the adipofascial anterolateral thigh flaps and vastus lateralis free tissue transfer (VLFTT), have been increasingly used in endoscopic skull base reconstruction.[13,14,15] The authors prefer the VLFTT as the primary choice for most skull base defects requiring endoscopic inset, and will provide surgical detail on the harvest of this flap.
- It is important to differentiate between free flaps used in open skull-based procedures versus primarily endoscopic cranial base reconstructions. As would be expected, endoscopic approaches have increased unique challenges that are not faced with an open approach. We will focus on free flaps used in endoscopic cranial base reconstruction.

19.3 Indications

- The primary goal of cranial base reconstruction is to provide durable separation between the extracranial and intracranial compartments.[16]
- This reconstruction can be done using a variety of reconstructive techniques including free graft, local flaps, and regional flaps.
- However, when these reconstructive options fail or are not a possibility, due to limitations such as lack of local or regional donor tissue, reconstruction utilizing free flaps can be considered.
- Free flaps also provide significant volume to obliterate dead space.

19.4 Limitations

- Much of the previous application of free flap reconstruction has been in the setting of open skull base resection including transcranial or transfacial approaches.
- As surgeons advance the complexity and extent of disease that can be resected through minimally invasive endoscopic surgery, there has been a concurrent need to develop minimally invasive reconstructive techniques.
- While open approaches provide a wide avenue for access, endoscopic resections significantly limit access to the skull base defect. As a result, the flap must be inset into a small space with minimal access.
- An additional challenge is the need for a flap with pedicle length reaching from the skull base to a recipient vessel in the neck.[13]
- Patients requiring free flap reconstruction for cranial base defects often have multiple risk factors for postoperative complications. These include previous failed reconstruction with free grafts and local or regional flaps, history of radiation, and in some cases, multiple revision surgeries.[17]
- There may also be areas of active infection, necrotic or unhealthy tissue, and/or cerebrospinal fluid (CSF) leaks.
- Beyond the challenges that exist at the skull base, there are limitations specific to the free microvascular flap.
- Critical features of the selected flap are that it must be thin, pliable, and with a long enough pedicle to reach the recipient vessels.
- Although techniques such as a vein graft can be utilized, it adds an additional variable to the reconstruction that may increase flap failure and complications.[18]

19.5 Surgical Technique (*Video 19.1*)

- We describe a technique of endoscopic cranial base reconstruction utilizing a sublabial approach with VLFTT.
- Although we describe our preferred transmaxillary procedure for access to the anterior skull base, there are a variety of other approaches that have been described including the

midface degloving, retropharyngeal, and transpalatal approach.[6,12,17,19,20,21]

19.5.1 Preparation of Recipient Site

- Endoscopic ablation should be performed in the traditional manner and approach. In the setting of secondary reconstruction, it is necessary to debride necrotic tissue and create a healthy platform at the skull base defect to onlay the free flap. As with free grafts, and local or regional flaps, sinonasal mucosa and/or previously placed tissue must be removed to healthy bone or dura that would allow for successful adherence and inosculation of the free flap tissue.
- We prefer the sublabial, transmaxillary approach for inset and access to the anterior cranial base, which will be described.[13,17] A sublabial incision at the ipsilateral side of the defect is made. From this incision, the anterior surface of the maxilla is exposed. The periosteum is elevated off the bone.
- An expanded anterior maxillotomy is performed in a manner similar to that of a Caldwell-Luc. The bone of the anterior wall of the maxillary sinus is removed completely in a "U-shaped" fashion, preserving the infraorbital nerve and piriform aperture.
- An endoscopic medial maxillectomy creates a passage for the free flap to pass from the anterior maxillotomy to the sinonasal cavity. It is important to maximize the anterior maxillotomy and medial maxillectomy to achieve a tension free inset and tunneling of the free flap.
- The recipient vessel is prepared. Typically, the facial artery and vein are reliable recipient vessels. A limited submandibular incision is made on the ipsilateral neck, just below the inferior border of the mandible. The submandibular gland is identified and the marginal mandibular branch of the facial nerve is preserved. The vessels are typically ligated just inferior to the nerve to maximize the length of the vessels. Two alternative recipient vessels include the facial vessels (exposed through a limited incision at the nasolabial fold) or the superficial temporal vessels (exposed through a preauricular incision).
- A tunnel is created from the neck incision to the sublabial and anterior maxillotomy, passing through the buccal space, deep to the buccinator muscle, and down to the neck.

19.5.2 Free Flap Harvest

- VLFTT (▶ Fig. 19.1a) is a modification of the anterolateral thigh free flap but without harvest of a cutaneous paddle. A line is drawn from the anterior superior iliac spine to the lateral patella. This marks the approximate location between the vastus lateralis and rectus femoris muscle.
- An incision on this line is made through the skin and subcutaneous tissue down to the rectus femoris muscle. The fascia over the rectus femoris muscle is incised and the muscle is retracted medially. In contrast to the anterolateral thigh flap, septocutaneous perforators to the cutaneous paddle can be sacrificed because the cutaneous paddle is not included in this flap.
- The pedicle of this flap is the descending branch of the lateral femoral circumflex artery. The pedicle is identified entering the vastus lateralis.
- An acoustic Doppler ultrasound probe can be used to trace the pedicle through the vastus lateralis. A narrow 3 cm strip of the vastus lateralis muscle is harvested along the course of the pedicle. It is important to harvest a long cuff of vastus lateralis to ensure coverage of the skull base defect and to add pedicle length to reach the recipient vessels. Enough tissue must be harvested to cover the defect and extend to the periphery to create an adequate seal. However, a flap that is too large will significantly obscure endoscopic visualization and make inset challenging.
- The descending branch of the lateral femoral circumflex artery is traced toward the main trunk of the lateral circumflex. The pedicle is traced until the branch to the rectus femoris is identified. This branch should be preserved and marks the limits of the pedicle dissection. Maximizing the length of the pedicle is important, given that it must span from the neck to the skull base. In our experience, up to 26 cm length of vastus lateralis and 8 cm pedicle length can be successfully harvested.
- The flap is harvested immediately prior to inset.
- The donor site is closed in multiple layers. Two drains are placed in the donor site. The vastus lateralis is sewn to the rectus femoris, followed by deep dermal and skin closure.

19.5.3 Free Flap Inset

- The free flap is passed through the sublabial incision, anterior maxillotomy, and into the maxillary sinus. The flap is then passed through the medial maxillectomy defect into the nasal cavity (▶ Fig. 19.1b).
- Next, the flap is positioned endoscopically. The distal portion of the flap is positioned toward the posterior extent of the skull base defect.
- The muscle is placed in an overlay fashion over the skull base defect. A Freer elevator is used to position the flap medially and superiorly to obliterate the communication between the sinonasal and intracranial cavity. The muscle is positioned directly over the defect.
- The muscle is then bolstered superiorly with nonabsorbable packing, such as an expandable sponge packing. Typically, two expandable sponges are used to displace the flap superiorly. It is important to pack the nose enough to support the flap and keep the tissue stable, but not enough to cause pressure and compromise perfusion to the free flap. A nasal trumpet is placed inferior to the packs to support the flap and provide a nasal airway.
- Following inset of the flap, the pedicle is tunneled from the sublabial incision, through the buccal space, deep to the buccinator, to the neck incision and recipient vessels. A Penrose drain can be helpful to guide the pedicle through the tunnel. It is important that this tunnel is large enough to prevent compression of the pedicle.
- Vein grafting may be considered if there is inadequate length of the pedicle.
- Microvascular anastomosis is performed in the standard fashion. It is important to complete the inset of the flap prior to reperfusion. Reperfusion can result in edema, enlargement, and displacement of the free flap tissue.
- The sublabial and neck incisions are irrigated and closed in a multilayered fashion. The gingivobuccal incision is closed in a

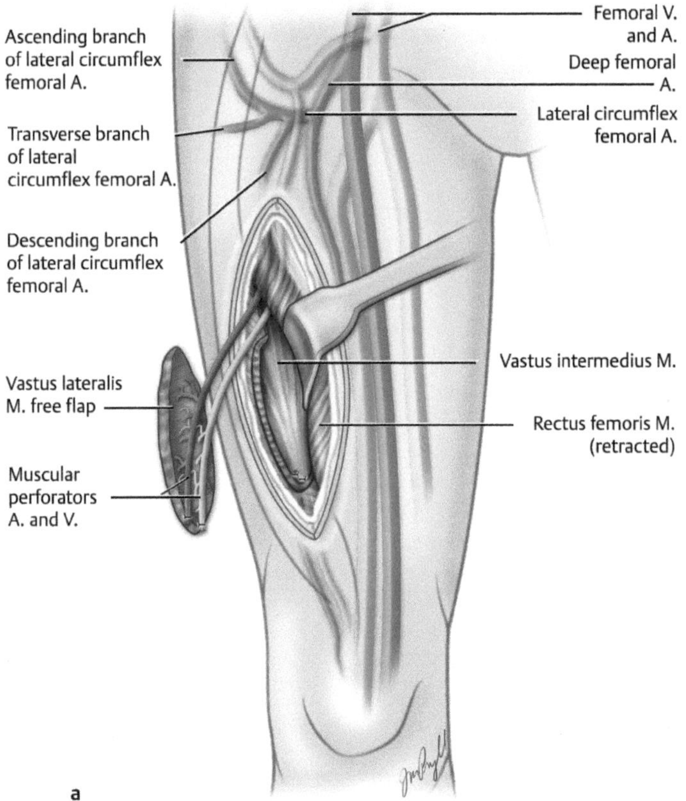

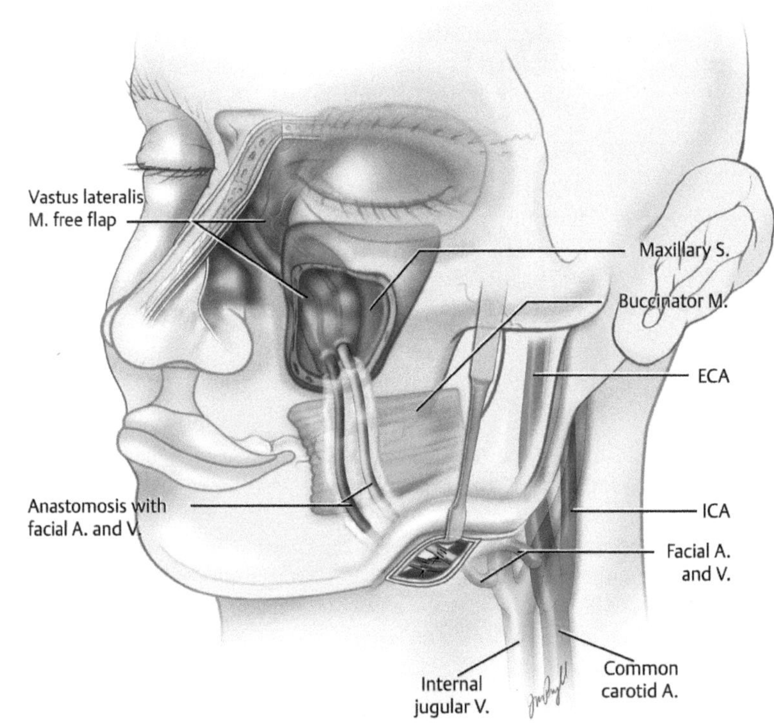

Fig. 19.1 **(a)** Illustration to show the anatomy of the vastus lateralis free tissue transfer (VLFTT). VLFTT is a modification of the anterolateral thigh free flap. The pedicle of this flap is the descending branch of the lateral femoral circumflex artery, which enters the muscle. A long (up to 26 cm) but narrow 3 cm strip of the vastus lateralis muscle is harvested along the course of the pedicle. **(b)** The free flap is passed through the sublabial incision, anterior maxillotomy, and into the maxillary sinus. The flap is then passed through the medial maxillectomy defect into the nasal cavity. Next, the muscle flap is endoscopically placed in an overlay fashion over the skull base. Following inset of the flap, the pedicle is tunneled from the sublabial incision, through the buccal space, deep to the buccinator, to the neck incision. The facial vessels are reliable recipient vessels, which can be accessed through a limited submandibular incision. A, artery; ECA, external carotid artery; ICA, internal carotid artery; M, muscle; S, sinus; V, vein.

watertight fashion to protect the flap pedicle from communication with the oral cavity. A drain is placed in the neck.

- An acoustic Doppler ultrasound is used to identify the arterial signal of the anastomosis. The signal should be easily identifiable at the neck or on the face as it is tunneled to the sinonasal cavity. This location is marked with a suture to allow for flap monitoring postoperatively.

19.6 Postoperative Care

- Nasal trumpets and packing remain for a minimum of 7 days.
- Prophylactic lumbar drains are typically not necessary.
- Prophylactic tracheotomy is typically not necessary with the transmaxillary approach. However, with a retropharyngeal and transpalatal approaches, which may contribute to obstruction of the airway, a tracheostomy may be needed.
- Patients are admitted to the neurointensive care unit for 24 hours.
- Noncontrasted brain computed tomography (CT) scans are performed immediately after surgery to rule out intracranial complications and to check the position of the flap.
- Additional imaging including magnetic resonance imaging (MRI) can be considered based on need, for example, to confirm complete oncologic resection.
- Free flap checks are performed through our institutions' standard protocol. Flaps are generally monitored through visual inspection as well as corroborating flow with an acoustic Doppler ultrasound probe. Given that there is no visible portion of the free flap, the flap is monitored only via Doppler.
- Patients are continued on antibiotics for a total of 7 days. There is no consistent recommendation on antibiotic regimen for endoscopic skull base surgeries. The duration of antibiotic prophylaxis largely varies by institution.[22] We recommend continuing some sort of antibiotic regimen while nasal packing is in place, until it is removed on postoperative day 7.
- Nasal saline sprays are started on postoperative day 1 to prevent nasal crusting.
- Nasal trumpet and nasal packing are left in place for a total of 7 days. The expandable sponge packing is saturated with saline prior to removal to prevent avulsing the flap upon removal. Once all nasal packing is removed, patients are instructed to continue nasal saline and begin nasal irrigation.
- Patients are discharged around postoperative day 7.
- Outpatient follow-up is scheduled about 1 week from time of discharge. Nasal endoscopy and debridement are performed in the postoperative period, which usually spans for 4 to 6 weeks from the time of surgery.

19.7 Complications

- Precise rates of complications following endoscopic cranial base free flap reconstruction are limited by their sparse numbers. Current estimates are mostly based on open free flap reconstructions rather than endoscopic.
- Free flap failure is a major complication of endoscopic cranial base free flap reconstruction. The literature supports low rates of free flap failure.[13] Free flap success rates in skull base reconstruction have been reported as 94%, although this is not specific for endoscopic approaches.[5,7]
- Inadequate separation of the sinonasal and intracranial cavities can lead to pneumocephalus, CSF leaks, and intracranial infections including meningitis and intracranial abscesses. In our cohort of four patients who underwent VLFTT for skull base reconstruction, one patient developed a postoperative acute bacterial meningitis and another developed an epidural abscess.[13] A similar case series on endoscopic cranial base reconstruction utilizing free flaps have also reported a high rate (two out of five patients) of infectious postoperative complications.[14] These results support the use of perioperative antibiotics. Incidence for infections including meningitis in one study of 1,000 patients who underwent endonasal endoscopic skull base surgery was reported at 1.8%. The most important risk factor for infection was the presence of a postoperative CSF leak.[23] Rates of CSF leaks in free flap cranial base reconstruction has ranged from 5 to 11.8%.[5,7,8]
- Nasal obstruction following surgery is considered a sequela rather than a complication. There is near complete nasal obstruction in the immediate postoperative period. The muscle flap does significantly atrophy with time and often undergoes mucosalization within the first 2 months.[13]
- Long-term sinonasal complications include development of mucoceles from obstruction of anatomical outflow tracts related to the flap or endonasal surgery.
- Aside from complications at the skull base, there are complications at the free flap donor site and neck incision site. This includes hematomas, seromas, and wound infections.

References

[1] Hachem RA, Elkhatib A, Beer-Furlan A, Prevedello D, Carrau R. Reconstructive techniques in skull base surgery after resection of malignant lesions: a wide array of choices. Curr Opin Otolaryngol Head Neck Surg. 2016; 24(2):91–97

[2] Ein L, Sargi Z, Nicolli EA. Update on anterior skull base reconstruction. Curr Opin Otolaryngol Head Neck Surg. 2019; 27(5):426–430

[3] Reyes C, Mason E, Solares CA. Panorama of reconstruction of skull base defects: from traditional open to endonasal endoscopic approaches, from free grafts to microvascular flaps. Int Arch Otorhinolaryngol. 2014; 18 Suppl 2: S179–S186

[4] Teknos TN, Smith JC, Day TA, Netterville JL, Burkey BB. Microvascular free tissue transfer in reconstructing skull base defects: lessons learned. Laryngoscope. 2002; 112(10):1871–1876

[5] Llorente JL, Lopez F, Camporro D, et al. Outcomes following microvascular free tissue transfer in reconstructing skull base defects. J Neurol Surg B Skull Base. 2013; 74(5):324–330

[6] Krane NA, Troob SH, Wax MK. Combined endoscopic and transcervical approach for free flap reconstruction of nasopharyngeal and clival defects: a case report. Microsurgery. 2019; 39(3):259–262

[7] Herr MW, Lin DT. Microvascular free flaps in skull base reconstruction. Adv Otorhinolaryngol. 2013; 74:81–91

[8] Macía G, Picón M, Nuñez J, Almeida F, Alvarez I, Acero J. The use of free flaps in skull base reconstruction. Int J Oral Maxillofac Surg. 2016; 45(2):158–162

[9] Rowe D, Emmett J. Reconstruction of the base of skull defect-lessons learned over 25 combined years. J Neurol Surg B Skull Base. 2016; 77(2):161–168

[10] Kang SY, Spector ME, Chepeha DB. Perforator based rectus free tissue transfer for head and neck reconstruction: new reconstructive advantages from an old friend. Oral Oncol. 2017; 74:163–170

[11] Schwartz MS, Cohen JI, Meltzer T, et al. Use of the radial forearm microvascular free-flap graft for cranial base reconstruction. J Neurosurg. 1999; 90 (4):651–655

[12] Kakarala K, Richmon JD, Durand ML, Borges LF, Deschler DG. Reconstruction of a nasopharyngeal defect from cervical spine osteoradionecrosis. Skull Base. 2010; 20(4):289–292

[13] Kang SY, Eskander A, Hachem RA, et al. Salvage skull base reconstruction in the endoscopic era: vastus lateralis free tissue transfer. Head Neck. 2018; 40 (4):E45–E52

[14] Rodriguez-Lorenzo A, Driessen C, Mani M, Lidian A, Gudjonsson O, Stigare E. Endoscopic assisted insetting of free flaps in anterior skull base reconstruction: A preliminary report of five cases. Microsurgery. 20 20; 40(4):460–467

[15] Chapchay K, Weinberger J, Eliashar R, Adler N. Anterior skull base reconstruction following ablative surgery for osteoradionecrosis: case report and review of literature. Ann Otol Rhinol Laryngol. 2019; 128(12):1134–1140

[16] Moyer JS, Chepeha DB, Teknos TN. Contemporary skull base reconstruction. Curr Opin Otolaryngol Head Neck Surg. 2004; 12(4):294–299

[17] Sinha P, Desai SC, Ha DH, Chicoine MR, Haughey BH. Extracranial radial forearm free flap closure of refractory cerebrospinal fluid leaks: a novel hybrid transantral-endoscopic approach. Neurosurgery. 2012; 71(2) Suppl Operative:ons219–ons225, discussion ons225–ons226

[18] Miller MJ, Schusterman MA, Reece GP, Kroll SS. Interposition vein grafting in head and neck reconstructive microsurgery. J Reconstr Microsurg. 1993; 9 (3):245–251, discussion 251–252

[19] Hackman TG. Endoscopic adipofascial radial forearm flap reconstruction of a clival defect. Plast Reconstr Surg Glob Open. 2016; 4(11):e1109

[20] London NR, Jr, Ishii M, Gallia G, Boahene KDO. Technique for reconstruction of large clival defects through an endoscopic-assisted tunneled retropharyngeal approach. Int Forum Allergy Rhinol. 2018; 8(12):1454–1458

[21] Vieira S, Nabil A, Maza G, et al. Salvage free tissue transfer for clival osteoradionecrosis after repeat proton beam therapy. World Neurosurg. 2020; 138:485–490

[22] Johans SJ, Burkett DJ, Swong KN, Patel CR, Germanwala AV. Antibiotic prophylaxis and infection prevention for endoscopic endonasal skull base surgery: our protocol, results, and review of the literature. J Clin Neurosci. 2018; 47:249–253

[23] Kono Y, Prevedello DM, Snyderman CH, et al. One thousand endoscopic skull base surgical procedures demystifying the infection potential: incidence and description of postoperative meningitis and brain abscesses. Infect Control Hosp Epidemiol. 2011; 32(1):77–83

Section VII

Challenging Cases

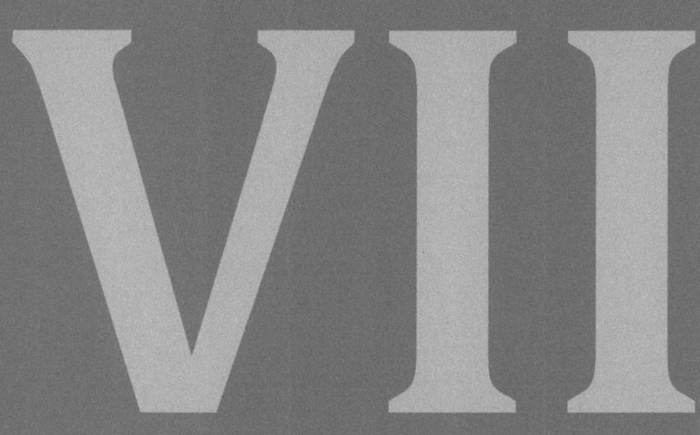

20 Free Flap Reconstruction

Adedamola Adepoju, Courtney Carpenter, Maria Peris-Celda, and Carlos D. Pinheiro-Neto

20.1 Case Description

20.1.1 Presentation

A 50-year-old female with a long history of cocaine abuse and consequent extensive erosion of hard palate, sinonasal structures, and anterior cranial base had a severe methicillin-resistant *Staphylococcus aureus* (MRSA) meningitis 10 years ago. She was operated at an outside hospital through a bifrontal craniotomy utilizing autologous bone graft from her calvarium for skull base cranial reconstruction. After the surgery, she referred chronic sinusitis symptoms for several years until she presented to our clinic complaining of nasal pain and purulent discharge. Nasal endoscopy showed severe inflammation of the nasal mucosa at the anterior cranial base with a small area of the exposed bone graft. There was no obvious cerebrospinal fluid (CSF) leak, and nasal discharge was sent for beta 2 transferrin test which was negative. A high-resolution computed tomography (CT) showed the autologous bone graft along the skull base from the posterior wall of the frontal sinus to the planum sphenoidale. The graft was stabilized anteriorly by a titanium plate across the anterior cranial base next to the posterior table of the frontal sinus. The plate bridged from the orbital roof on one side to the orbital roof on the contralateral side and was fixed to both orbital roofs and to the bone graft with titanium screws (▶ Fig. 20.1). The patient underwent endoscopic endonasal surgery for debridement and coverage of the exposed bone with a vascularized flap of a remnant middle turbinate. The exposed bone graft had areas of soft bone, which were debrided and sent for microbiology and pathology. There was no dural defect or CSF leak. The tissue culture was positive for MRSA and pathology confirmed osteomyelitis. The infectious disease team recommended complete removal of the bone graft and hardware.

20.1.2 Surgical Procedure (*Video 20.1*)

Endoscopic endonasal approach was performed to expose the anterior cranial base including a wide Draf III frontal sinusotomy. The bone graft was drilled out until it was thin enough to be dissected from the dura with a Cottle dissector and rongeurs. The bone graft was separated from the titanium plate anteriorly with rongeurs. Once the bone graft was completely removed, the titanium plate was detached from the orbital roofs. First, both lamina papyraceae were partially removed and the periorbita dissected from the orbital roofs. The lateral dissection was progressed until exposure of all screws. The orbital roof was drilled around the screws until the plate was detached and removed. At the end of the resection, a large area of exposed dura was present (3.2 × 2.1 cm) with a low-flow CSF leak at the posterior edge of the defect next to the planum sphenoidale.

A vastus lateralis free tissue transfer (VLFTT) was used for skull base reconstruction. The transposition of the flap to the nasal cavity was performed through the maxillary sinus. A right sublabial incision was performed, and a wide anterior maxillotomy was completed to expose the maxillary sinus. In this patient's specific case, there was no need for medial maxillectomy since the medial wall of the maxilla was completely eroded due to cocaine abuse. A right-sided submandibular neck incision was performed to expose the facial artery and vein. The pedicle of the flap was transposed from the sublabial incision to the neck after a tunnel was dissected through the buccal space. This tunnel was deep to the superficial musculoaponeurotic system (SMAS) and platysma.

First a Penrose drain was placed through the dissected tunnel. Then the vascular pedicle was marked for orientation to avoid twisting and was carefully inserted in the lumen of the Penrose drain located at the sublabial incision. The pedicle transposition was completed with gentle and steady pulling of the other end of the Penrose drain which was located in the neck. This allowed the vascular pedicle that was protected inside the lumen of the Penrose to slide through the facial tunnel from the sublabial incision to the neck incision. The flap was transposed to nasal cavity through the maxillary sinus, and the microvascular anastomosis was completed with the facial artery and vein in the neck (▶ Fig. 20.2). The inset of the flap to cover the entire anterior cranial base defect was performed under endoscopic visualization, with attention to avoid blockage of the frontal sinus outflow. Oxidized cellulose pieces were used along the borders of the flap in contact to the skull base followed by dural sealant. To support the reconstruction, absorbable packing was placed in contact to the flap followed by nonabsorbable packing along the floor of the nasal cavity bilaterally.

20.1.3 Postoperative Course

The patient did well postoperatively and was treated with intravenous antibiotics for 6 weeks. Follow-up nasal endoscopy 18 months after the surgery showed the free flap well healed to the skull base, no evidence of infection and sinus outflow patent (▶ Fig. 20.3). CT scan showed no evidence of pneumocephalus or any collection between the flap and the brain (▶ Fig. 20.4). Patient had no further episode of CSF leak, meningitis, sinusitis, or facial cellulitis.

20.2 Challenges

- No intranasal flaps were available due to the destruction of sinonasal structures, including the hard palate, from cocaine abuse.
- Pericranial flap was not available due to previous craniotomy for anterior cranial base reconstruction.
- Poor recipient site for any tissue transfer due to compromise of the overall vascularization of the nasal cavity from cocaine abuse.
- Requirement of removal of contaminated hardware fixed to the intracranial surface of the orbital roofs using an endoscopic endonasal route.

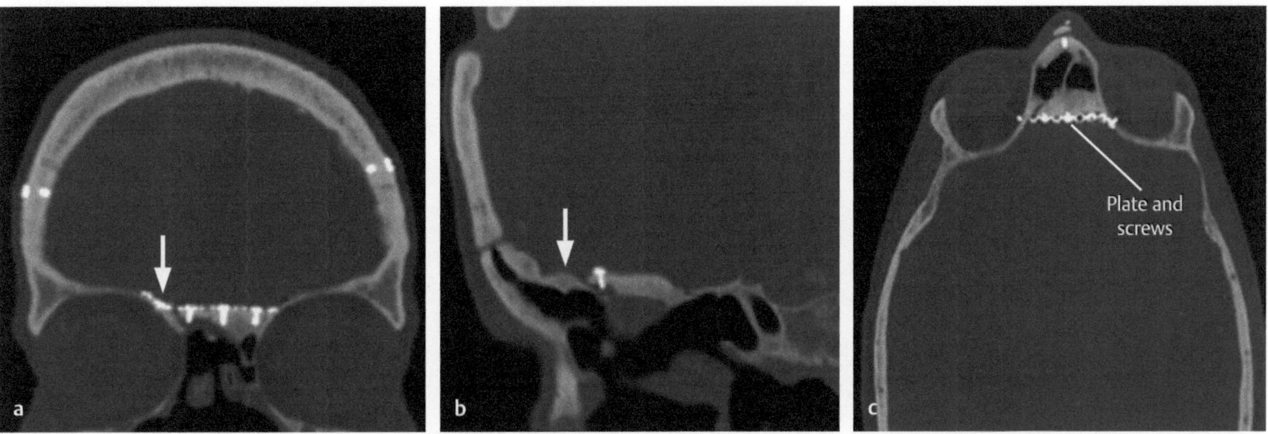

Fig. 20.1 Noncontrast computed tomography (CT) scan showing the anterior cranial base defect reconstructed with a bone graft fixed with plate and screws. **(a)** Coronal view. Note the plate fixed to the orbit (*arrow*). **(b)** Sagittal view. Hyperostotic bone along the anterior cranial base (*arrow*). **(c)** Axial view.

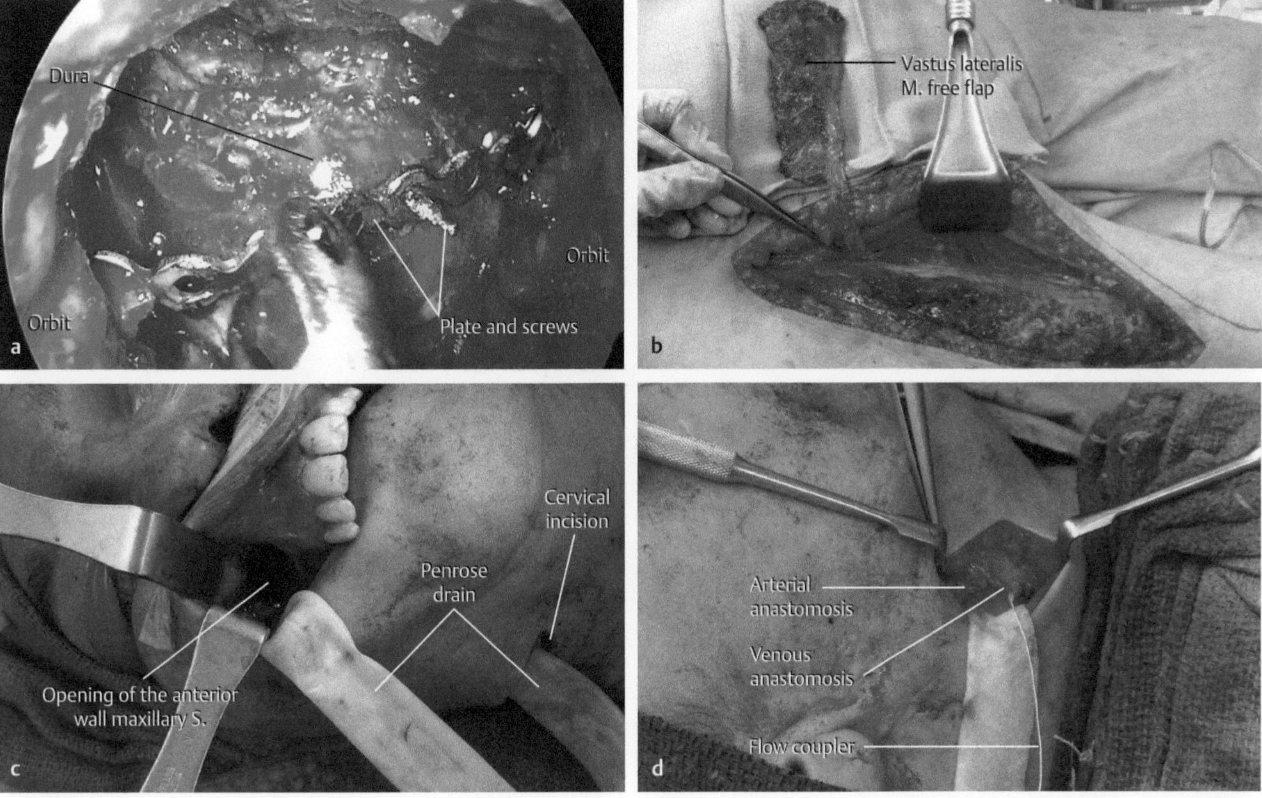

Fig. 20.2 **(a)** Intraoperative picture obtained with a 0-degree endoscope during the removal of infected hardware and bone. **(b)** Harvest of the vastus lateralis muscle free flap. **(c)** Right sublabial approach and anterior maxillotomy for transposition of the free flap into the nasal cavity. Observe that the Penrose drain was passed from the cervical incision to the sublabial incision. **(d)** Microvascular anastomosis with facial artery and vein. M, muscle; S, sinus.

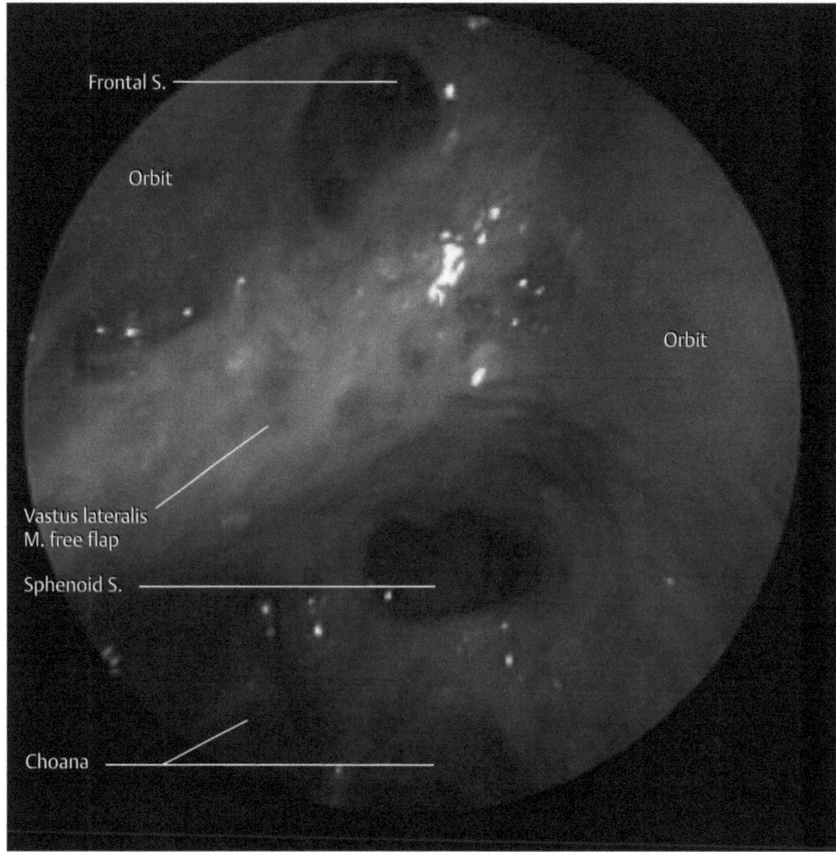

Fig. 20.3 Eighteen-month postoperative nasal endoscopy in clinic showing the vastus lateralis muscle free flap well mucosalized and healed to the anterior cranial base. Observe the patent drainage pathways of frontal and sphenoid sinuses. M, muscle; S, sinus.

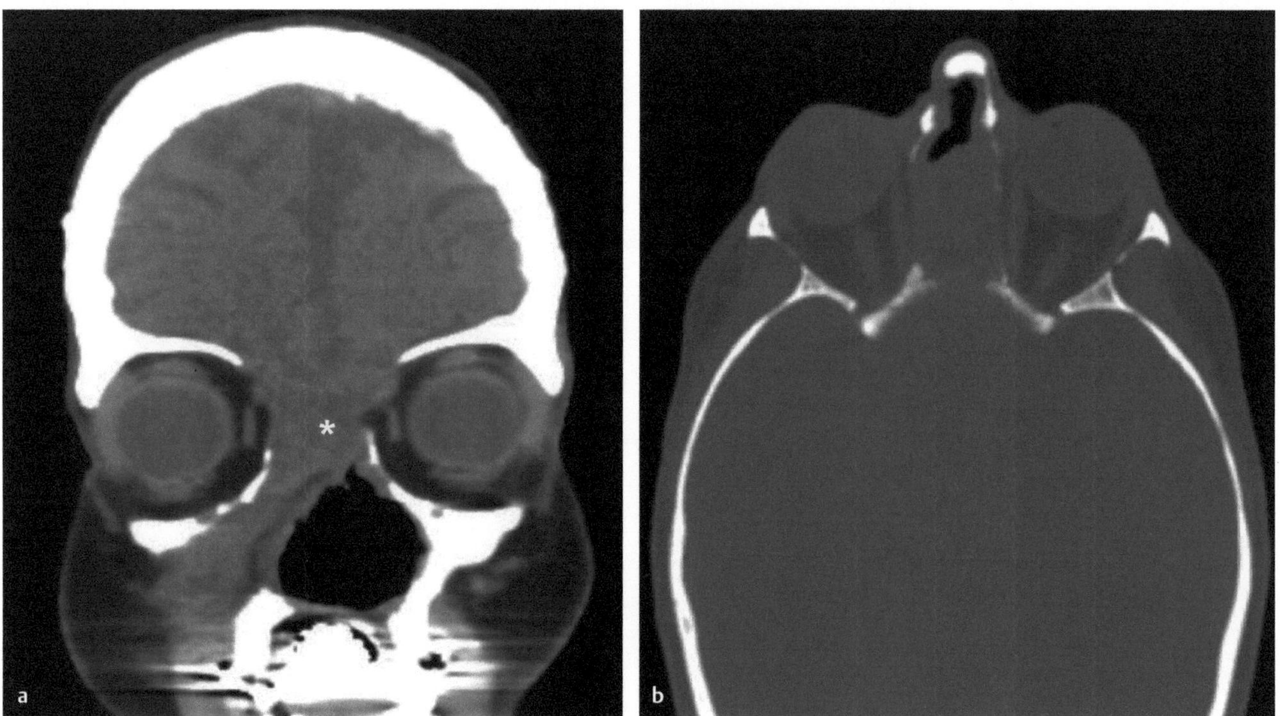

Fig. 20.4 Eighteen-month postoperative computed tomography (CT) scan showing the flap covering the anterior cranial base. **(a)** Coronal view. *Asterisk* = vastus lateralis muscle free flap. **(b)** Axial view. Note the opening to the frontal sinus anterior to the flap.

20.3 Discussion

The use of free flap from anterolateral thigh for skull base reconstruction requires an experienced skull base team, including a microvascular surgeon immersed in endoscopic skull base surgery.[1] The harvest of the free flap must be coordinated with preparation of the recipient site along the skull base. The transposition of the flap to the anterior skull base is an important step. Inadequate opening through the anterior and medial walls of the maxillary sinus can compress the flap. Revascularization edema of the flap should be accounted when evaluating the adequacy of the transmaxillary corridor.

The removal of the infected bone graft and hardware through an endoscopic endonasal approach required familiarity with dissection in the coronal plate of the orbit and experience with angled endoscopes since the plate was lateral and very anterior at the orbital roof. The transcranial removal of the hardware was an option; however, it would have increased the morbidity of the surgery, particularly in this patient who had prior craniotomy.

20.4 Alternatives

Alternative options for reconstruction are scarce in this case:

- Exclusive graft reconstruction is contraindicated for this patient due to active infection. The large defect and poor vascularization of the recipient site from vascular damage due to cocaine abuse are also factors against graft reconstruction.
- No intranasal flaps were available.
- The only regional flaps available were temporoparietal fascia (TPF) flap (used more often for posterior cranial base defects) and buccinator myomucosal flap (limited clinical applicability in skull base reconstruction). Both flaps were not ideal for such large anterior cranial base defect, particularly in this patient with poor vascularization of the recipient site.
- Considering the patient's history, a more robust reconstruction with rich vascularization was recommended.

20.5 Conclusions

Skull base reconstruction is challenging in cases of reoperations, history of cocaine abuse, and lack of intranasal tissue for vascularized flap reconstruction. Familiarity and experience with different flap reconstruction techniques require a multidisciplinary endoscopic skull base team.

Reference

[1] Hanasono MM, Sacks JM, Goel N, Ayad M, Skoracki RJ. The anterolateral thigh free flap for skull base reconstruction. Otolaryngol Head Neck Surg. 2009; 140(6):855–860

21 Galeal-Frontalis Muscle Flap

Adedamola Adepoju, Tyler Kenning, Maria Peris-Celda, and Carlos D. Pinheiro-Neto

21.1 Case Description

21.1.1 Presentation

A 55-year-old female with a history of Factor V Leiden and a large olfactory groove meningioma presented with progressive anosmia and ageusia. She underwent subtotal resection at an outside institution through a bifrontal craniotomy with frontal sinus cranialization. Pathology demonstrated a WHO grade 2 meningioma. She developed cerebrospinal fluid (CSF) leak in the immediate postoperative period that was repaired with reopening of the bifrontal craniotomy. She received proton beam radiation for residual tumor at the cribriform plate. Eight years later, the patient was referred to our service after developing tumor progression at the anterior cranial base that extended into the olfactory cleft and over the orbital roof (▶ Fig. 21.1). She underwent a combined endoscopic endonasal superior ethmoidal approach and a left eyebrow approach with supraorbital craniotomy for tumor resection. Besides the tumor resection, all dura of the anterior cranial base and left orbital roof was removed. The anterior edge of the defect was very anterior at the anterior table of the frontal sinus due to prior frontal sinus cranialization. Temporalis muscle and fat grafts were used along the anterior edge of the defect to decrease the dead space intracranially. After that, the skull base was reconstructed with an inlay dural synthetic substitute and fascia lata graft. A right nasoseptal flap (NSF) was harvested for onlay reconstruction. There was a small gap anteriorly that was not covered optimally by the NSF. Alloderm was placed to cover the gap at the anterior edge.

Four weeks later, she developed clear nasal drainage. Nasal endoscopy showed a small defect anterior to the anterior edge of the NSF with CSF flow. She underwent endoscopic endonasal cranial base exploration and repair of the defect with a plug of muscle graft from the rectus abdominis. A week later, she presented with another CSF leak and extensive pneumocephalus with no new neurological deficits. Nasal endoscopy revealed persistent anterior cranial defect with CSF leak. The area that was initially covered with Alloderm did not heal appropriately (▶ Fig. 21.2).

21.1.2 Surgical Procedure

Bifrontal craniotomy was performed for exploration of the anterior cranial base defect and reconstruction with a galeal-frontalis muscle flap. Subperiosteal dissection of the scalp flap was extended to the nasion. After the removal of the bone flap from the previous craniotomy, the dura was carefully dissected from the NSF until identification of the planum sphenoidale. A galeal-frontalis muscle flap was harvested from the scalp with a broad pedicle anteriorly and was mobilized to cover the anterior cranial base. The flap covered the orbital roof bilaterally and extended to the planum sphenoidale. The most concerning area along frontal sinus outflow was nicely sealed with this flap. Enough bone was removed from the bone flap to prevent compression of the flap pedicle. The scalp was gently mobilized posteriorly without pulling on the flap for closure. Because of the absence of galea in the anterior scalp flap, no multilayer closure was performed. Instead, generous Prolene sutures were used through the epidermis, dermis, and subcutaneous fat for a single-layer closure of the scalp.

21.1.3 Postoperative Course

The CSF leak and the pneumocephalus were resolved (▶ Fig. 21.3). There was no facial discoloration or change in contouring of the face. Several months later, she had a recurrent tumor at the tuberculum sellae compressing the right optic canal. She underwent endoscopic optic nerve decompression and resection of the tumor. A left NSF was harvested for the reconstruction of the suprasellar defect.

21.2 Challenges

- Prior radiation and surgery.
- Prior frontal sinus cranialization, which extended the anterior limit of the defect to the anterior table of the frontal sinus beyond the reach of the NSF.
- The use of the pericranium flap from prior surgery eliminated this option for reconstruction.
- Extensive dural and osseous resection at the cranial base.

21.3 Discussion

This case is an example of endoscopic skull surgery following a traditional craniotomy and skull base reconstruction. A revision craniotomy with broader exposure of the anterior cranial base could have been performed for the recurrent tumor. However, the absence of the pericranial flap was an extra challenge for the open reconstruction. Also the transcranial approach would not provide the best access to the ethmoidal region considering the aggressive nature of this atypical meningioma. The resection of the tumor through the endonasal route alone would limit the access to the supraorbital portion of the tumor. Thus, the combined use of the endoscopic endonasal and the supraorbital craniotomy allowed maximum tumor resection and avoided opening the previous bicoronal approach.

A crucial factor that made this case challenging was the extent of the frontal sinus cranialization, which made the anterior edge of the defect extremely anterior at the level of the anterior table of the frontal sinus. The NSF was not sufficient to provide coverage. At that time, we had not started using the extended dissection of the pedicle and its release from the pterygopalatine fossa[1] (Chapter 6). The improvement of the flap reach obtained with that technique may have prevented the postoperative CSF leak at the anterior border of the NSF. The absence of the posterior wall of the frontal sinus imposes a remarkable challenge for reconstruction. There is a lack of support anteriorly for grafts placed intracranially. Besides that, the space present intracranially after the tumor resection and frontal sinus cranialization creates a "column" of CSF anteriorly that pressures the anterior edge of the reconstruction.

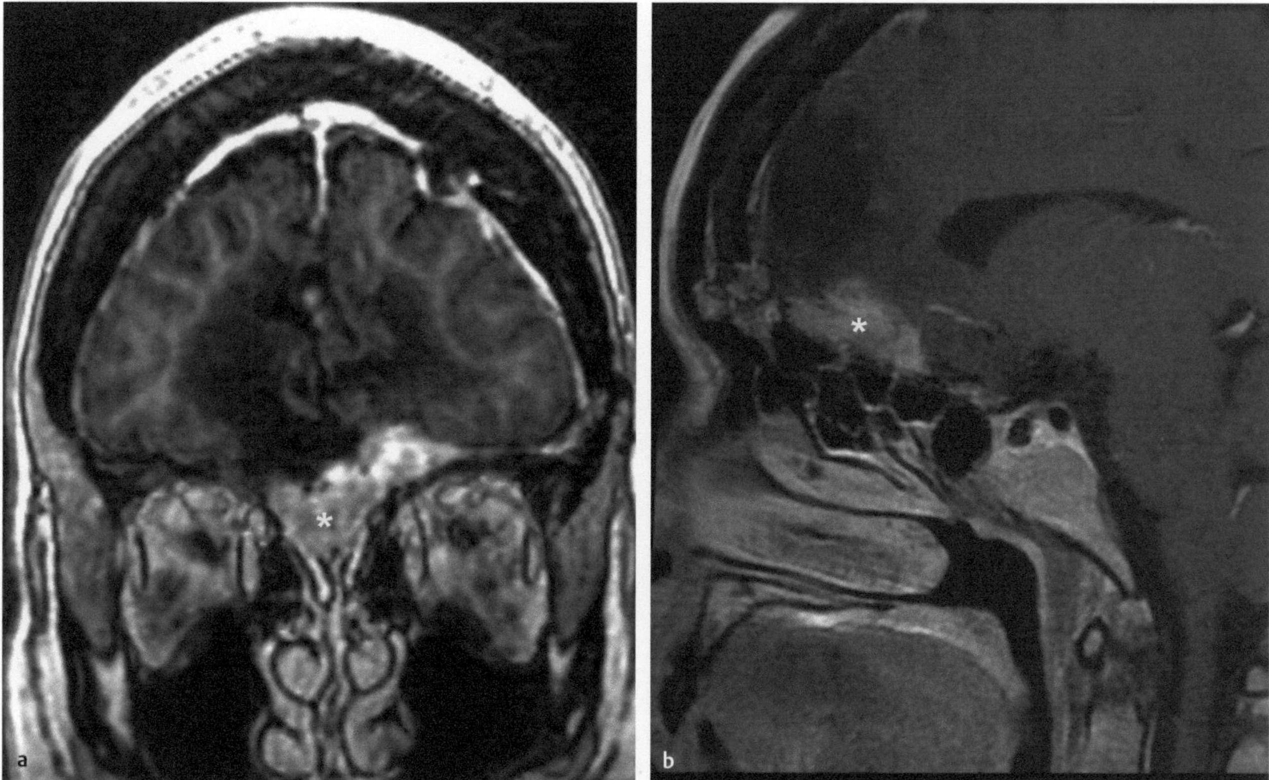

Fig. 21.1 Preoperative magnetic resonance imaging (MRI) T1 with contrast. **(a)** Coronal view showing the meningioma (*asterisk*) involving the olfactory cleft and extending along the left orbital roof. **(b)** Sagittal view. Note the tumor (*asterisk*) extending anteriorly toward the frontal bone.

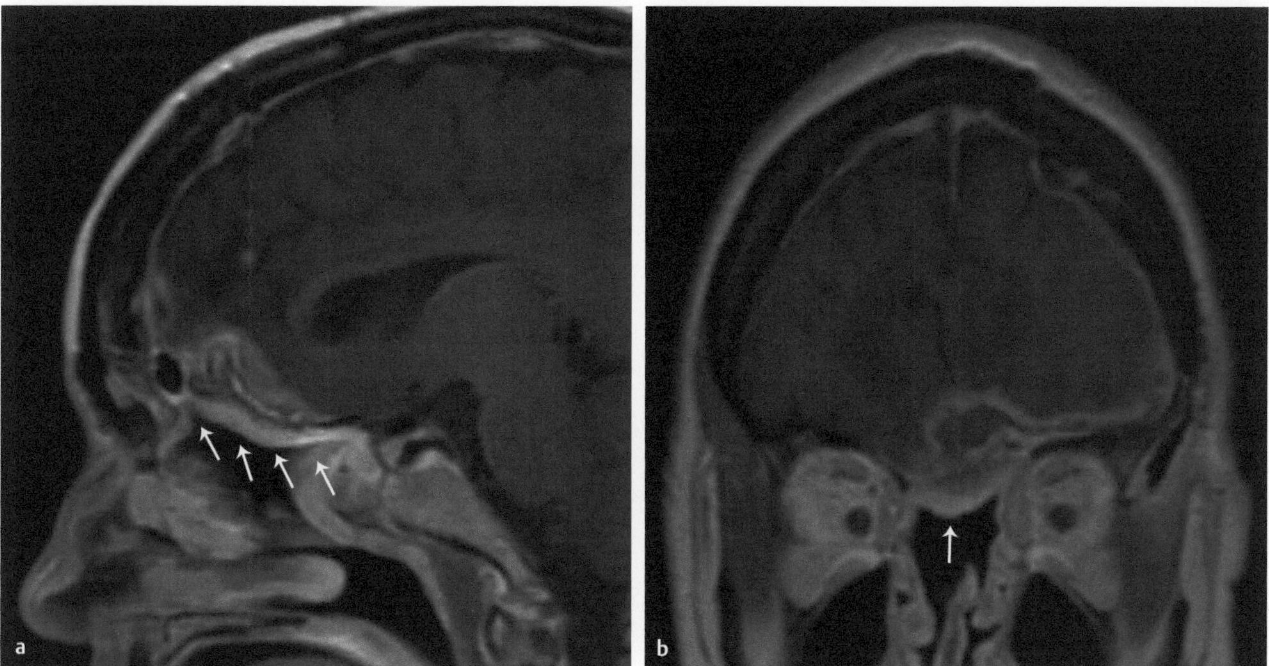

Fig. 21.2 Magnetic resonance imaging (MRI) T1 with contrast 5 weeks after the tumor resection. The patient presented with postoperative cerebrospinal fluid (CSF) leak. **(a)** Sagittal view. Observe the nasoseptal flap (NSF) enhanced with contrast (*white arrows*). *Yellow arrow* shows a gap between the anterior edge of the NSF and the anterior margin of the defect, responsible for the CSF leak and formation of a pneumocephalus right above the defect. **(b)** Coronal view showing the NSF enhanced with contrast and covering the anterior skull base from orbit to orbit.

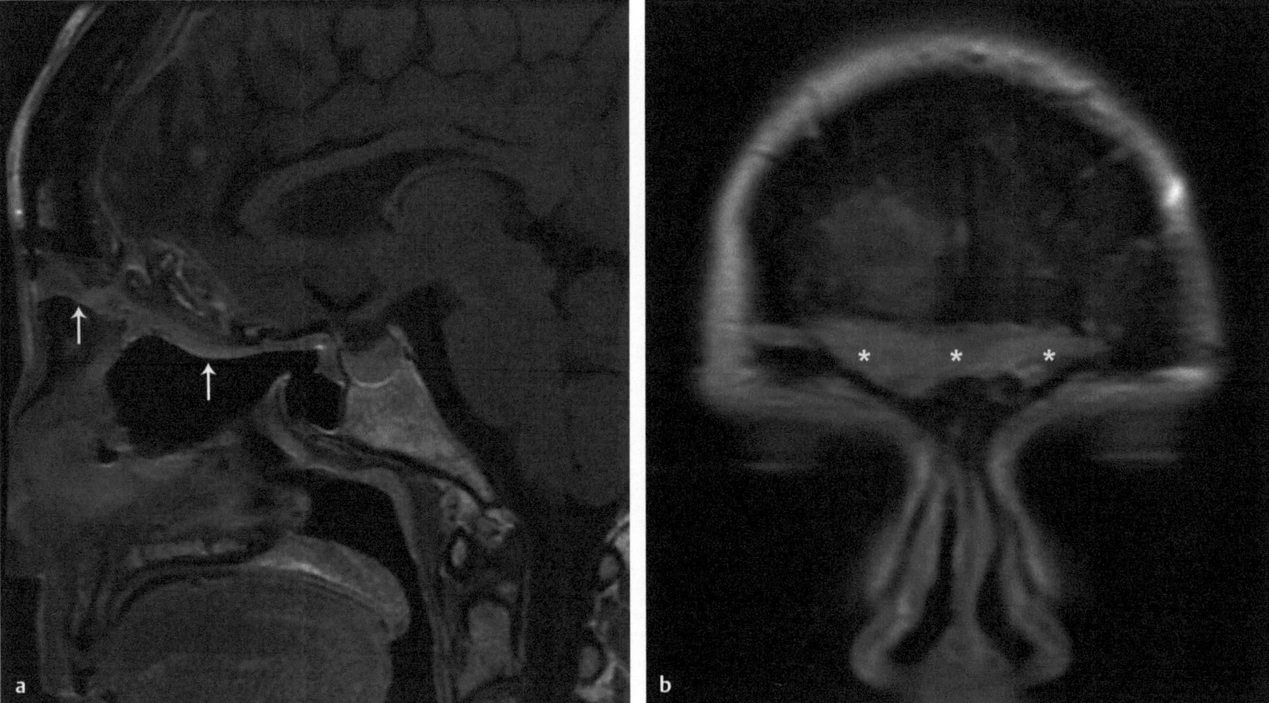

Fig. 21.3 Three-month postoperative magnetic resonance imaging (MRI) T1 with contrast following the galeal-frontalis muscle flap reconstruction. **(a)** Sagittal view. Observe the flap (*yellow arrow*) passing across the frontal osteotomy and covering the most anterior aspect of the cranial base. *White arrow* shows the nasoseptal flap. **(b)** Coronal view showing the lateral extension of the thick galeal-frontalis muscle flap (*asterisks*) and how it fills the region where the frontal sinus was cranialized.

In most cases of large anterior cranial base defects, when the NSF is not available, a pericranial flap is the next option.[2,3] However, the pericranium, in this case, was used in the previous transcranial reconstruction. Therefore, a less commonly used but equally effective flap from the galea was harvested to cover the anterior cranial base. The galeal flap has similar vascularity as the pericranium flap. It is thicker than the pericranium flap, which may help in minimizing brain sagging through the cranial defect.[4,5] There are few factors that can determine the use of the galeal flap. One is the thickness of the scalp. Thin scalps are associated with thinner galea and higher risk of skin necrosis compared to a thicker scalp.[4] The other factor is the technical experience. The flap is dissected along the subcutaneous tissue where there is no defined surgical plane. The galea continues with the frontalis muscle anteriorly which is also separated from the skin of the forehead. Complications related to the galeal flap are the risk of injury of the skin and resulting facial scars, skin necrosis, loss of frontalis muscle action, and consequent changes in facial expression. The galeal flap, like the pericranial flap, is associated with a prolonged period of crusting during the mucosalization of its endonasal surface. This requires several visits to the clinic for nasal debridement.

Our patient had a superior ethmoidal approach with preservation of part of the ethmoid and contralateral septal mucosa.[6] Several months later, she presented with a recurrent tumor at the tuberculum sellae compressing the right optic nerve. The tumor was resected endoscopically and the defect was reconstructed with the contralateral NSF.

21.4 Alternatives

- Since the right NSF was initially used for reconstruction, the repair of the persistent anterior cranial base defect could have been performed with the contralateral NSF with pedicle dissection within the pterygopalatine fossa. This would have increased the mobilization of the flap and coverage at the anterior edge of the defect. However, harvesting a contralateral NSF before mucosalization of the right side would have increased remarkably the risk of postoperative septal deformities due to lack of mucoperichondrium bilaterally.
- Anterior-based lateral nasal wall flap or posterior-based lateral nasal wall flap with pedicle dissection within the pterygopalatine fossa. Both are potential good options for salvage reconstruction. However, considering the patient's history of radiation, failure of previous endoscopic repair, location of the defect, and cranialization of the frontal sinus, a more robust reconstruction anteriorly was indicated.
- This extreme anterior defect would have been a far reach for the temporoparietal fascia flap.
- Even though this patient had multiple potential options available, the galeal-frontalis muscle flap offered the best wide coverage at the critical area of this patient's defect. The inlay inset of the galeal-frontalis muscle flap from anterior to posterior and covering both orbital roofs provided an excellent and reliable reconstruction at the space between the anterior table of the frontal sinus and the edge of the NSF previously used. The wide base of the flap created a stable and efficient tent effect anteriorly against the CSF pressure. Similar degree of reliable tent effect would not have been possible to be achieved with a sole endonasal reconstruction.

21.5 Conclusions

Skull base reconstruction is challenging in cases of multiple reoperations and prior radiation. Most of the postoperative CSF leaks can be successfully managed with less-invasive techniques including endoscopic repair with grafts and/or intranasal flaps. For high-risk patients, especially if a less-invasive technique was attempted first and failed, it is recommended to go up in the ladder of reconstruction instead of insisting on less-invasive endonasal approaches. In this case, the opening of the previous bifrontal craniotomy, which was avoided for tumor resection, was performed for the reconstruction after the failure of the first attempt of endoscopic endonasal repair. An unusual flap was used: Galeal-frontalis muscle flap. In an extreme situation, a paramedian forehead flap with de-epithelization of the skin is also an option to seal very anterior skull base defects. This case also illustrates the importance of preserving nasal structures in endoscopic endonasal skull base surgery. A contralateral NSF was later used for reconstruction after resection of a recurrent turberculum sellae meningioma.

References

[1] Peris-Celda M, Pinheiro-Neto CD, Funaki T, et al. The extended nasoseptal flap for skull base reconstruction of the clival region: an anatomical and radiological study. J Neurol Surg B Skull Base. 2013; 74(6):369–385

[2] Patel MR, Shah RN, Snyderman CH, et al. Pericranial flap for endoscopic anterior skull-base reconstruction: clinical outcomes and radioanatomic analysis of preoperative planning. Neurosurgery. 2010; 66(3):506–512, discussion 512

[3] Price JC, Loury M, Carson B, Johns ME. The pericranial flap for reconstruction of anterior skull base defects. Laryngoscope. 1988; 98(11):1159–1164

[4] Snyderman CH, Janecka IP, Sekhar LN, Sen CN, Eibling DE. Anterior cranial base reconstruction: role of galeal and pericranial flaps. Laryngoscope. 1990; 100(6):607–614

[5] Ito E, Watanabe T, Sato T, et al. Skull base reconstruction using various types of galeal flaps. Acta Neurochir (Wien). 2012; 154(1):179–185

[6] Peris Celda M, Kenning T, Pinheiro-Neto CD. Endoscopic superior ethmoidal approach for anterior cranial base resection: tailoring the approach for maximum exposure with preservation of nasal structures. World Neurosurg. 2017; 104:311–317

22 Necrotic Pericranial Scalp Flap

Carl H. Snyderman and Paul A. Gardner

22.1 Case Description

22.1.1 Presentation

A 62-year-old male presented with a recurrent squamous cell carcinoma of the anterior cranial base 1 year following endoscopic sinus surgery and radiochemotherapy. Imaging demonstrated tumor involvement of the anterior cranial base without involvement of the orbits (▶ Fig. 22.1). There was dural invasion but no intradural extension.

The patient was morbidly obese with type 2 diabetes mellitus and hypertension. Endoscopic examination confirmed the extent of the disease. Due to the extent of prior sinus surgery, local intranasal flaps were not an option for reconstruction. Metastatic workup was negative, and the patient was considered a suitable candidate for surgery (endonasal resection of anterior cranial base with extracranial pericranial flap reconstruction).

22.1.2 Surgical Procedure

An endoscopic endonasal transfrontal/transcribriform/transplanum approach with resection of anterior cranial base (bone, dura, and olfactory bulbs/tracts) was performed. All dural and olfactory margins of resection were negative by frozen section.

A three-layer reconstruction of the anterior cranial base was performed, culminating with a vascularized, extracranial pericranial flap (▶ Fig. 22.2). A collagen substitute was placed as an inlay graft between the brain and dura. A generous fascia lata graft was used as an extradural onlay graft. Where possible, a fold of the graft was tucked into the epidural space, between dura and bone and also over the orbital roof. A bicoronal scalp incision provided access for elevation of a unilateral pericranial flap based on the right-sided supraorbital and supratrochlear vessels. The bone of the nasion was drilled to create a window for introduction of the flap below the plane of the skull base (extracranial pericranial flap).[1,2] The flap pedicle was slightly displaced to one side to maintain patency of the Draf III frontal sinusotomy, but carefully tucked up against the inferior aspect of the posterior table of the frontal sinus. The reconstruction was supported with Gelfoam and Merocel tampons. A lumbar spinal drain was placed with drainage of cerebrospinal fluid (CSF) at a rate of approximately 10 mL/h for 72 hours.

22.1.3 Postoperative Course

Computed tomography (CT) on postoperative day 0 revealed moderate pneumocephalus, consistent with postoperative changes (▶ Fig. 22.3a). The lumbar spinal drain was removed on postoperative day 3. Due to a change in mental status, a follow-up CT was obtained on postoperative day 4 which demonstrated increased air with evidence of tension pneumocephalus (▶ Fig. 22.3b). There was no clinical evidence of a CSF leak with the nasal packing in place.

22.2 Challenges

This patient presented multiple challenges simultaneously:

- Acute mental status change—differential diagnosis, evaluation.
- Tension pneumocephalus—risk factors, management, prevention.
- Flap necrosis—reconstructive options.

22.3 Discussion

Due to increasing pneumocephalus and altered mental status, the patient was placed on 100% oxygen via a nonrebreather face mask and returned to the operating room. Endoscopic examination of the surgical site demonstrated a necrotic pericranial flap with air between the fascia lata and flap (▶ Fig. 22.4). The necrotic flap was debrided endoscopically and the fascia lata appeared to be intact. The bicoronal incision was reopened to assess the residual pericranium. It appeared that the bony window at the nasion was insufficient and the flap pedicle was compressed due to postoperative tissue edema. The flap pedicle was further debrided and the bony opening enlarged. A pericranial flap was harvested from the contralateral side and transposed through the opening to cover the fascial lata. Prior to packing the nasal cavity, a nasal trumpet was inserted to prevent tension pneumocephalus (▶ Fig. 22.5). A lumbar spinal drain was reinserted.

Follow-up CT scans showed resolving pneumocephalus (▶ Fig. 22.6). Endoscopic examinations following removal of packing confirmed viability of the flap and healing without CSF leak.

Multiple factors contributed to the failure of the reconstruction. A root cause analysis is a useful tool to investigate the contributing factors and create a learning opportunity (▶ Fig. 22.7).

- Morbid obesity with obstructive sleep apnea increases the risk of tension pneumocephalus from higher upper airway pressure. This separates the layers of the reconstruction, delaying vascularization and increasing the risk of infection and flap necrosis.
- Morbid obesity and obstructive sleep apnea also increase intracranial pressure and risk of a postoperative CSF leak.
- Prior irradiation therapy may impede vascularization.
- A unilateral pericranial flap has a narrower pedicle (susceptible to torsion) and less vascularity than a bilateral flap. Overdissection of the flap during harvest may compromise the blood supply.
- A bulky flap pedicle may become compressed by a small bony opening at the nasion, especially with postoperative edema of the flap pedicle.

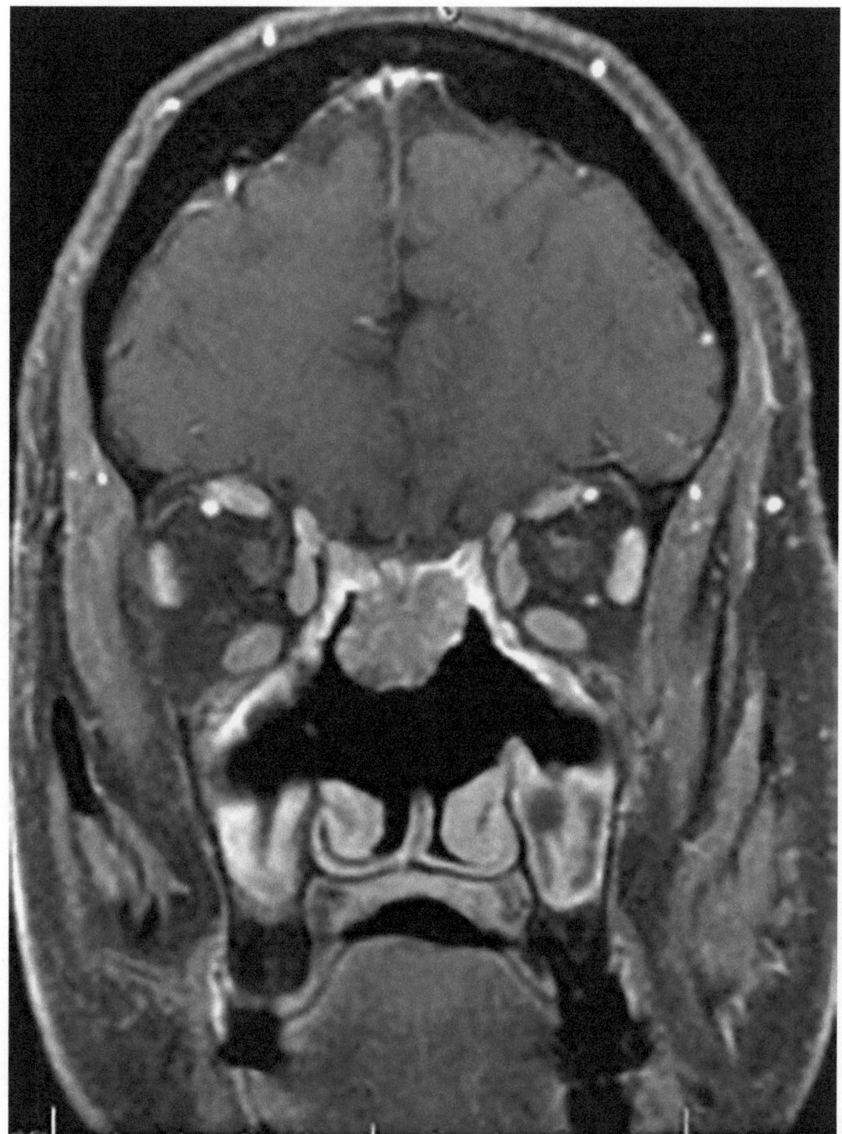

Fig. 22.1 Coronal T1 magnetic resonance imaging (MRI) demonstrates recurrent tumor located centrally at the anterior cranial base without intracranial or orbital invasion. There has been extensive removal of sinus structures with loss of vascular pedicles for a nasoseptal flap or lateral nasal wall flap.

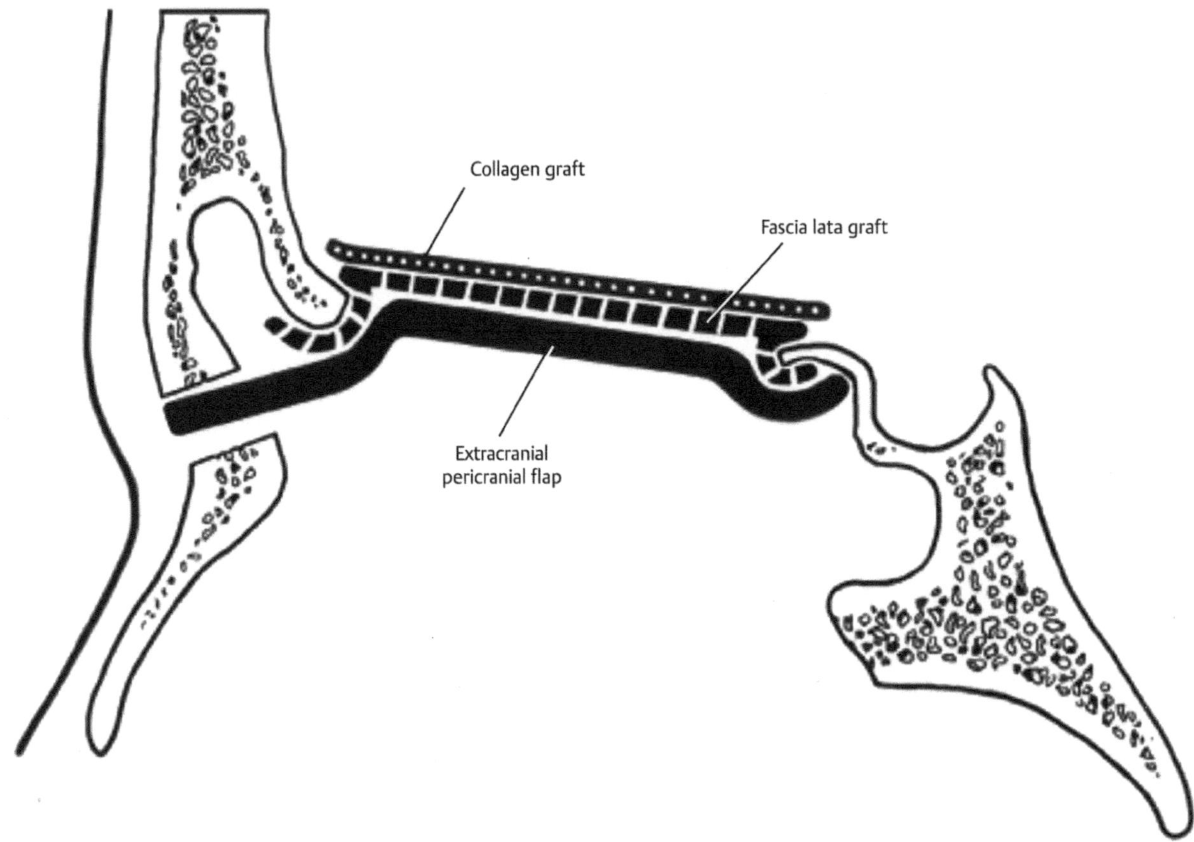

Fig. 22.2 Drawing showing a three-layer reconstruction of the anterior cranial base including an extracranial pericranial flap.

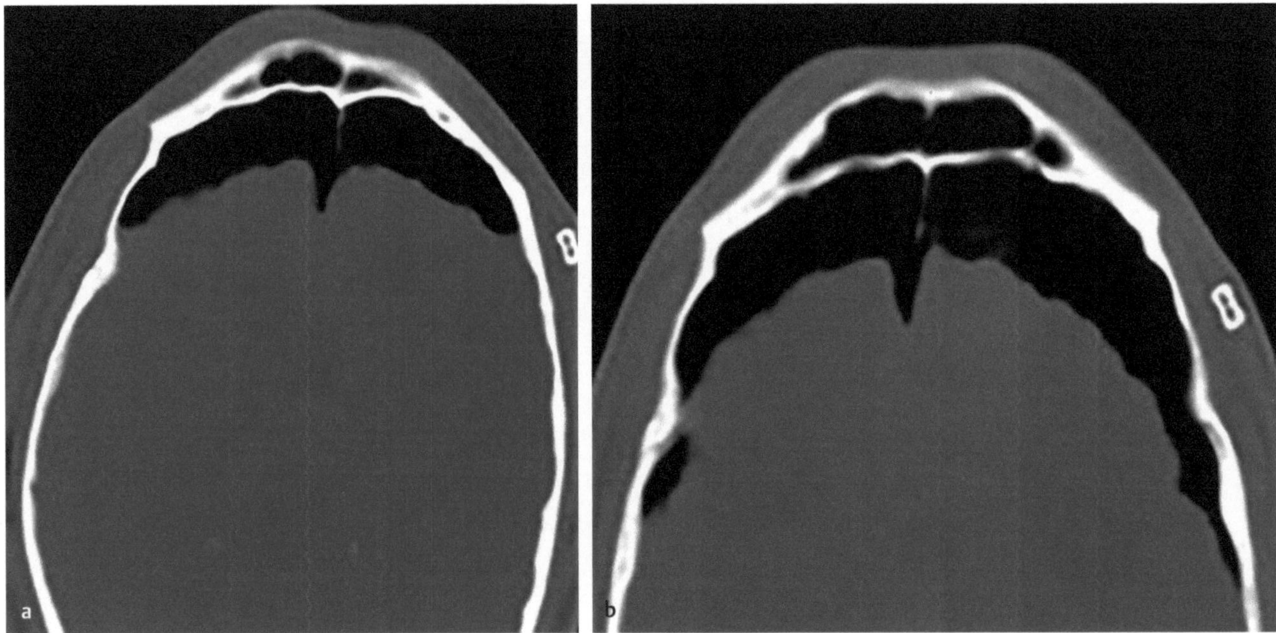

Fig. 22.3 **(a)** Computed tomography (CT) on postoperative day 0 revealed moderate pneumocephalus, consistent with postoperative changes. **(b)** CT obtained on postoperative day 4 demonstrated increased air with evidence of tension pneumocephalus.

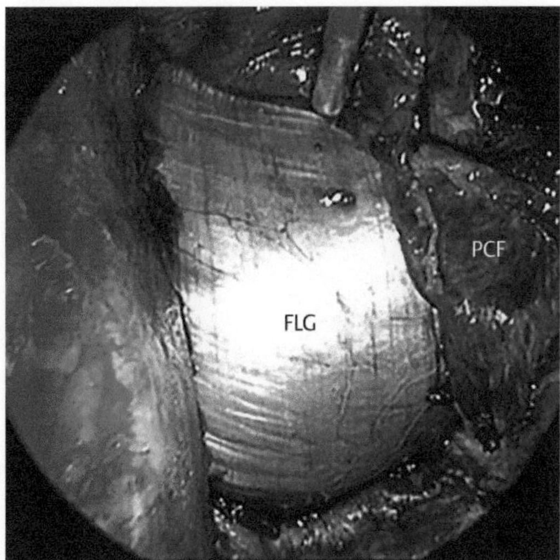

Fig. 22.4 The nonviable pericranial flap (PCF) was completely debrided to expose intact fascia lata graft (FLG).

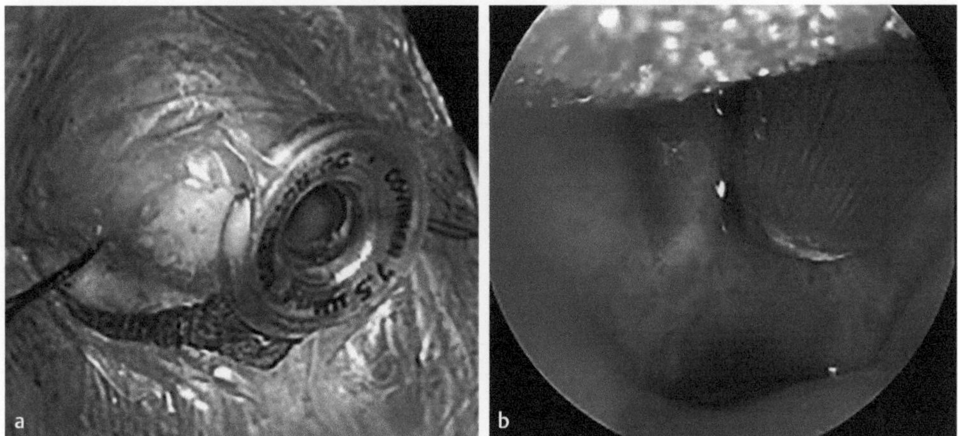

Fig. 22.5 **(a)** Nasal trumpet was placed inferior to nasal packing. Strings are from nasal packing. **(b)** Nasopharyngeal end of nasal trumpet prevents generation of increased intranasal air pressure, thereby potentially decreasing the risk of tension pneumocephalus.

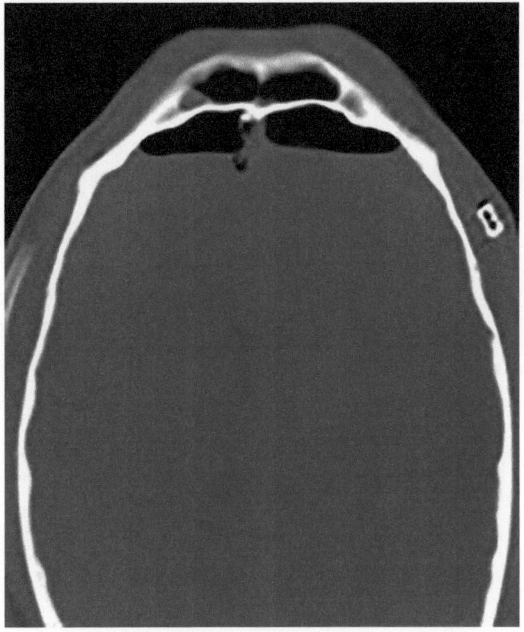

Fig. 22.6 Follow-up computed tomography (CT) scan shows resolving pneumocephalus.

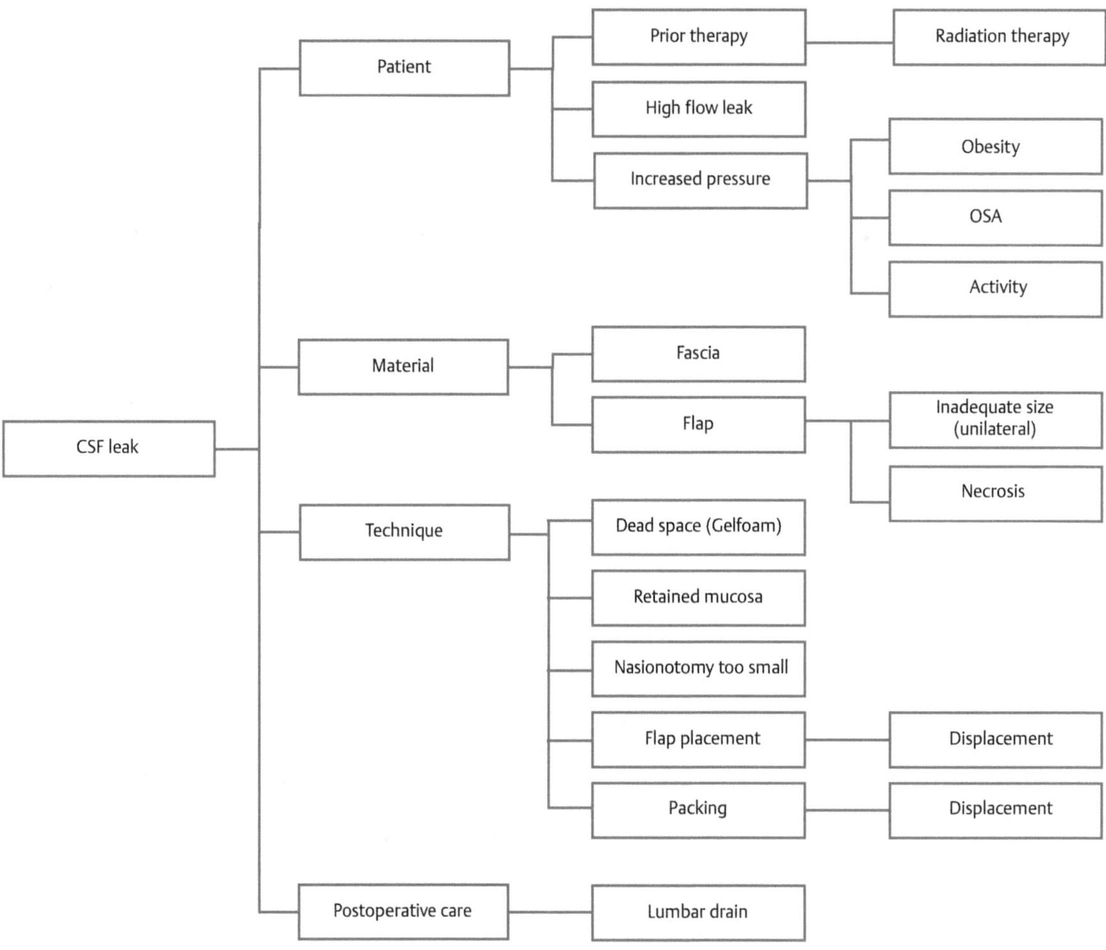

Fig. 22.7 Root cause analysis.

22.4 Alternatives

Alternative reconstructive options are limited in this patient due to extensive prior surgery. Possibilities include:

- Nonvascularized secondary reconstruction using additional layer of fascia lata and possible fat grafts around periphery.
- Microvascular free flap.
- Temporalis myofascial flap and temporoparietal fascial flap are unlikely to reach.

22.5 Conclusions

- The extracranial pericranial flap is the preferred vascular flap for reconstruction of the anterior cranial base when a nasoseptal flap is not an option.
- Although a bilateral flap may be necessary for repair of large defects, a unilateral pericranial flap is usually adequate and preserves the option of a second flap if needed.
- A large bony opening is necessary to prevent compression of the vascular pedicle with an extracranial pericranial flap. Location at the nasion will create no long-term deformity regardless of size.
- Increasing pneumocephalus on serial postoperative CT scans indicates a dural fistula even in the absence of CSF rhinorrhea.
- Tension pneumocephalus may be prevented by placing a nasopharyngeal airway.
- Avoid placing nonvascularized tissues/materials (Gelfoam, tissue glue, adipose tissue, bone graft, and alloplastic graft) between tissue layers. The layers of reconstruction (fascia lata, flap) should be in contact to promote early vascularization. The intranasal surface of the flap should be supported with packing to obliterate the dead space.
- The optimal management of a postoperative dural defect is early surgical intervention.

References

[1] Zanation AM, Snyderman CH, Carrau RL, Kassam AB, Gardner PA, Prevedello DM. Minimally invasive endoscopic pericranial flap: a new method for endonasal skull base reconstruction. Laryngoscope. 2009; 119(1):13–18

[2] Patel MR, Shah RN, Snyderman CH, et al. Pericranial flap for endoscopic anterior skull-base reconstruction: clinical outcomes and radioanatomic analysis of preoperative planning. Neurosurgery. 2010; 66(3):506–512, discussion 512

23 Necrotic Nasoseptal Flap

Carl H. Snyderman and Paul A. Gardner

23.1 Case Description

23.1.1 Presentation

A 45-year-old male presented with headache and diplopia. Physical examination revealed a unilateral right sixth nerve palsy. Computed tomography (CT) and magnetic resonance imaging (MRI) demonstrated a lesion of the middle and lower clivus with imaging characteristics of a chordoma (▶ Fig. 23.1). There was significant dural penetration without involvement of intracranial vessels. Physical examination including nasal endoscopy demonstrated evidence of prior endoscopic sinus surgery with narrowed vascular pedicles for a nasoseptal flap (NSF) (▶ Fig. 23.2).

23.1.2 Surgical Procedure

At the beginning of the surgery, Doppler was used to confirm presence of the posterior septal branches of the sphenopalatine artery. Indocyanine green (ICG) fluoroscopy provided additional confirmation and the side with the best vascularity (right) was selected for elevation of an NSF (▶ Fig. 23.2).[1]

An endoscopic endonasal transclival approach to the posterior cranial fossa was performed with complete drill-out of the clivus from the floor of the sella to foramen magnum. Laterally, bone was removed to the paraclival segment of the internal carotid arteries, requiring mobilization of the flap pedicle, and the sixth cranial nerves were decompressed in Dorello canal. The periosteal and meningeal layers of the dura were resected along with the intradural tumor.

A standard full transclival reconstruction was performed with inlay collagen graft, onlay fascia lata graft, fat graft, and vascularized NSF (▶ Fig. 23.3). An inferiorly based rhinopharyngeal mucosal flap overlapped the fascial lata graft inferiorly.[2] The reconstruction was supported with Gelfoam and Merocel tampons. A lumbar spinal drain was placed with drainage of cerebrospinal fluid (CSF) at a rate of approximately 10 mL/h for 72 hours.

23.1.3 Postoperative Course

Early postoperative MRI was performed to assess the completeness of tumor resection. There was no evidence of residual tumor, but lack of enhancement of the distal NSF was noted (▶ Fig. 23.4). The lumbar spinal drain was removed after 3 days and nasal packing was removed at 1 week following surgery.

Three weeks after surgery, the patient presented with fever, increasing headache, and neck pain. A foul odor was noted from the nasal cavity. Endoscopic examination revealed a necrotic NSF with minimal purulence (▶ Fig. 23.5). MRI again demonstrated lack of enhancement of the NSF but no purulent collection. CSF studies were consistent with meningitis but cultures were negative.

Endoscopic debridement of the necrotic flap was performed in the operating room. Purulence with partial fat graft necrosis was noted deep into the flap. Fat and fascia lata grafts were removed, but the inlay collagen graft was intact (▶ Fig. 23.6). There was no evidence of active CSF leak. An ipsilateral lateral nasal wall (inferior turbinate) flap was harvested and placed over a new fascia lata graft (▶ Fig. 23.7). The inferior edge of the fascia lata was sutured to the edge of the rhinopharyngeal flap using a V-Loc suture.[3] ICG fluoroscopy and postoperative imaging confirmed excellent vascularity of the lateral nasal wall flap.

The patient was treated with antibiotics for possible meningitis and had an uneventful recovery.

23.2 Challenges

This patient has both diagnostic and therapeutic challenges:

- Early recognition of necrotic flap with associated extradural infection.
- Diagnosis of meningitis.
- Secondary reconstruction using vascularized lateral nasal wall flap.

23.3 Discussion

- Large transclival defects including the dura are best reconstructed with a four-layer repair, including inlay collagen graft, onlay fascial graft, adipose tissue graft to fill the clival defect and prevent pontine herniation, and a vascularized flap (▶ Fig. 23.3).
- The inferior edge of the repair is most susceptible to failure. An inferiorly based rhinopharyngeal flap allows tucking of the inferior edge of the fascia lata deep into the mucosa. The inferior margin of graft or flap can also be secured with a running V-Loc suture.[3]
- This case highlights the rare complication of NSF necrosis.[4] Risk factors for NSF necrosis are prior surgery, lack of enhancement on postoperative MRI, and the use of a fat graft. Prior surgery is a risk factor due to narrowing of the NSF vascular pedicle. It is unclear if fat graft necrosis with infection is a contributing factor, though there does seem to be an association, perhaps relative to clival defects (see following text). Intraoperative Doppler and ICG fluoroscopy are useful in evaluating the residual vascularity intraoperatively.
- Clival defects can be particularly susceptible to flap necrosis due to frequent flap pedicle manipulation and dissection. The pedicle itself is often overlying the pterygoid bone which must be removed for full tumor and petroclival access.
- Patients with delayed NSF necrosis can present with symptoms and signs of meningitis but without a CSF leak. A foul nasal odor may be noted.
- Debridement of nonviable tissue with secondary vascularized flap reconstruction is recommended.

23.4 Alternatives

In patients who have had prior surgery and the NSF flap pedicle is narrowed, there are several reconstructive options:

- Nonvascularized reconstruction.
- NSF reconstruction if Doppler or ICG fluoroscopy demonstrate preserved posterior septal arteries.

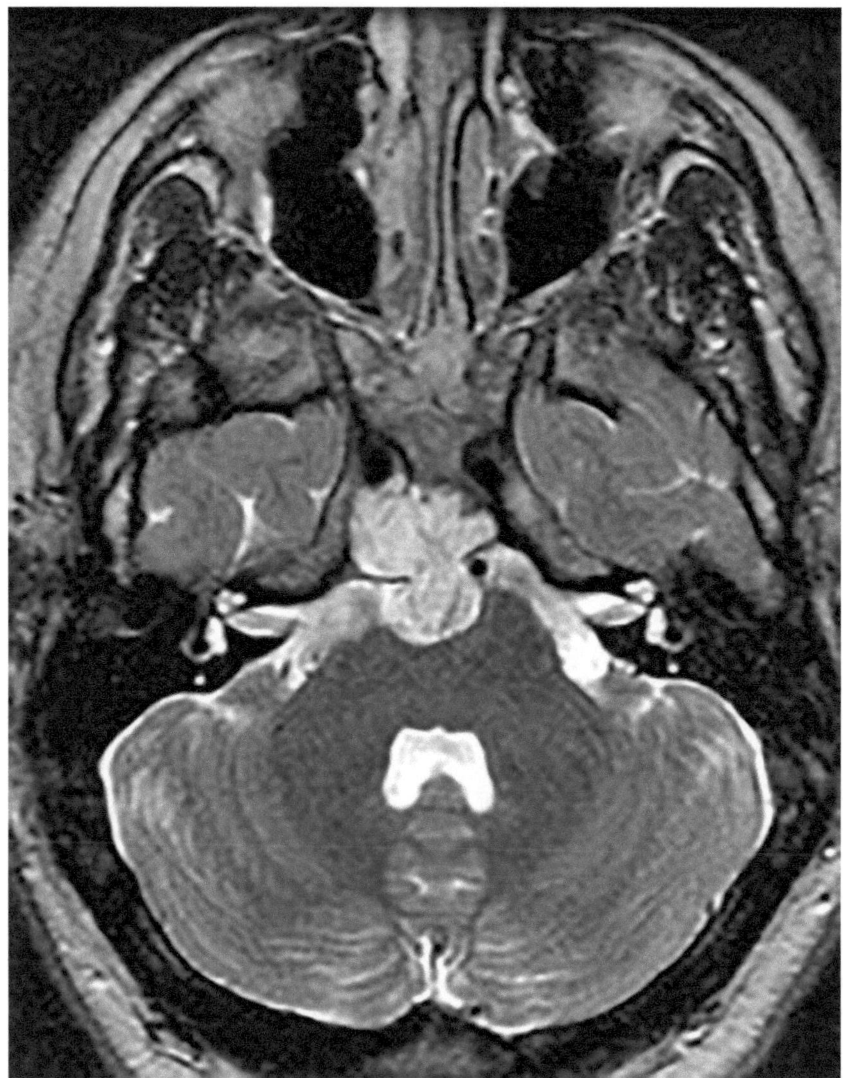

Fig. 23.1 T2 axial magnetic resonance imaging (MRI) demonstrates a clival chordoma with intradural extension. The basilar artery is displaced to the left. The tumor is compressing the right abducens nerve posterior to the paraclival internal carotid artery.

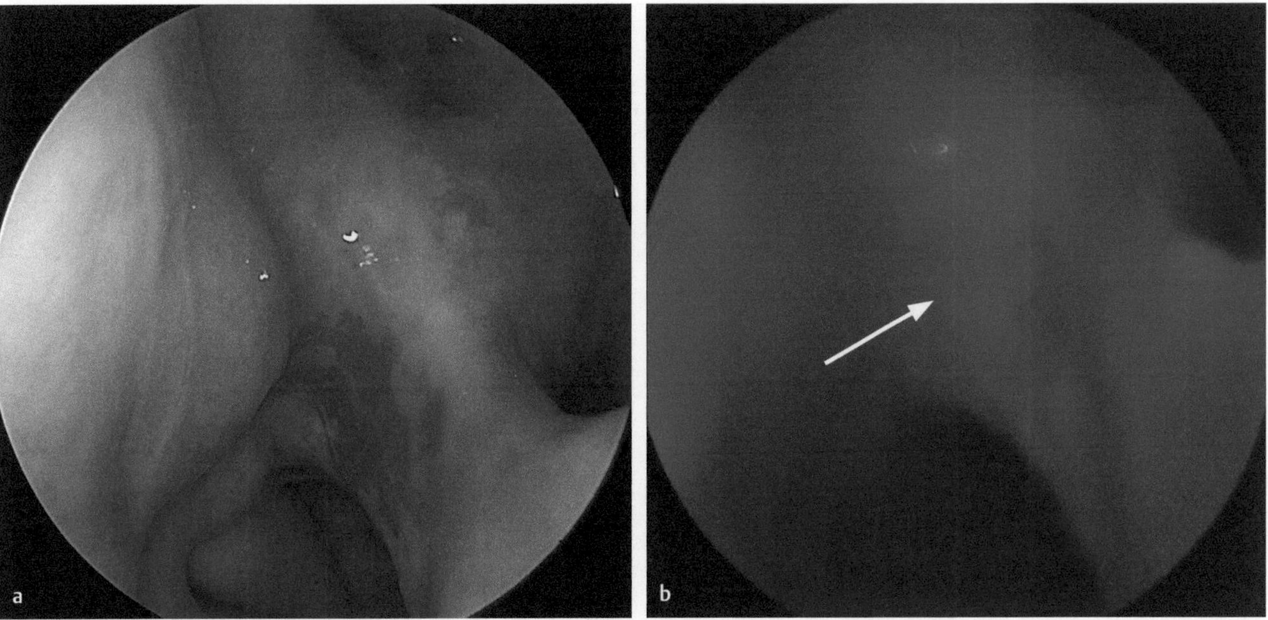

Fig. 23.2 (a) Nasal endoscopy (*right side*) demonstrates a narrowed vascular pedicle for a nasoseptal flap. Doppler probe can be used to detect posterior septal branches of the sphenopalatine artery. **(b)** Indocyanine green fluoroscopy demonstrates adequate vascularity of the vascular pedicle (*arrow*).

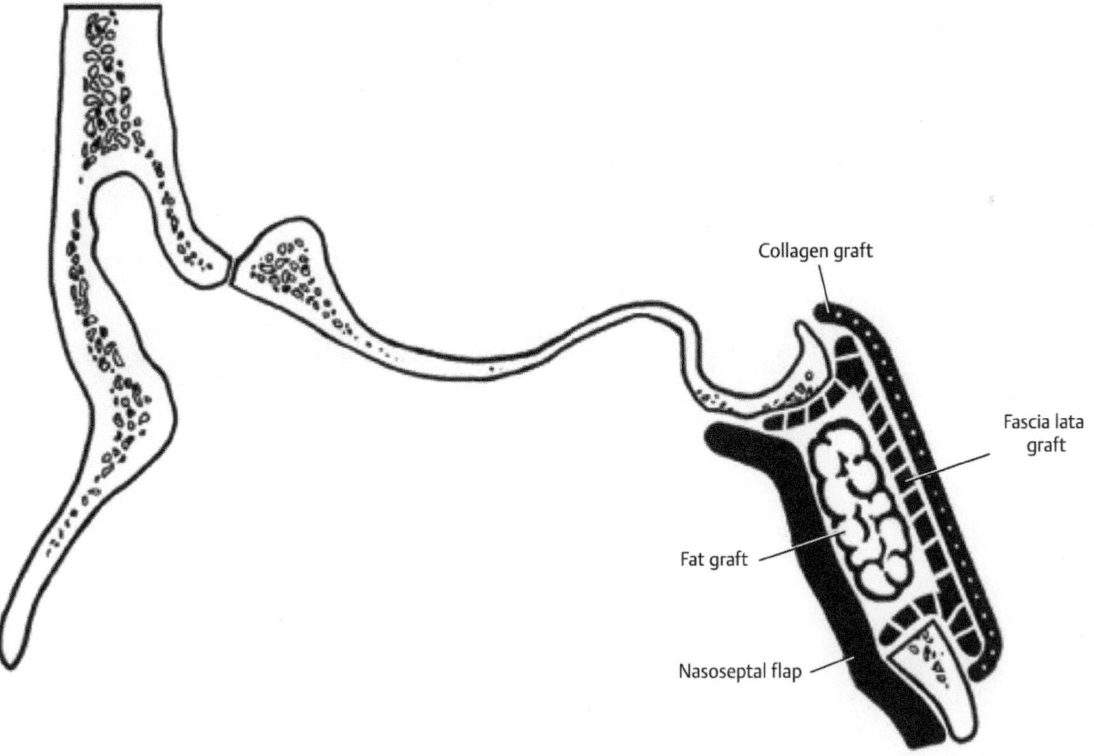

Fig. 23.3 The clival defect is reconstructed using a four-layer technique. Intradural collagen graft is covered with an extradural fascia lata, bolstered with fat graft to prevent pontine encephalocele. The entire reconstruction is then covered with a vascularized nasoseptal flap.

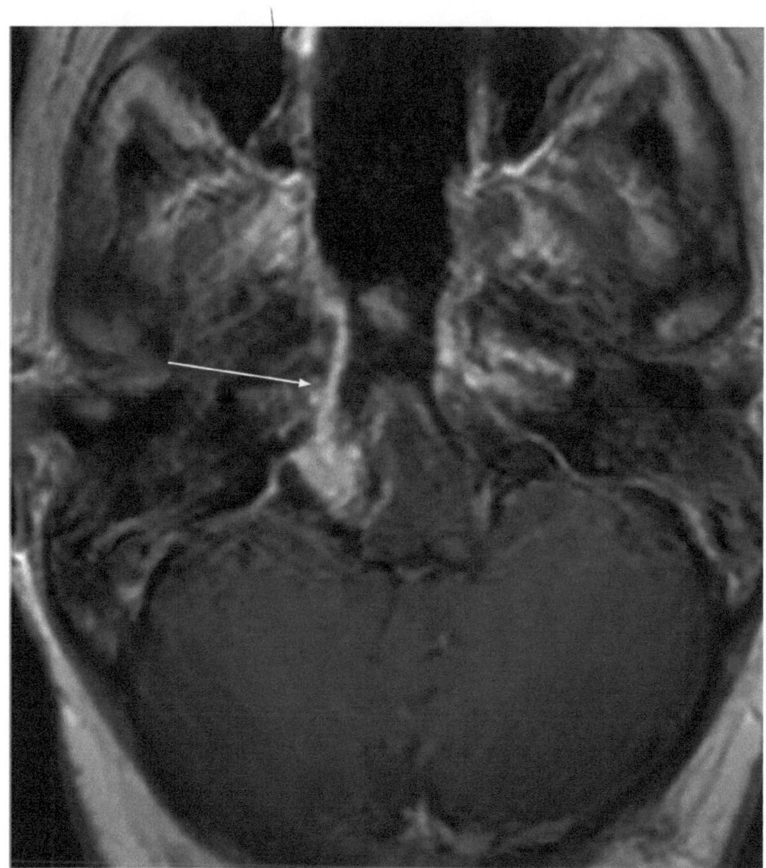

Fig. 23.4 Axial T1-weighted, postcontrast magnetic resonance imaging (MRI) demonstrates enhancement of only the proximal portion (*arrow*) of a right-sided nasoseptal flap.

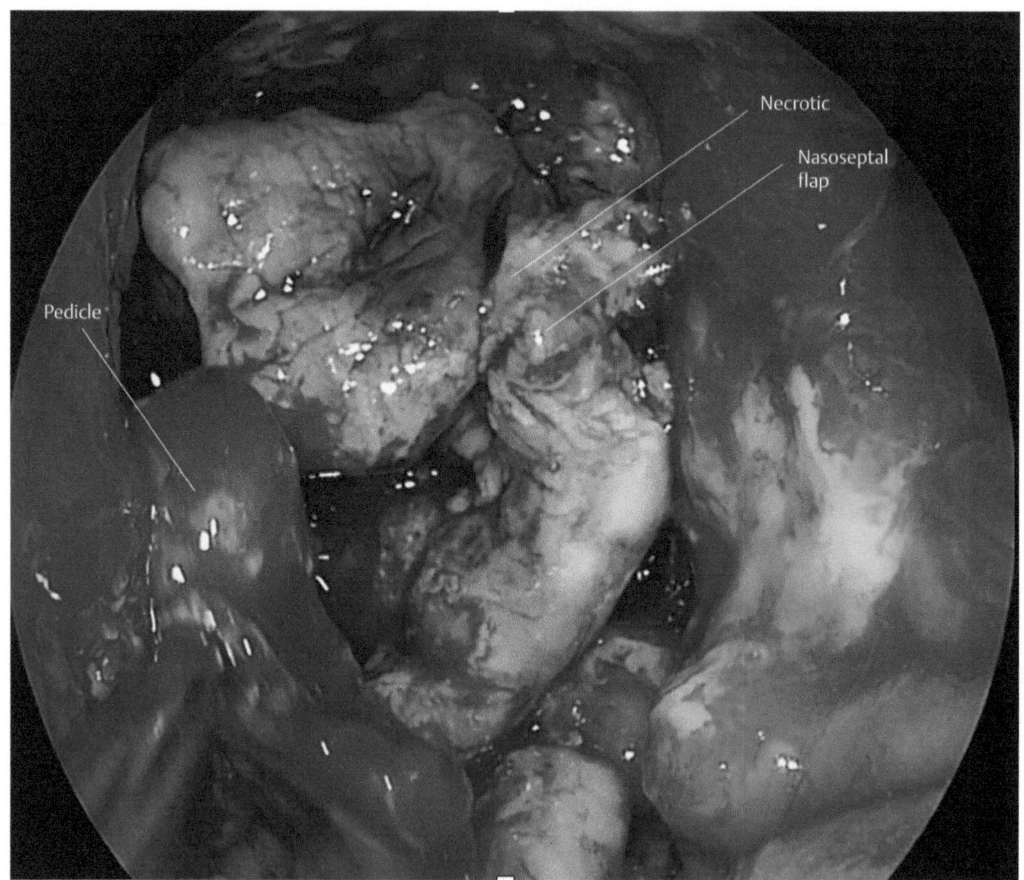

Fig. 23.5 Endoscopic endonasal view showing that the distal portion of the right-sided nasoseptal flap is necrotic with purulence deep into the flap.

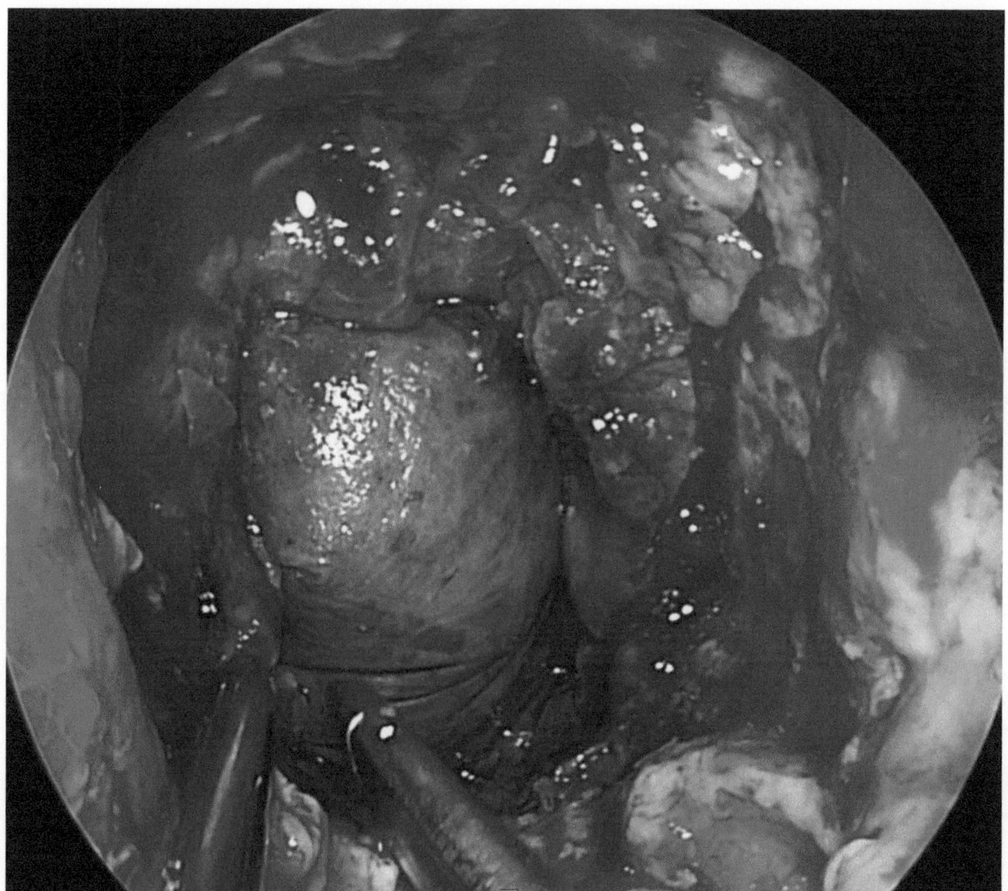

Fig. 23.6 Following debridement of the necrotic nasoseptal flap, fat, and fascia lata grafts, the inlay collagen graft is noted to be intact.

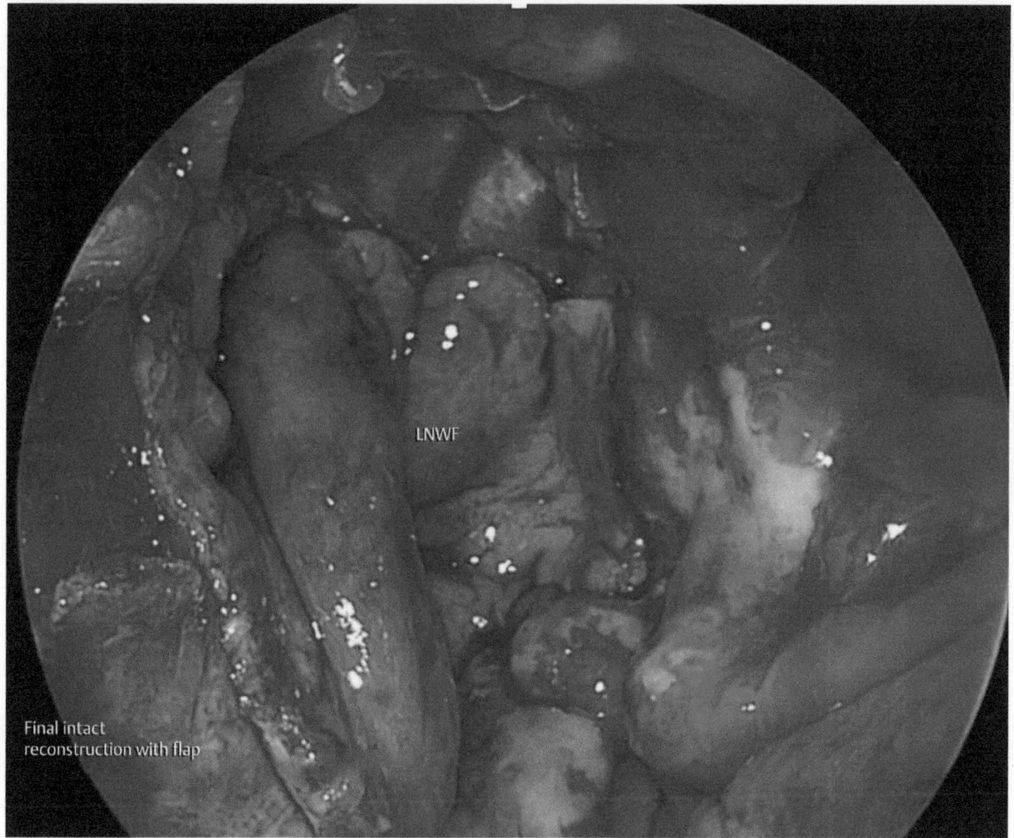

Fig. 23.7 The exposed intradural graft was covered with a new fascia lata graft and a right-sided vascularized lateral nasal wall flap (LNWF).

- Lateral nasal wall flap reconstruction. This can be extended to include mucosa from the nasal floor and nasal septum as needed.

23.5 Conclusions

- Patients with risk factors for NSF necrosis should be followed closely postoperatively for symptoms and signs of infection.
- Intraoperative evaluation with ICG endoscopic angiography, with or without postoperative contrast MRI, can be used to detect nonviable flaps.
- Delayed NSF necrosis should be suspected in patients who develop delayed symptoms of meningitis.
- Prompt surgical debridement and repair with vascularized tissue should be performed along with antibiotic therapy to prevent progression of infection.

References

[1] Geltzeiler M, Nakassa ACI, Turner M, et al. Evaluation of intranasal flap perfusion by intraoperative indocyanine green fluorescence angiography. Oper Neurosurg (Hagerstown). 2018; 15(6):672–676
[2] Champagne PO, Zenonos GA, Wang EW, Snyderman CH, Gardner PA. The rhinopharyngeal flap for reconstruction of lower clival and craniovertebral junction defects. J Neurosurg. 2021:1–9
[3] Zwagerman NT, Geltzeiler MN, Wang EW, Fernandez-Miranda JC, Snyderman CH, Gardner PA. Endonasal suturing of nasoseptal flap to nasopharyngeal fascia using the V-Loc™ wound closure device: 2-dimensional operative video. Oper Neurosurg (Hagerstown). 2019; 16(2):40–41
[4] Chabot JD, Patel CR, Hughes MA, et al. Nasoseptal flap necrosis: a rare complication of endoscopic endonasal surgery. J Neurosurg. 2018; 128(5):1463–1472

24 What to Do When a Nasoseptal Flap Is Not Perfusing?

Jamie J. Van Gompel, Janalee Stokken, and Salomon Cohen Cohen

24.1 Case Description

24.1.1 Presentation

A 65-year-old gentleman presented to his local physician with rapid changes in vision. Visual field testing demonstrated substantial visual field deficits (▶ Fig. 24.1). He subsequently underwent a magnetic resonance imaging (MRI) of the brain which showed a 3.3 cm third intraventricular tumor with extension to the pituitary stalk and with mass effect on the optic chiasm (▶ Fig. 24.2 and ▶ Fig. 24.3). He denied any headache but had gained 45 pounds in the past 5 months. He was found to be panhypopituitary on laboratory testing.

24.1.2 Surgical Procedure

Surgery was discussed not only for tissue diagnosis but also for decompression of the optic apparatus. Given the location of the chiasm on FIESTA (fast imaging employing steady-state acquisition) imaging (▶ Fig. 24.3), an endonasal transtuberculum route was chosen. After thorough preoperative discussion, he was taken for a lumbar drain placement. Then he was positioned for an endonasal approach. A nasoseptal flap was prepared, the right middle turbinate was removed, as well as an ethmoidectomy was performed. After a bilateral sphenoidotomy, approach to the sella was performed. Then, all the intersinus septae were drilled down and the sphenoid sinus demucosalized. The landmarks were identified, and the bone over the pituitary gland, the tuberculum, and the planum was drilled out. After this opening was made, there was bleeding from the circular sinus, which was then packed with hemostatic foam. Then, area above and below this was opened, this region was bipolar cauterized, and the circular sinus was crossed without difficulty. Then the diaphragm was opened. The superior hypophyseal artery branches were identified and pushed upwards in order to preserve them across the chiasm. It should be noted that the whole anterior portion of the tumor was covered in stalk. Therefore, a portion of this had to be resected. Multiple fragments were sent to pathology and found to be adamantinomatous craniopharyngioma. Then, the tumor was internally debulked and a gross total resection was performed, which was confirmed with 0, 30, and 45 degree endoscope inspection. The stalk itself was intact. Fascia lata graft and fat were harvested from the left thigh. A fascia lata graft and DuraGen were placed inlay, and the nasoseptal flap was then placed and was felt to look very healthy in the operative theater.

24.1.3 Postoperative Course

At this point in time, the patient was extubated and did well for the first day. An MRI demonstrated a complete resection, but the nasoseptal flap did not enhance (▶ Fig. 24.4).

The patient was dismissed from the hospital 5 days after surgery with no evidence of CSF leak. He then presented with a rapidly progressive CSF leak that occurred at 7 days postoperatively, which was tested for beta-2 transferrin and found to be positive. It seems to be more frequent with flap necrosis for the CSF leak to present 1 to 2 weeks after surgery rather than immediately. It can also look like a low-grade meningitis. Here, given the suspicion for flap failure, he was immediately taken to the operative theater. The prior flap appeared dark, necrotic, and thrombosed. New fascia lata was used in the repair, and the dural substitute and fascia lata were replaced, and a left-sided nasoseptal flap was raised and placed. He underwent 3 days of lumbar drainage again. This flap healed without issue (▶ Fig. 24.5). Delayed automated visual fields showed complete recovery of vision (▶ Fig. 24.5). Further, MRI demonstrated a complete resection (▶ Fig. 24.6). He is now 30 months after surgery, has not received radiation, and is without recurrence. He is on complete pituitary replacement with 1-deamino-8-D-arginine vasopressin (DDAVP) as well. He has not developed hypothalamic obesity.

24.2 Challenges

- High-flow postoperative CSF leak.
- Nasoseptal flap necrosis.
- 30-day return to the operative theater.

24.3 Discussion

Our surgical team discussed the MRI findings as there was concern about the flap, given it did not perfuse on the MRI postoperative day 1. A transtubercular approach with a craniopharyngioma in the third ventricle is among the highest risk cases for postoperative CSF leak. We believed a good multilayer repair was performed, but should one take the patient back for revision of the flap and placement of the left-sided nasoseptal flap? Obviously, an immediate concern is the repair may work and the patient may not need another operation; further, repeat surgery within 30 days is tracked nationally. Our group has experience with chordomas that have invaded both nasoseptal flaps or extensive skull base malignancies done solely through the nose, where multilayer fascial repairs have done well without CSF leak. In this case, we felt that we would continue lumbar drainage at 10 mL every 2 hours for 3 days after the initial surgery. We further believed that the defect was overall quite small, and the nonperfused nasoseptal flap would serve as a free graft, with the exception of a large area of demucosalization, as planned, to allow the graft to heal to the bone. In this case, it failed, and recognizing the lack of perfusion on the postoperative MRI was important to heighten our awareness to the potential CSF leak.

24.4 Alternatives

A variety of approaches could have been considered in this case. At the time, FDA approval was not provided for the indocyanine green endoscopes. However, probably 6 to 12 months after this

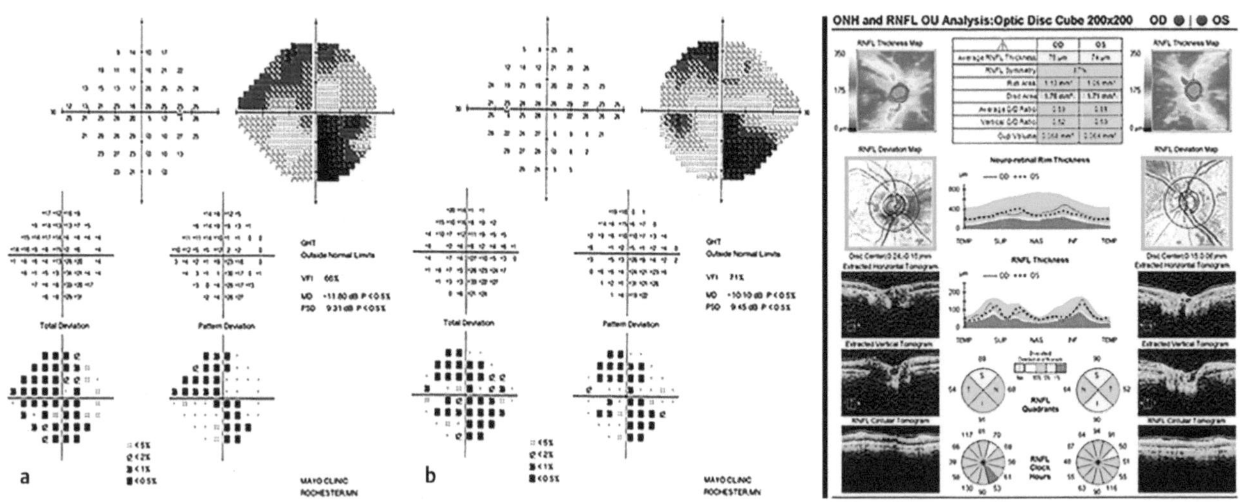

Fig. 24.1 Automated visual fields of the **(a)** right and **(b)** left eyes. Optical coherence tomography of the optic nerve suggesting recoverable visual fields *(green and yellow quadrants)*.

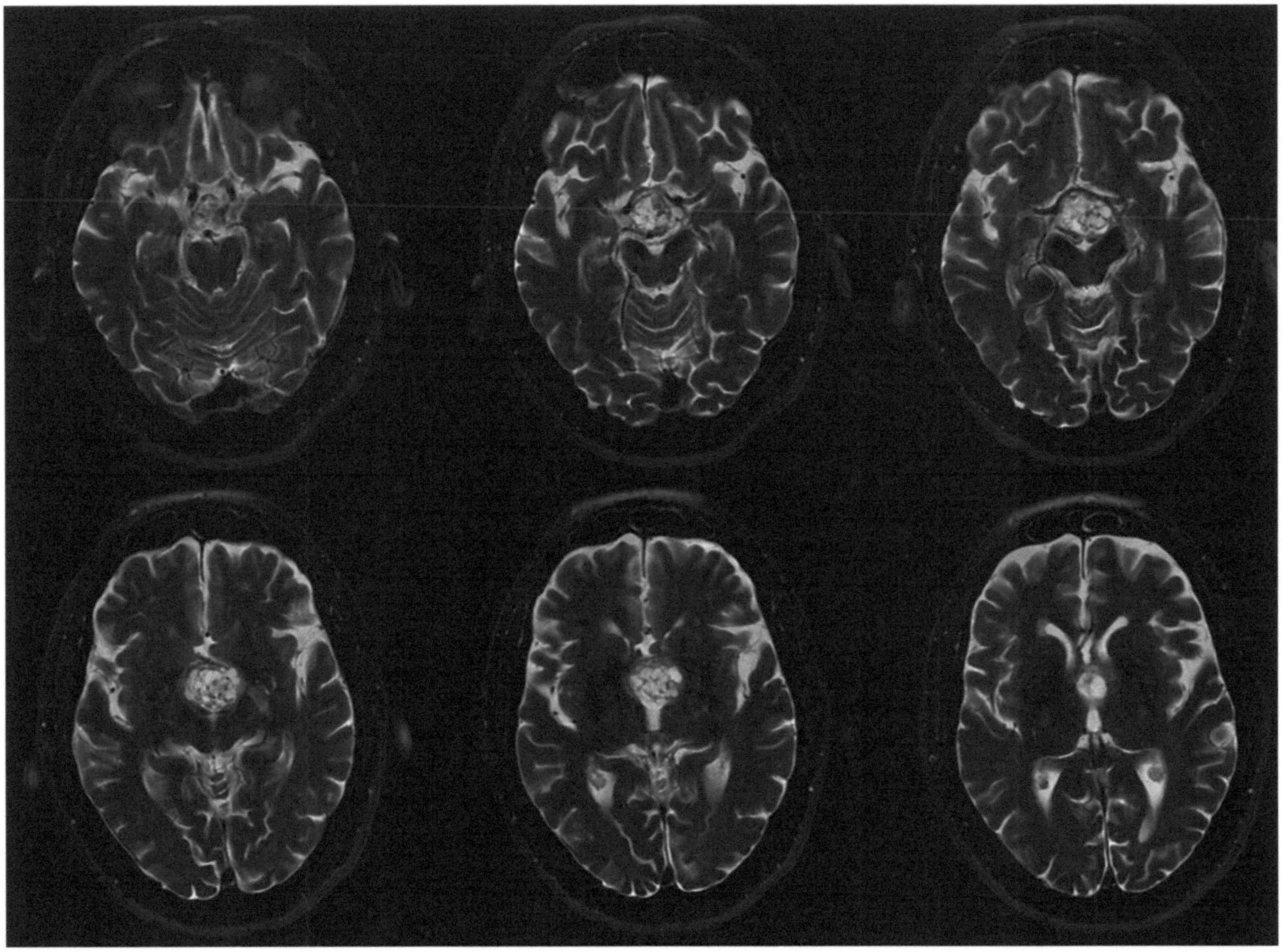

Fig. 24.2 Serial axial T2 magnetic resonance imagings (MRIs) demonstrating a third ventricular mass.

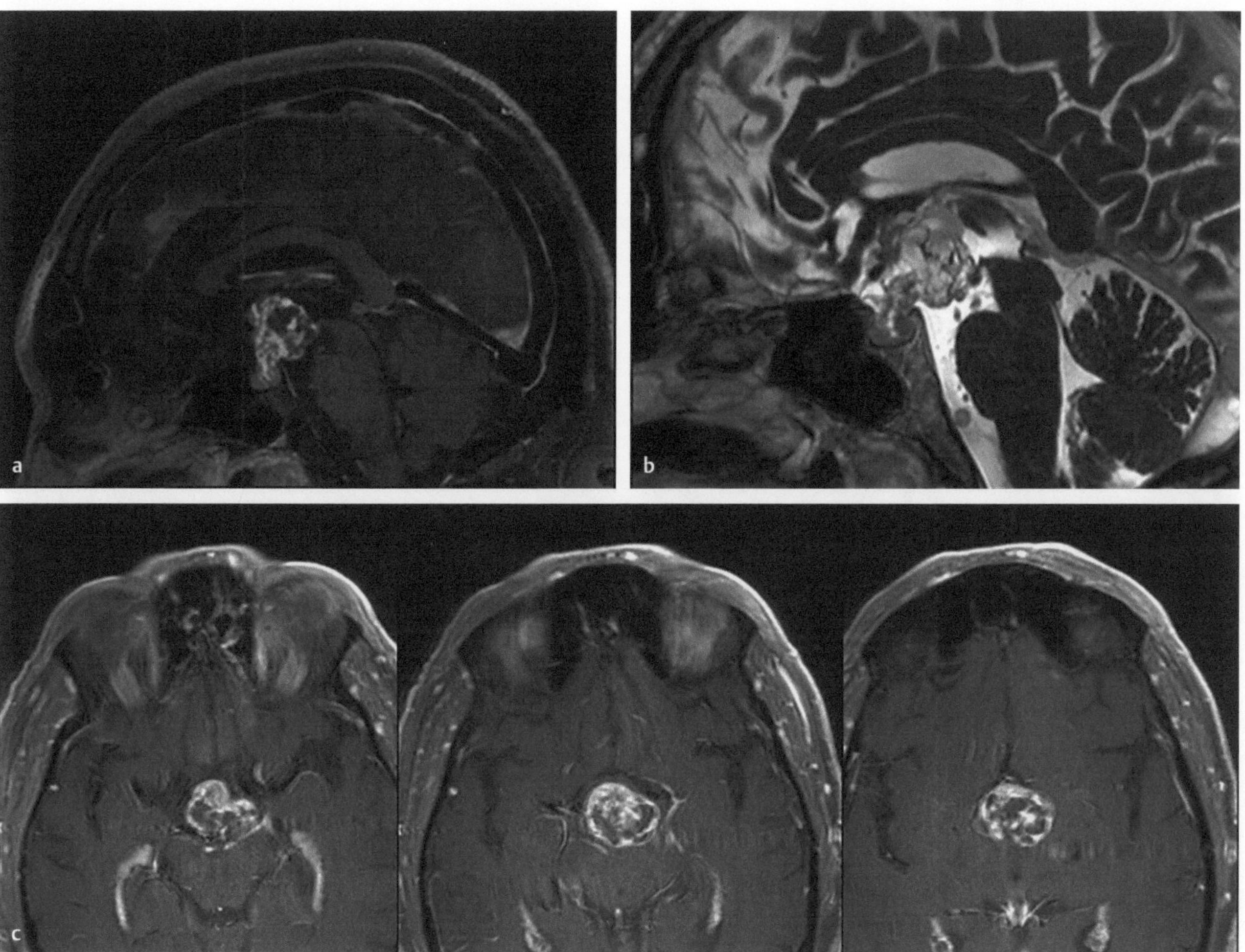

Fig. 24.3 **(a)** Sagittal T1 contrast-enhanced magnetic resonance imaging (MRI), **(b)** sagittal FIESTA (fast imaging employing steady-state acquisition) imaging, **(c)** serial axial T1 with contrast all demonstrating a mass consistent with a craniopharyngioma which is mostly in the third ventricle.

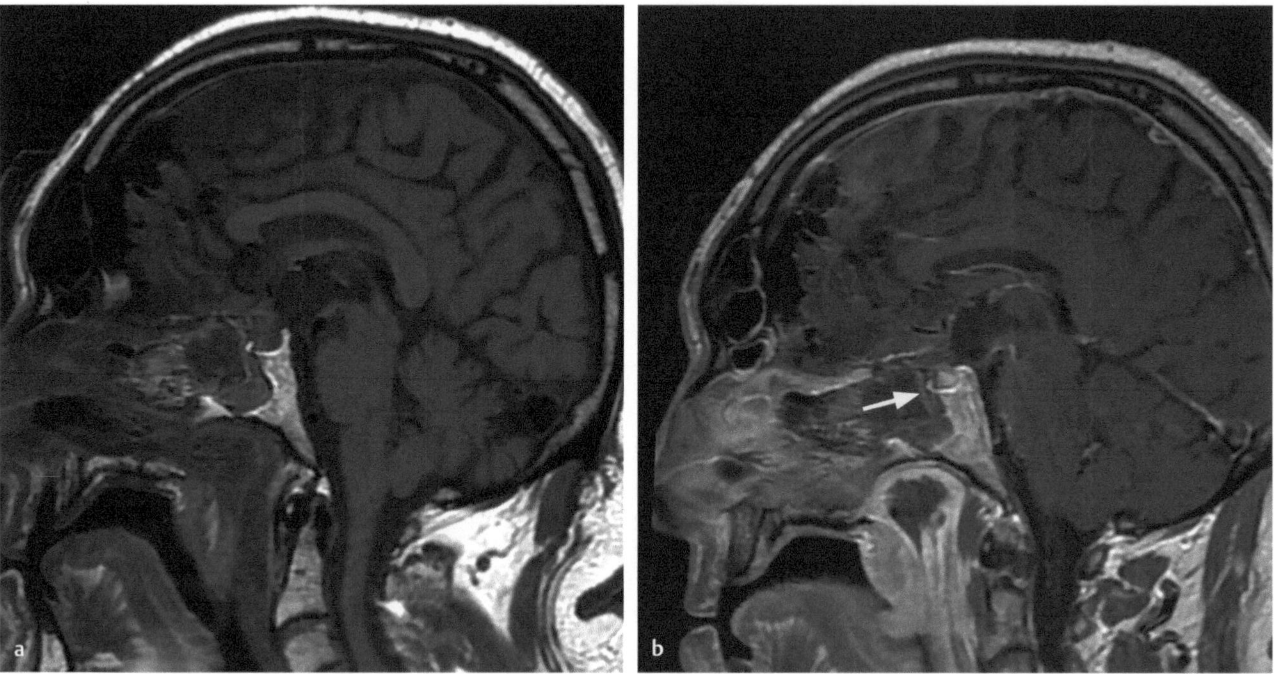

Fig. 24.4 Sagittal T1 magnetic resonance imaging (MRI) **(a)** without and **(b)** with contrast demonstrating lack of enhancement of the nasoseptal flap (*arrow*).

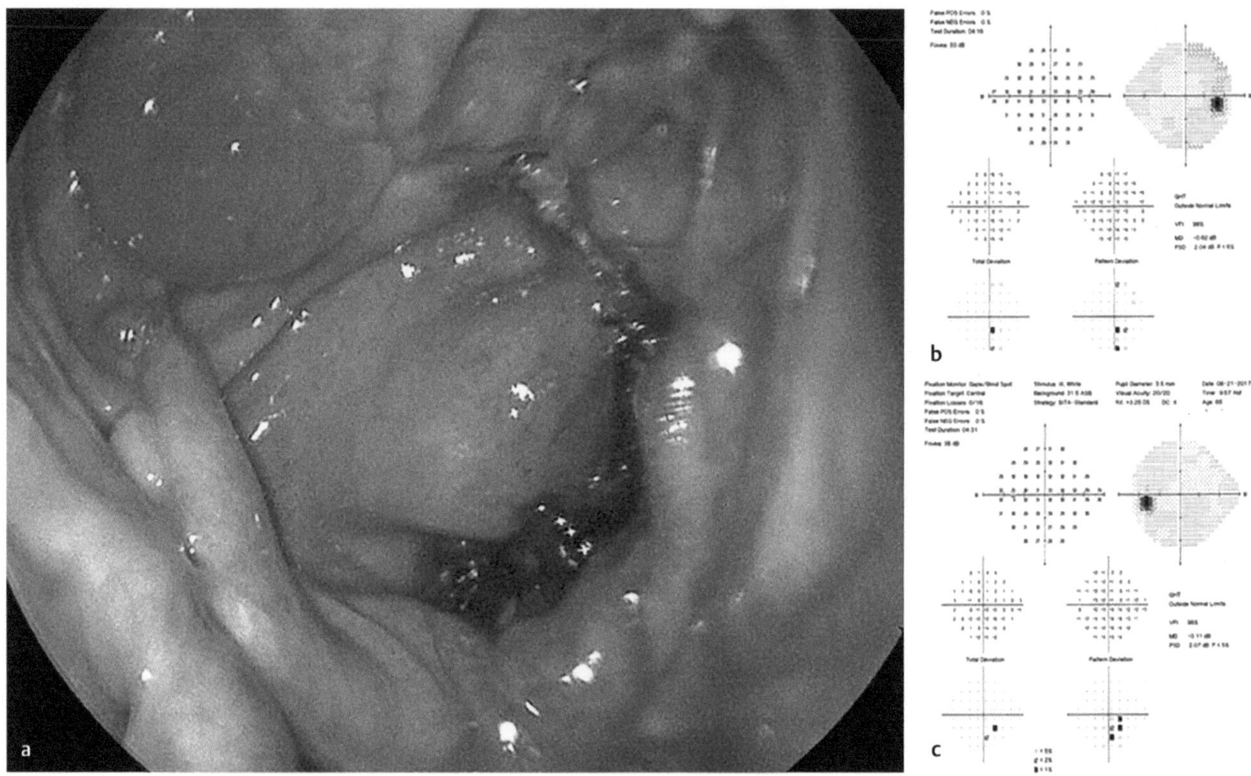

Fig. 24.5 **(a)** Picture of healing revision nasoseptal flap. **(b)** Right and **(c)** left automated visual fields demonstrating complete visual recovery after surgery.

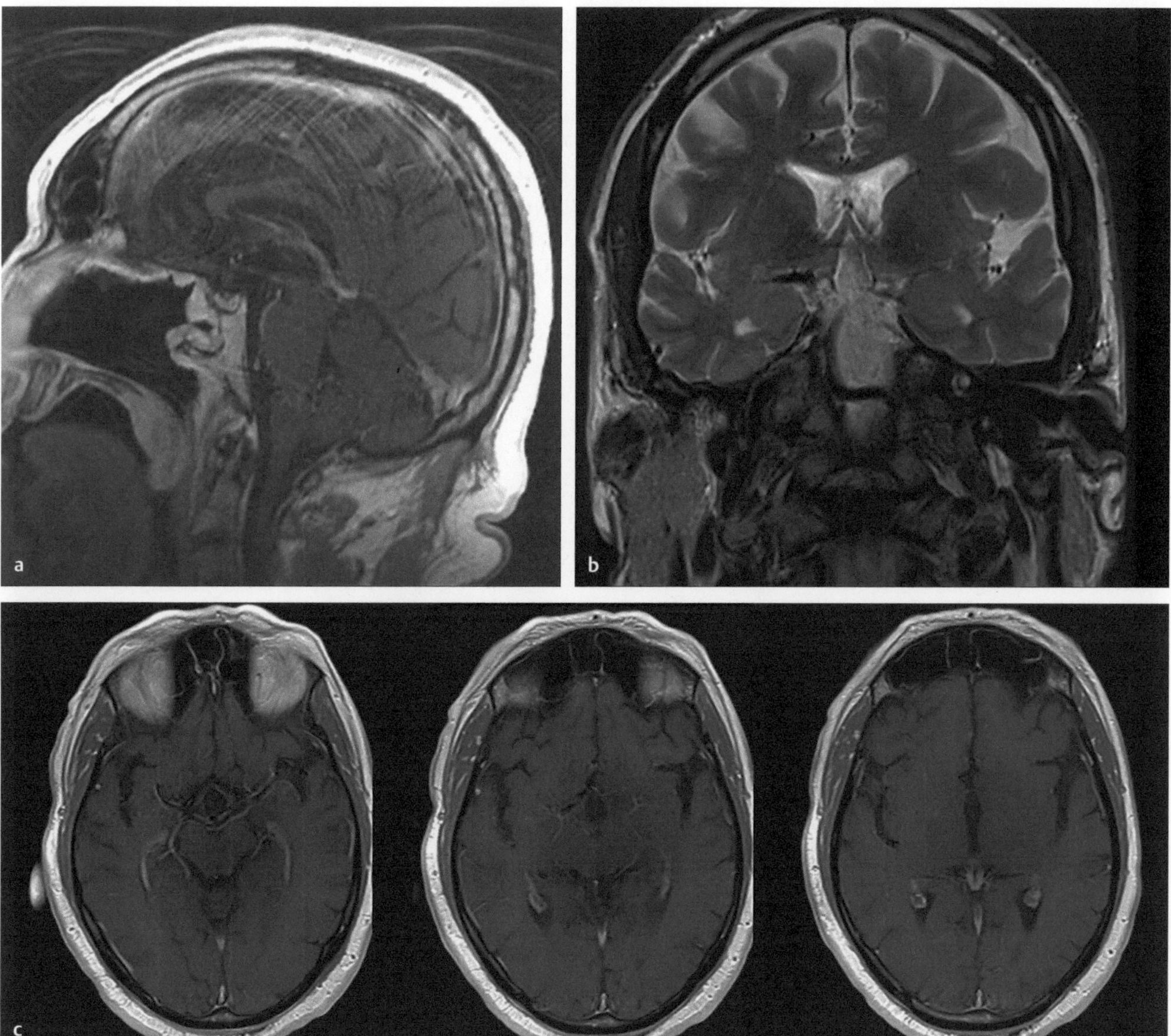

Fig. 24.6 (a) Sagittal contrast-enhanced magnetic resonance imaging (MRI), (b) coronal T2, and (c) axial contrast-enhanced MRI demonstrating complete resection of the adamantinomatous craniopharyngioma.

case, these endoscopes were approved and became one of the approaches to check the flap perfusion before you leave the operative theater. One can also try to insinuate the nasoseptal artery with a Doppler; however, this can lead to a false sense of security, given it is difficult to insinuate out further into the flap and it could be thrombosed distally and still have flow proximally. Further, we could have elected to proceed back to the operative theater as soon as we recognized the flap was not perfused, but we decided to give this repair a chance to work as, although this has been recognized to contribute to a higher chance of flap failure, for years we have repaired with nonvascularized repairs and were able to have successful outcomes.

24.5 Conclusion

Pay attention to your postoperative imaging, and in cases where there is no evidence of flap perfusion on MRI, have a low index of suspicion for return to the operative theater for revision of the repair.

25 Persistent Subcutaneous/Epidural Pneumocephalus Following Skull Base Surgery

Michael J. Link, Maria Peris-Celda, and Garret W. Choby

25.1 Case Description

25.1.1 Presentation

The patient is a 54-year-old man from Puerto Rico, who in 2014 was noted to develop progressive left-sided proptosis and headache. Imaging to investigate this complaint revealed a complex extra-axial, likely highly vascularized tumor involving the left sphenoid wing, orbit, and overlying temporalis muscle. The patient is a Jehovah's Witness and due to concern of possible intraoperative blood loss, he underwent a formal cerebral angiogram and embolization of the external carotid artery supply to the tumor. He then underwent a left frontotemporal craniotomy and subtotal resection of the tumor, all performed elsewhere. By report, the pathology was consistent with a WHO grade 1 meningioma. He did well following surgery but in 2016 developed recurrent proptosis and new-onset left head pain and diplopia, and imaging showed significant progression of residual tumor along the sphenoid wing, orbit, and infratemporal fossa. He again underwent subtotal resection by reopening his frontotemporal craniotomy, again at his home institution, without complication and the pathology report showed WHO grade 1 meningioma. Over the subsequent 1 year, he reported progressive visual loss in the left eye, left facial numbness, and increasing left head pain. Unfortunately, all of the prior imaging, pathology specimens, and operative notes were destroyed when Hurricane Maria devastated Puerto Rico in September, 2017.

Upon initial presentation to Mayo Clinic in Rochester, Minnesota in January, 2018, he had a well-healed frontotemporal incision, moderate temporalis atrophy, 20/60 vision in the left eye with moderate left optic atrophy confirmed on optical coherence tomography (▶ Fig. 25.1), trigeminal sensory loss in all three divisions, and a mild left third nerve palsy without ptosis. He preferred to keep his left eye closed and his gait was slightly wide-based.

Imaging confirmed a large infiltrative tumor, consistent with residual/recurrent meningioma involving the left sphenoid wing, anterior clinoid, orbit, cavernous sinus with extension to the sphenoid sinus, and infratemporal fossa (▶ Fig. 25.2).

25.1.2 Surgical Procedure

We proceeded to the operating room and reopened the prior frontotemporal bone flap, performed an orbitozygomatic (OZ) osteotomy, anterior clinoidectomy, and achieved a very aggressive subtotal resection of the tumor. We removed the lateral wall of the cavernous sinus but did not remove tumor from within the cavernous sinus. The patient had a very pneumatized skull base, and we necessarily entered his large left frontal sinus with our OZ osteotomy as well as entered a posterior ethmoid air cell when decompressing the left optic canal and entered the lateral left sphenoid sinus in the anterolateral triangle between V2 and V3 and removed gross tumor from the lateral sphenoid. The dura and skull base were reconstructed using autologous fat and fascia lata harvested from the left lateral thigh. The opened sinuses were excluded from the intracranial space by removing mucosa, placing free fascia lata into the sinus, packing a large pledget of fat over this, and then covering the fat with an additional piece of fascia lata and Tisseel fibrin sealant (Baxter, Deerfield, Illinois, USA). The OZ process was reattached using plates and screws, but the free frontotemporal bone flap was sent for decalcification and pathologic analysis as it appeared grossly involved by tumor. A titanium mesh cranioplasty (Stryker, Kalamazoo, Michigan, USA) was then performed. Pathologic analysis of the resected tumor confirmed a WHO grade 2 meningioma. The patient did well following surgery and was discharged on postoperative day (POD) 4.

25.1.3 Postoperative Course

He returned on POD 14 continuing to do well but was noted to have marked fullness at the surgical site most suggestive of a large pseudomeningocele. A noncontrast computed tomography (CT) scan surprisingly showed no extradural cerebrospinal fluid (CSF) collection but rather a large amount of subcutaneous, epidural air, without intradural air, and no evidence of hydrocephalus (▶ Fig. 25.3a–d). The patient denied any rhinorrhea or drainage from the incision. Provocative maneuvers, having the patient lean forward and Valsalva, did not result in any rhinorrhea. He was experiencing no headache. It should be noted that his family described regular loud disruptive snoring while sleeping, although there was no formal diagnosis of obstructive sleep apnea (OSA). A conservative approach was elected with simple observation, but serial CT scans showed persistence of a large subcutaneous/epidural air collection. We tried aspirating the air one time with an 18-gauge needle after sterile preparation but it reaccumulated within 24 hours. The air collection was persistent 8 weeks after surgery (▶ Fig. 25.3e–h).

25.1.4 Surgical Repair

Ultimately, we felt the best approach was to reinforce the skull base endoscopically from the paranasal sinuses to try and prevent further ongoing pneumocephalus. Therefore, 2 months following the original tumor resection, an endoscopic endonasal transsphenoidal and left transpterygoid approach were performed to widely visualize the left lateral recess of the sphenoid sinus, and transethmoidal approach to the left frontal recess was performed. A right-sided vascularized nasoseptal flap was raised at the beginning of the exposure and left protected in the nasopharynx. A free mucosal graft from the floor of the nasal cavity was also harvested. The face of the sphenoid was removed and an ethmoidectomy was performed and we could

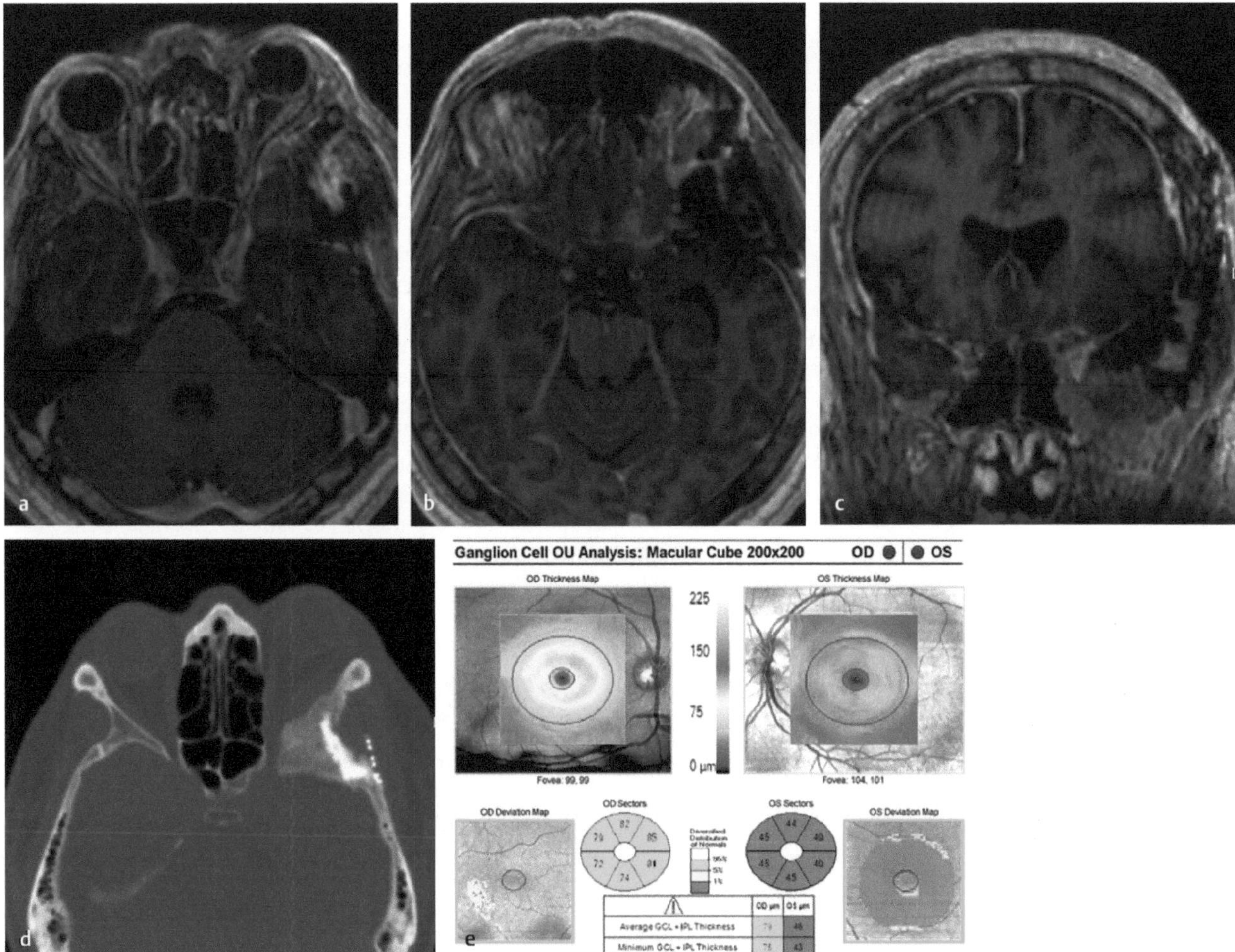

Fig. 25.1 Preoperative magnetic resonance imaging (MRI) **(a–c)** and computed tomography (CT) scan **(d)** show hyperostosis and enhancement involving the left sphenoid wing. Tumor involvement of the periorbita causes left eye proptosis. The tumor also extends through the cavernous sinus into the left sphenoid sinus. Prior bone cement and cranial fixation hardware from prior surgery are seen in **(d)**. Note hyperpneumatization of both squamous temporal bones on the CT scan. **(e)** Preoperative optical coherence tomography shows significant thinning of the ganglion cell layer in the left eye measuring only 48 µm compared to the normal right eye, 79 µm.

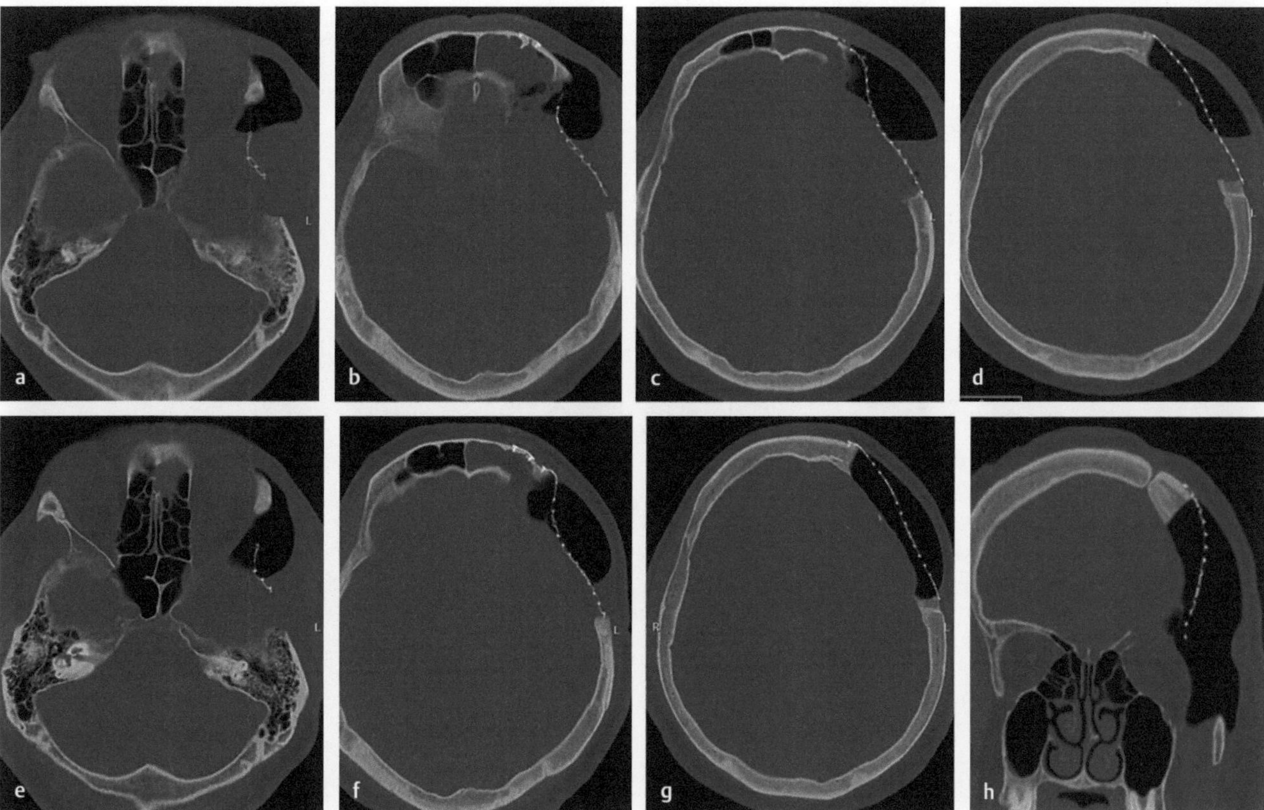

Fig. 25.2 (a–d) Noncontrast head computed tomography (CT) on postoperative day (POD) 14 to evaluate for possible pseudomeningocele due to "swelling" in region of left pterion shows extensive epidural, subcutaneous pneumocephalus with no obvious communication with air in the paranasal sinuses. Note extensive fat and fascia packing in the large left frontal sinus. The air was aspirated with a needle. **(e–h)** Two months after surgery, the epidural and subcutaneous air persisted; decision was made to perform endoscopic endonasal exploration and reconstruction.

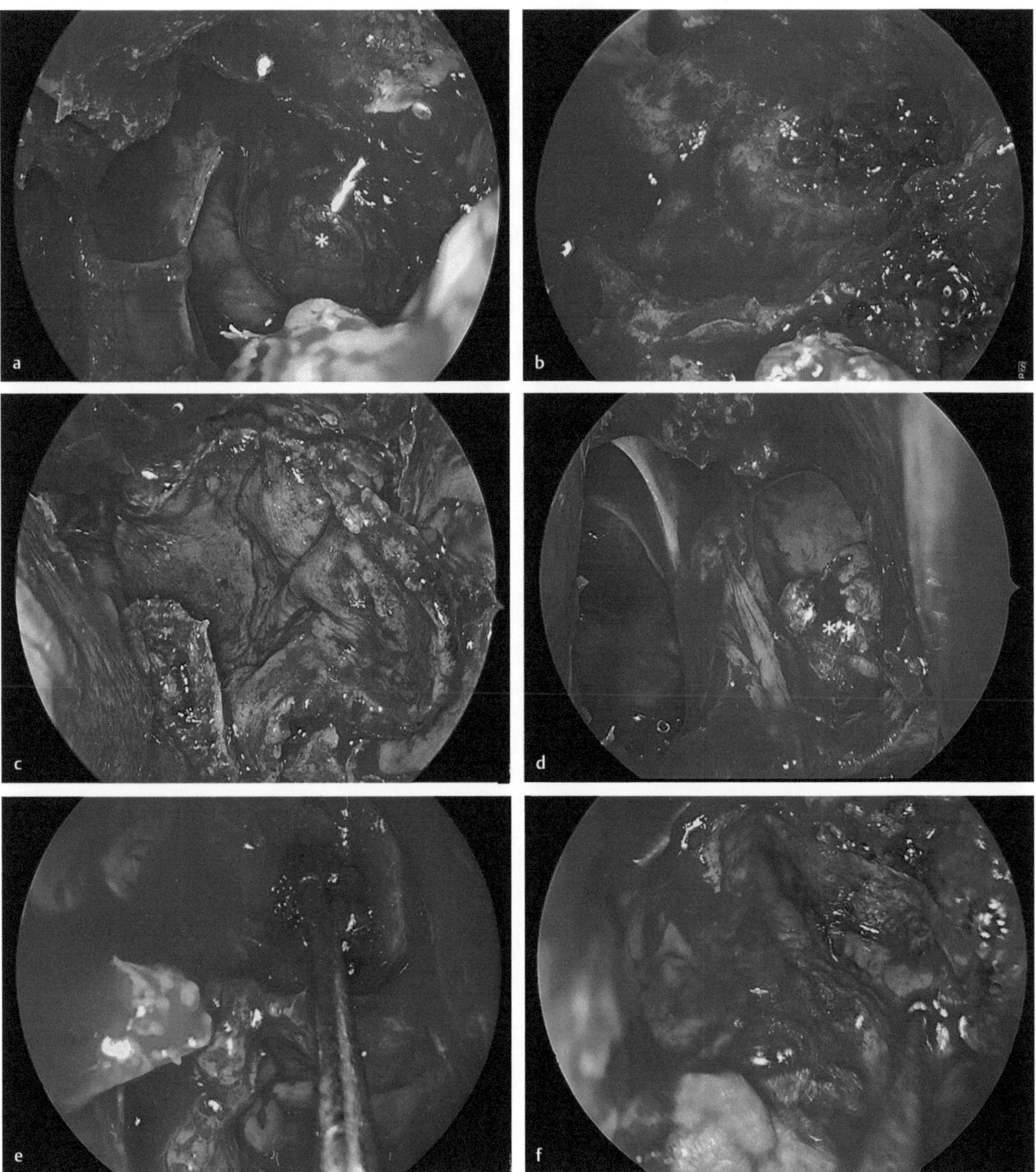

Fig. 25.3 Endoscopic endonasal repair and postoperative imaging. **(a)** View of the sphenoid sinus after a left transpterygoid approach with residual tumor (*). **(b)** View after tumor resection, the repair placed intracranially is identified. Additional fat graft was placed and covered with a right-sided nasoseptal flap transposed through a posterior septectomy **(c)**. **(d)** After opening the frontal recess, the fat placed intracranially was identified (**). Additional fat and oxidized cellulose was placed in the recess before covering it with a free mucosal graft **(e, f)**.

(Continued)

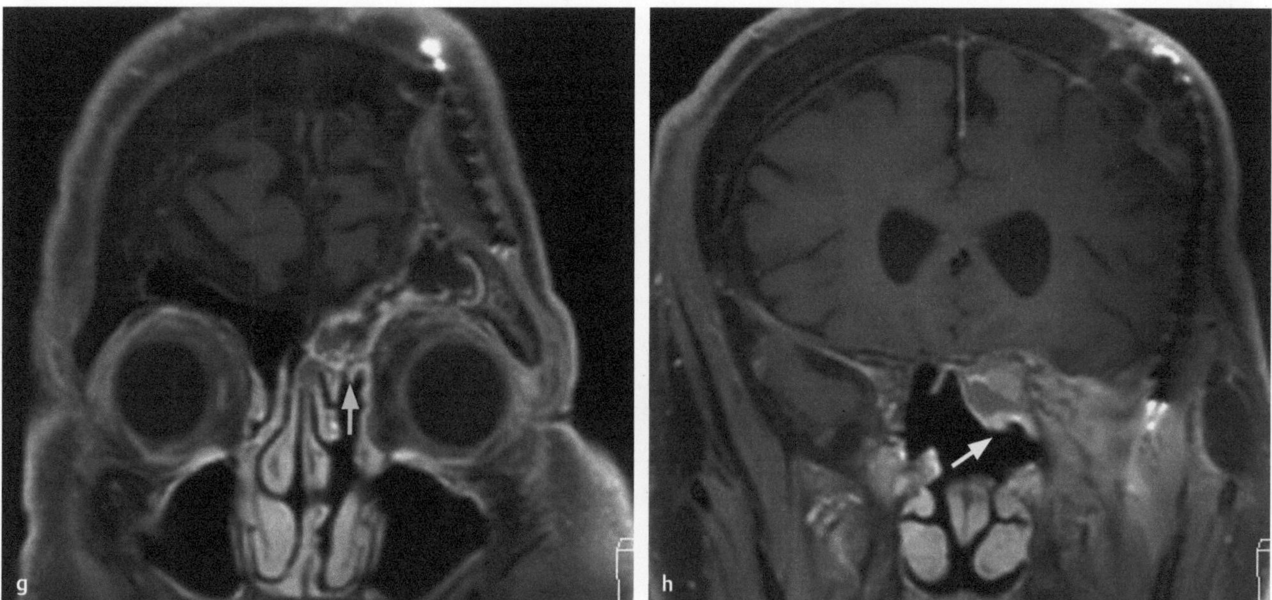

Fig. 25.3 *(Continued)* **(g)** Postoperative coronal magnetic resonance imaging (MRI) T1 with contrast after the endoscopic repair, note the covered frontal recess with a free mucosal graft (*green arrow*). **(h)** Nasoseptal flap placed posteriorly to cover the sphenoid sinus defect (*yellow arrow*).

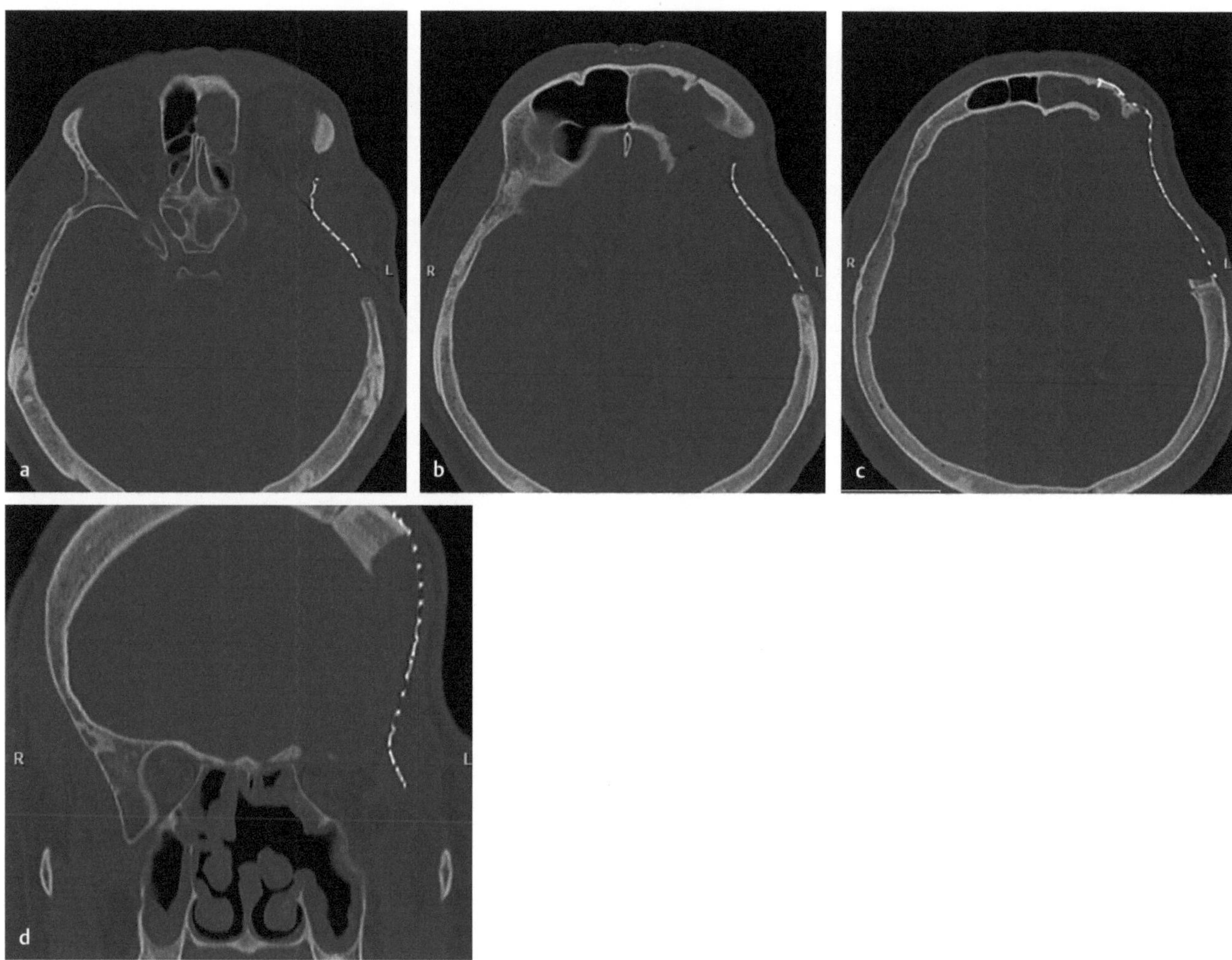

Fig. 25.4 Axial **(a–c)** and coronal **(d)** postoperative computed tomography (CT) scans demonstrating the resolution of the pneumocephalus 1 month after surgery.

identify our fat graft placed transcranially in the ethmoid cell at the initial operation. The frontal recess was widely opened and once again the fat and fascia lata in the frontal sinus were easily inspected in this previously obliterated left frontal sinus. We then worked laterally in the transpterygoid corridor, identifying the sphenopalatine artery and coagulating and dividing it and pushing the contents of the pterygopalatine fossa inferiorly. The base of the pterygoid was drilled, identifying and preserving V2, and we had an excellent view of the lateral sphenoid sinus. Residual tumor in the sphenoid sinus was removed, and the fat and fascia lata deep to this were identified. There was no egress of CSF from any of the prior surgical sites with intraoperative Valsalva. A fat graft was harvested from the abdomen and additional fat was placed in the frontal recess and covered with the free mucosal graft, with the mucosal side toward the nasal cavity. Additional fat was also placed in the lateral sphenoid sinus and then the entire exposed sphenoid sinus was covered with the vascularized nasoseptal flap.

Once again, he did well following the procedure and was discharged on POD 2. Follow-up showed resolution of the subcutaneous air on examination, confirmed on imaging. Given his loud snoring and suspected OSA, he was also provided a mandibular advancement oral device to reduce his snoring during the postoperative period. He has subsequently done well with no signs of CSF leak, infection, or recurrent pneumocephalus (▸ Fig. 25.4). He has remained well now 2 years following surgery and was recommended to have radiotherapy for the residual tumor but has declined.

25.2 Challenges

This was a particularly challenging problem because there was no clear site of air communication with the surgical site or reason why it persisted. Clearly, there had to be some connection between the paranasal sinuses and the epidural space that somehow functioned as a one way valve such that air could be entrained into the wound but not vented. Since there was no discernable CSF leak, we did not feel it was urgent but were worried it could pose an infection risk to the OZ process and nonvascularized tissues of free fat, fascia lata, and titanium mesh.

25.3 Discussion

This case demonstrates the relatively rare circumstance of persistent intracranial, extradural pneumocephalus caused by a persistent communication between the paranasal sinuses and a recent surgical site following an extensive transcranial skull base approach for resection of an aggressive recurrent sphenoid wing, anterior clinoid, orbital, central skull base meningioma. Likely, a one-way valve mechanism allowed air to be entrained through the skull base, resulting in a "pseudomeningocele" appearance that surprisingly on CT showed a large collection of epidural subcutaneous intracranial air.

25.4 Alternatives

The alternative option would have been to reopen the cranial incision and pack additional fat or free muscle grafts into the opened paranasal sinuses from above. We felt this carried increased risk of infection or wound-healing problems, considering it would have been the fourth operation through that incision. Most importantly, we were worried we had overlooked an opening into one of the sinuses and we could not do better at sealing off the skull base from above any better than we had done at the time of the initial operation. Therefore, even though we did not have a way to definitively identify the source of air entry into the wound site, we felt we had the best opportunity to eliminate it by widely exposing the skull base from the endonasal side and reinforcing it with a combination of free fat graft, free mucosal graft, and vascularized nasoseptal flap.

25.5 Conclusions

Rarely, when the skull base is breached and there is communication between the intracranial space and the paranasal sinuses, it can result in a one-way valve mechanism in which air can become trapped intracranially. If the dura is competent, the air remains extradural but poses a potential risk of infection as well as a cosmetic problem. Sealing the skull base from the endonasal side offers an efficient and low-risk strategy to resolve the problem as this case illustrates.

26 Recalcitrant Cerebrospinal Fluid Leak

Abdulaziz Alrasheed, Akina Tamaki, Daniel Prevedello, Stephen Y. Kang, Enver Ozer, Mathew Old, Nolan Seim, Amit Agrawal, and Ricardo L. Carrau

26.1 Case Description

26.1.1 Presentation

A 36-year-old female with a history of Factor V Leiden and clival chordoma, who previously underwent multiple endoscopic and open resections with left internal carotid artery sacrifice, as well as two separate treatments with proton beam. She developed a spontaneous cerebrospinal fluid (CSF) leak following gamma knife treatment for progressive disease. Multiple attempts to repair the CSF leak with local flaps and free radial forearm free flap at an outside facility failed to seal the fistula. Eventually, she underwent ventriculoperitoneal shunting and was referred to our care for the management of the persistent CSF leak complicated by pneumocephalus and meningitis (▶ Fig. 26.1 and ▶ Fig. 26.2).

26.1.2 Surgical Procedure (*Video 26.1*)

The patient first underwent a repair with a bath-plug technique using a free abdominal fat graft and repositioning a previously harvested inferior turbinate flap as an overlay. However, 2 weeks later, she presented with a CSF leak. She then underwent a repair using galeopericranial flap reconstruction with buccal fat pad flap. This rare combination of flaps was needed to cover the entire defect. Unfortunately, 10 days later, she presented again with CSF leak due to necrosis of the distal pericranial flap. Therefore, we elected to proceed with free flap reconstruction of the clival defect using vastus lateralis free flap transferring its pedicle via a retropharyngeal corridor. Free flap reconstruction of the skull base is complex, and it is even more demanding when performed by endoscopic assistance. Furthermore, this particular case presented two additional difficulties: the retropharyngeal corridor had been previously used for the radial forearm free flap; and this flap was occupying the posterior aspect of the skull base defect as well as the posterior wall of the nasopharynx down to the level of Passavant's ridge. The pedicle of the radial forearm had to be preserved and its skin lining had to be eliminated to allow the healing of the muscle flap around the defect. The most inferior aspect of the radial forearm flap was exposed via a transoral approach using a Dingman retractor and superior displacement of the soft palate. We then incised the junction of the flap and the mucosa of the posterior nasopharyngeal wall, identified the pedicle, and dissected it off the mucosa. The skin was eliminated using a radiofrequency bipolar electrocautery that facilitated burning the skin off the flap down to the deep dermis. Once this was accomplished, the vastus lateralis free flap was inserted via the retropharyngeal tunnel, conformed to the skull base to widely cover the areas around the defect, and anastomosed to the neck vessels in standard fashion.

26.1.3 Postoperative Course

She recovered well after the surgery, with no subsequent CSF leak; postoperative magnetic resonance imaging (MRI) with gadolinium showed well-vascularized free flap covering the skull base defect (▶ Fig. 26.3). She continued to do well at 11 months follow-up.

26.2 Challenges

Challenges arising from this case could be attributed to three main factors: the first is related to the limited availability reconstructive options, which had been exhausted by previous surgeries and attempts to repair the defect; the second is related to poor wound healing due to the extensive radiation effects; and third is the location of defect at the most posterior aspect of the planum sphenoidale. With multiple procedures in the past as well as radiotherapy, it was evident she had a nonhealing defect secondary to skull base radionecrosis and no option to harvest a robust local flap for reconstruction.

26.3 Discussion

The skull base reconstructive ladder includes simple grafts, pedicled flaps, and free flaps. The failure of all the available pedicled flaps (options limited by previous surgeries) and the presence of skull base necrosis (poor healing due to the sparse recipient site blood supply) left us with limited choices. In these dire situations, we strongly advocate the use of a muscular flap, such as the vastus lateralis or the serratus anterior flap that best conform to the skull base.

26.4 Alternatives

Nasoseptal, lateral wall, and temporoparietal flaps had been previously used or rendered nonviable.

26.5 Conclusion

Microvascular free flaps are an established alternative for the reconstruction of skull base defects and should be considered in the setting of complex reconstruction.

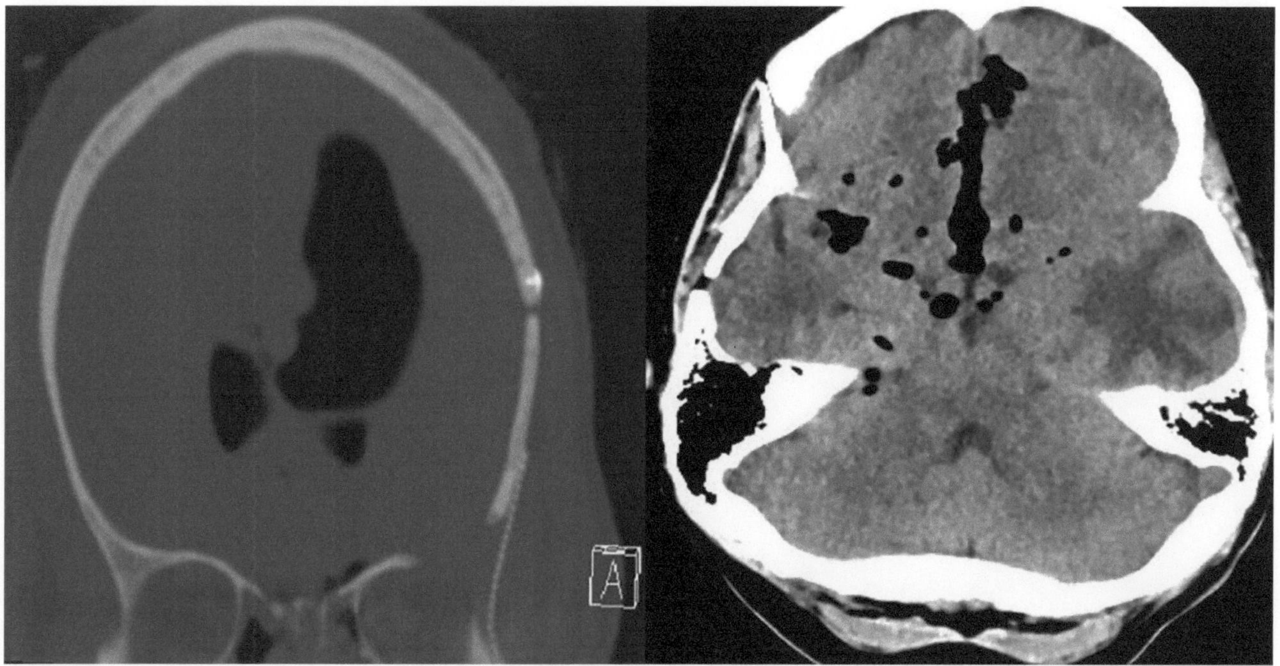

Fig. 26.1 Computed tomography (CT) scan of the brain with evidence of pneumocephalus.

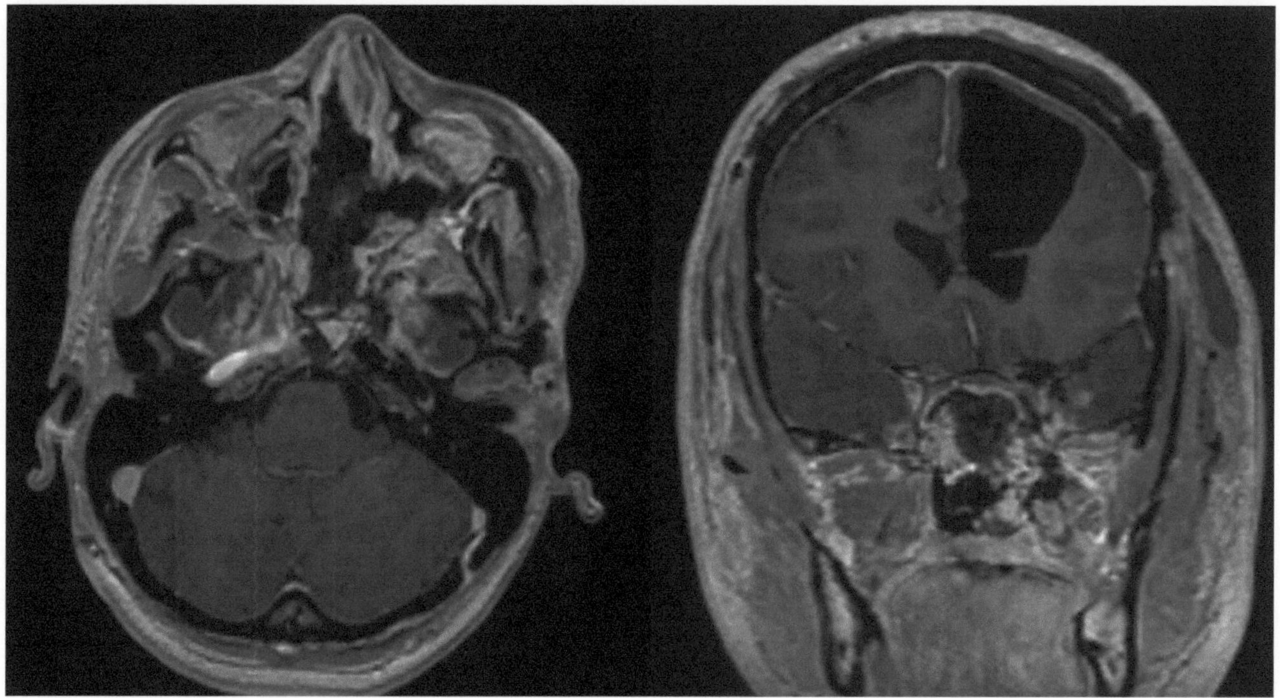

Fig. 26.2 Preoperative magnetic resonance imaging (MRI) showing clival defect and pneumocephalus.

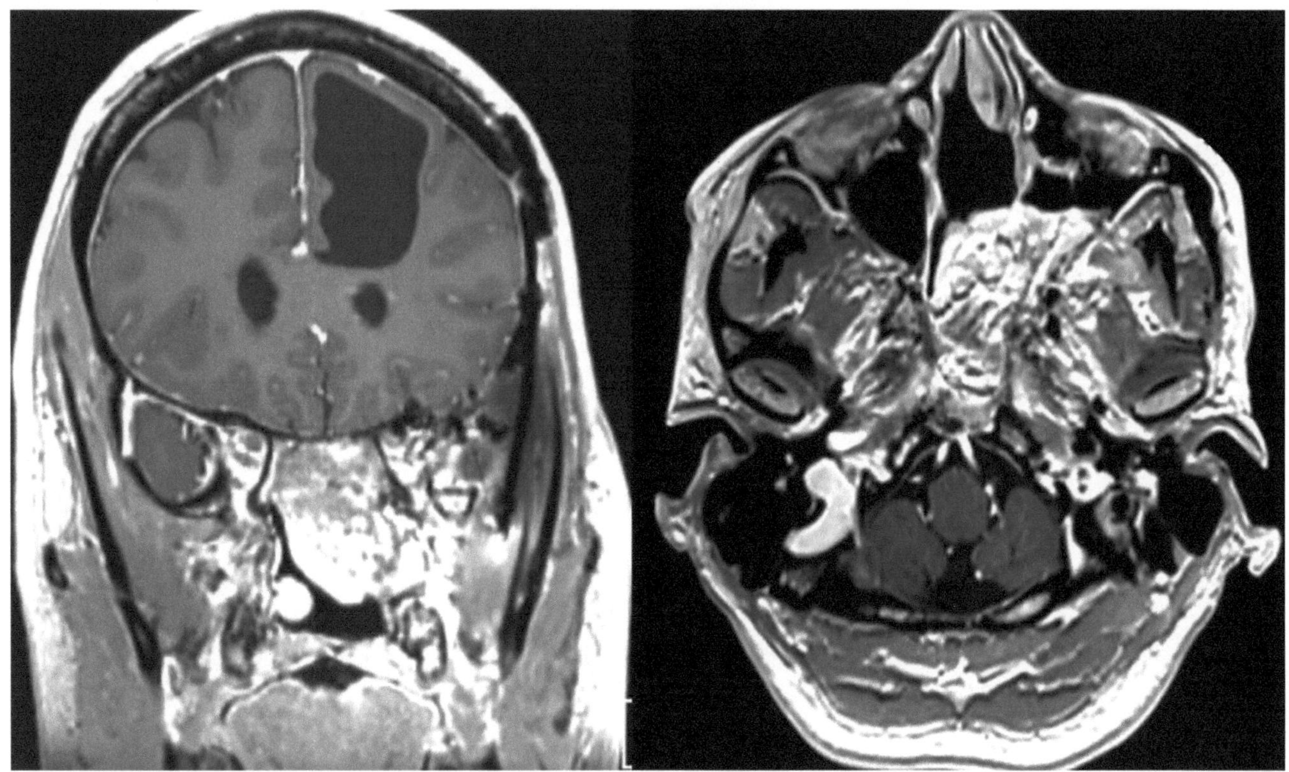

Fig. 26.3 Postoperative magnetic resonance imaging (MRI) with the vascularized free flap covering the skull base defect.

Index

Note: Page numbers set **bold** or *italic* indicate headings or figures, respectively.